D1308723

STRAIGHT TALK ON STUTTERING

Second Edition

STRAIGHT TALK ON STUTTERING

Information, Encouragement, and Counsel for Stutterers, Caregivers, and Speech-Language Clinicians

By

LLOYD M. HULIT, Ph.D.

Professor Emeritus of Speech Pathology and Audiology
Illinois State University
Normal, Illinois

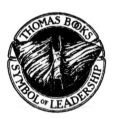

CHARLES C THOMAS · PUBLISHER, LTD.
Springfield · Illinois · U.S.A.

Published and Distributed Throughout the World by

CHARLES C THOMAS • PUBLISHER, LTD.
2600 South First Street
Springfield, Illinois 62704

©2004 by CHARLES C THOMAS • PUBLISHER, LTD.

ISBN 0-398-07519-0 (hard)
ISBN 0-398-07520-4 (paper)

Library of Congress Catalog Card Number: 2004046002

Printed in the United States of America
SM-R-3

Library of Congress Cataloging-in-Publication Data

Hulit, Lloyd M.
    Straight talk on stuttering : information, encouragement, and counsel for
stutterers, caregivers, and speech-language clinicians / by Lloyd M. Hulit.--
2nd ed.
        p. cm.
    Includes bibliographical references and index.
    ISBN 0-398-07519-0 -- ISBN 0-398-07520-4 (pbk.)
    1. Stuttering. 2. Stuttering in children. 3. Stuttering--Treatment. I. Title.

RC424.H869 2004
616.85'54--dc22
                                                                    2004046002

To the loving memory of my parents, Sarah Ellen and Lloyd Darl Hulit, and my brother, Mark James Hulit,

And to the sources of my greatest joys and pride, Pamela, Yvonne, Carmen, Scot, John, Christopher, Lance, Benjamin, Peyton, and Brianna

PREFACE

This book is not for everyone. It was written for people who stutter and for those who interact with people who stutter, including caregivers, teachers, and speech-language pathologists.

I have tried to write this book in a *reader friendly* manner, and I have tried to make it as practical as possible. Even though it is a reasonably thorough review of what we know about stuttering, there is a heavy emphasis on what I would consider to be *bottom-line conclusions,* not on the details of the theoretical speculations and the research findings that have driven us to these conclusions. I do not pretend that this presentation is free of my own life experiences with stuttering because that would not be true. I am a stutterer. I am a clinician who specializes in the treatment of stuttering. I am a teacher who is passionate about helping others learn about stuttering. These perspectives have heavily influenced how I have written this book. In the pages that follow, I offer my insights, opinions, and advice, but I am careful to indicate that I am addressing the reader, not as a guru of truth, but as a person who has gained some understanding about stuttering through my professional and personal experiences with this disorder.

The second edition of *Straight Talk on Stuttering* is divided into two parts. The first part includes basic information about the disorder. In these chapters, I address common questions people have about stuttering, such as *What is stuttering?, What causes it?, How does it develop?, Can it be prevented?, Are there things parents can do to help a child who is stuttering?, How has stuttering been treated in adults?,* and *Are there things the adult stutterer can do to help himself?* In the first part of this edition, I have included a new chapter entitled *Living with Stuttering.* This chapter includes ten suggestions about living victoriously with stuttering. It is a very personal, stutterer-to-stutterer account of lessons I have learned and want to share with those who have carried stuttering into adolescence and adulthood. The second part of the book is a description of the therapy approach I use with adults and children who stutter. This part includes another new chapter, *Evaluating People Who Stutter.*

In writing this book, I have not avoided the technical language speech-language pathologists use in reference to stuttering, but I have taken great care to make sure that each technical term is adequately explained the first time I use it. In addition, there is a glossary at the end of the book that includes definitions of many of the terms that might be unfamiliar to some readers.

Before beginning the journey through the pages of this book, the reader should know that stuttering is an utterly fascinating communication disorder. Because it is surrounded by so much mystery, so many unanswered questions, and so many myths and misperceptions, it can be a frustrating disorder to study, treat, and endure. I have tried to dispel the myths, correct the misperceptions, answer as many questions as I believe are answerable, and above all else, I have tried to weave a message of *hope* for all people who stutter, a message I believe is absolutely justified.

Lloyd M. Hulit, Ph.D.

CONTENTS

Page

Preface vii

Part One

UNDERSTANDING STUTTERING

Chapter

1. Introduction 5
2. Stuttering: Up Close and Personal 14
3. In Search of a Definition 29
4. The Behaviors of Stuttering 48
5. What Causes Stuttering? 70
6. Stutterers Are Ordinary People Too 91
7. The Development of Stuttering 107
8. Can Stuttering Be Prevented? 117
9. Helping the Stuttering Child 131
10. Treating the Adult Stuttering: A Brief History 145
11. Self-Help for the Adult Stutterer 157
12. Stuttering in the Future 166
13. Living with Stuttering 169

Part Two

TREATING PEOPLE WHO STUTTER:
ADULTS AND CHILDREN

14. Charles Van Riper Therapy: An Introduction 195
15. Motivating the Adult Stutterer 203
16. Identification 212
17. Desensitization 221
18. Modification 227

19.   Stabilization 240
20.   Therapy for Children Who Stutter: An Introduction 247
21.   Therapy for the Young Beginning Stutterer 255
22.   Therapy for the Young Advanced Stutterer 270
23.   Interviewing and Counseling 281
24.   Evaluating People Who Stutter 295

References 317
Glossary 319
Index 325

STRAIGHT TALK ON STUTTERING

Part One

UNDERSTANDING STUTTERING

Chapter 1

INTRODUCTION

What the World Needs Now

Burt Bacharach is one of the most prolific songwriters of his generation. One of his best known songs is *What the World Needs Now Is Love,* recorded by Jackie DeShannon in 1968. When I wrote the first edition of this book, I thought about the lyrics of this song. When the time came to write the second edition, I decided to include a few of Bacharach's words to make a point about the book you are beginning to read. Actually, after browsing through this first paragraph, you may decide NOT to read the book, but I ask that you at least finish this first chapter before abandoning my message. Consider a few of Bacharach's lyrics: *What the world needs now is love, sweet love . . . Lord, we don't need another mountain . . . There are oceans and rivers enough to cross.* The general idea is that there are many things in life that are overstocked, but there can never be enough love. One could make the argument that what the world does not need is another book about stuttering, and on some level, I would have a difficult time refuting that assertion. There are plenty of books about stuttering—enough to fill a library devoted to this one subject. In the early years of speech-language pathology as a profession, there was more written about stuttering than all other communication disorders combined. That is no longer true, but it is interesting that a disorder affecting only about 1 percent of the world's population at a given time still commands considerable interest.

So why did I write *Straight Talk on Stuttering* in the first place, and why am I writing a second edition? Because while it is true that there are plenty of books about stuttering, this one offers a different view than most. I have written about stuttering from a personal perspective, which is NOT unique, but it is a personal perspective shaped by four decades as a teacher and clinician as well as a lifetime of experience with the disorder itself, and that does separate my presentation from most others.

In order to appreciate what this book has to offer, therefore, it is important that you know I am a stutterer. There was a time in my life when I considered myself a stutterer, first, last, and always. When I was an adolescent, it was difficult for me to place my stuttering in any meaningful personal context because it seemed almost larger than my life. Fortunately, I can now put my stuttering into proper perspective. It is one small part of who I am. More accurately, it is one small part of what I do and has nothing to do with my essential personhood. This perspective has been gained, in large measure, as I have learned to control my stuttering so that it no longer controls me.

One of my qualifications as author of this book, therefore, is that I am a stutterer. I have lived with this disorder most of my life, certainly all of the life I can remember. I want to make it clear, however, that my experience as a stutterer is the least of my qualifications. I am also a clinician, counselor, and a teacher. In these roles, I have learned infinitely more about stuttering than I have as a stutterer. The problem with trying to understand stuttering from the inside is that you see only one point of view, and even that point of view is distorted by the incredibly personal nature of the disorder. Stutterers tend to want others to understand stuttering the way they have experienced it. If every stuttering experience were the same, we would only need one view, one understanding, but stuttering experiences are as vastly different as people are different. There is some common ground, however, and we will best understand the disorder if we look for the common ground stutterers share. I have found some of that common ground in my work as researcher, clinician, and teacher. It is that understanding of stuttering I want to share with you.

Despite the countless books, portions of books, and journal articles written by psychologists, psychiatrists, philosophers, physicians, physicists, rhetoricians, speech-language pathologists, and by stutterers themselves, despite all the research, all the theorizing and speculation, despite all the analysis and discussion, stuttering remains one of the most misunderstood of communication disorders. Much of the misunderstanding is justified. We have simply not been able to put together many facts about stuttering, which means that much of what we think we know is based on shreds of evidence about which there has been much conjecture. Some of the misunderstanding is not justified. Many writers over the centuries have mistaken their personal biases for *truths* and have written about stuttering as though the puzzle has been solved. No matter what you may have been led to believe, this puzzle has not been solved. There is still infinitely more about stuttering we do not know than we do know. In many important respects, it is as much an enigmatic mystery today as it was 100 years ago.

One of the indisputable facts about stuttering, as I have already noted, is that there are hundreds of books on the subject you could read, but most readers would not find the majority of these books particularly helpful. Many of these books are too theoretical to be of much practical value. Others are so steeped in research data and analysis that the reader loses sight of the essential questions about stuttering because the authors of these books become so absorbed in discussing the strengths and weaknesses of research design and the nuances of statistical interpretation that the essential questions are either ignored or obscured. Many books on stuttering are so obviously biased toward a single theoretical interpretation of the disorder that the reader gains an extremely narrow view of a very complicated, life-pervasive problem. Some authors overreact to some of the problems I have identified here, and in an attempt to make stuttering understandable, they provide descriptions that are entirely too simplistic.

In my work as a clinician and counselor, I have found that adult stutterers and the parents of young stutterers want and need information that is best provided in material that can be read and pondered. I can give a client a great deal of information in a one-hour session, but it is not likely that much of the information I share will be retained for long. There is also the real danger that what I have said will be remembered incompletely and incorrectly. According to the common maxim, *A little knowledge is a dangerous thing.* I have no doubt that this is true, and I am even more convinced that a little knowledge that is warped by failed memory, distorted perception, or incomplete understanding is even more dangerous.

In my work as a teacher of future speech-language clinicians who will work with stutterers, I have become increasingly sensitive to the problems students experience in trying to understand this disorder. They are frustrated by the fact that there are no clear answers to the most basic questions about stuttering. While I am convinced it is professionally inappropriate and irresponsible to provide simplistic answers to complex questions, I am even more convinced that students who are considering the issues surrounding stuttering prior to their first clinical experiences with people who stutter need to understand, in the clearest possible language, what the questions are. They also need to know, in the context of all that has been written about stuttering, what the most responsible answers to these questions seem to be.

I have tried to write a book for stutterers, the parents of stutterers, and for speech-language pathologists in training and in practice that describes stuttering in plain English, an explanation of the disorder that does not go unreasonably beyond what we actually know about stuttering. I have tried to provide practical advice for clients, parents, and clinicians who must deal with stuttering on a daily and personal basis and who are not particularly interested in the great, and often esoteric, debates waged by the experts, debates incidentally that have so far not moved us very close to the *truth* about stuttering.

There is also a very personal reason for my writing this book. I want to convey the message that stuttering is not nearly as funny as it is depicted in cartoons and comedic movies, nor is it necessarily as tragic as some stutterers allow it to be. My stuttering was most devastating when I was in elementary school. It was not the most severe at that time, but it had the most profound influence on my life during those years. Children are especially vulnerable to criticism and teasing when they are 6 to 13 years old, and I was no exception. Children, and even some adults, cannot tolerate being different, and there is no doubt that people who stutter are set apart from people who do not. People are, by their human nature, social and communicative beings. The individual whose ability to talk is limited by any speech or language disorder is penalized in many ways. He may be ostracized, teased, or mocked. He may be perceived as incompetent or stupid, the object of pity or scorn. As is potentially true of anyone with a speech or language disorder, the stutterer loses some of his communicative ability, but he might suffer more than other communicatively disordered people because his disorder can be seen as well as heard, and because it often catches listeners unaware, provokes shock, and sometimes laughter. It should not be difficult to understand how the stutterer comes to feel persecuted and why he might come to think of himself as a stutterer, first, last, and always. Many stutterers do, in fact, allow stuttering to dominate their lives, to define who they are as people, but the key word here is *allow.*

Some years ago, I watched a television interview with a young girl, about nine years old, who was dying of cancer. She was being interviewed because she had an extraordinarily positive attitude for someone who was facing death, and particularly for someone so young. The interviewer wanted to know the source of this attitude. When he posed the question, the little girl reflected for a moment, obviously giving this very serious question the thought it deserved. Her answer became part of my personal perspective on life and on my speech disorder, and I will never forget it. She said that when she first found out she was dying, she was frightened and angry. During every waking hour of those first weeks and months after her diagnosis, she was consumed with terrible thoughts about the cancer that was inside her. As time passed, however, she came to an understanding of her illness that significantly changed her attitude and the quality of the life she had left. It was an insight that was as profound as it was simple. She came to understand that the cancer did not own her. She owned the cancer, and she had control of her life, no matter how short that life might be. Cynics might suggest that this little girl could not have reached this determination without the help of adults. I would submit that it does not matter if this was a self-discovery or a facilitated discovery because it was obvious that she understood the difference between owning the cancer and the cancer owning her, and it was obvious that knowing the difference made a difference in the way she chose to live her last days in a failing body. There are at least two important lessons for the stutterer in this little girl's story.

First, the stutterer often was a *woe be unto me* attitude about his stuttering, believing that nothing could be worse than the agony of stuttering. One does not have to look very far to discover that such an attitude about stuttering is preposterous. There are many conditions with which a person might be afflicted that are far worse than stuttering. I do not want to be unduly harsh on stutterers who choose to wallow in self-pity because I have spent time in the self-pity pit myself, but it is crucial that the stutterer recognize at some point in his life that he has not been struck by life's cruelest blow. I would rather not stutter, of course, but when I step back from my speech disorder and view it within the total tapestry of human problems, it is not nearly as tragic, not nearly as life-altering, and certainly not as horrific as I tend to imagine it when I view it only from the inside out.

The second lesson to be learned from the dying girl concerns ownership. We all have the potential to be slaves to something about ourselves we do not like. If I am unusually short, I can become so obsessed with my shortness that everything I do is affected by my perception of myself as *short*. I cannot play basketball because I am too short. I cannot ask that special girl for a date because I'm too short, and surely she could not like a short person. I'm not even going to ask for that promotion I know I deserve because the boss does not like short people. On the other hand, I can refuse to be a victim of my shortness. I can choose to view my shortness as one part of who I am and go about the business of living my life without always thinking first about the shattering shame of shortness.

The person who stutters also needs to do some serious thinking about what owns whom or who owns what and how the difference can make a difference in the living of his life. No one can dispute that stuttering is a disorder of speech, but the person who stutters can make a choice about his disorder. He can choose to make the stuttering a handicap, or he can choose to own the disorder, and once he has claimed ownership, he can choose to seize control over his disordered fluency. I want to make a final point here about stuttering and choice. The stutterer can choose to be fluent. The process toward becoming fluent is difficult, sometimes painful, and usually long, but it is possible. The stutterer can make the choice. People who are blind, deaf, paraplegic, or who are terminally ill with cancer or AIDS can, like the stutterer, choose to own their conditions, but they cannot choose to overcome them to the same extent that the stutterer can choose to overcome his stuttering.

These lessons lead quite naturally to the first specific, practical piece of advice I want to offer to all people, including parents, siblings, friends, teachers, and speech-language clinicians, who interact with stutterers. Do not pity the stutterer. Do not mock, tease, ridicule, or torment the stutterer in any way, but please do not pity him. Your pity is not constructive and may directly feed the fires of the stutterer's feelings of inadequacy and despair. If he perceives that he is helpless, that he is the prisoner of a tongue that cannot flit about his mouth with the dexterity required of normal speech, or lips that either stick together or remain paralyzed in an open position, or a larynx that has a broken *on/off* switch, your pity will only reinforce his belief that his speech mechanism is broken. Your pity supports his self-deprecating complaint that he ". . . just can't help it!" No matter the stutterer's age, he needs your unqualified acceptance. He needs whatever understanding you can muster. He needs your support and encouragement, but he absolutely, positively does not need your pity, and as surprising as it may seem to some people, most stutterers abhor pity more than they despise the teasing and mocking, more even than the stuttering itself.

The longer I live with my own stuttering, the longer I study the disorder, and the longer I work with stutterers and the parents of stutterers, the more convinced I become that the single most important key to success in dealing with this disorder is *understanding*. Clients and/or their parents are often looking for easy, miraculous cures when they come to speech-language pathologists for help. There are no miracle cures in the treatment of stuttering. There are no tricks, no shortcuts to long-term success. The successful treatment of stuttering is grounded in motivation, dedication, commitment, patience, courage, and understanding. If you are reading this book as an adult stutterer, I hope to give you a basic understanding of the disorder so that you might be prepared to face it objectively, with courage, and with a determination to modify what can be modified. If you are reading this book as the parent of a young stutterer, you need to understand the disorder well enough that you can separate the stuttering from the child. If you are a clinician, you must understand the disorder more thoroughly than the client in your care because it will be your responsibility to guide the client and/or his parents on the journey from fluency disorder to fluency order. The guide must always know the trail better than those who are being led. No matter your role in dealing with the stuttering problem, you must know that if the stutterer understands his disorder, at whatever level is appropriate to his age, motivation and commitment to the therapy method being utilized will follow. Conversely, if he does not understand stuttering, he is likely to believe that it is a condition beyond his control, and as long as he believes that stuttering is beyond his control, there is no reasonable hope for improvement.

The second chapter of this book, **Stuttering: Up Close and Personal,** includes my own stuttering story and some personal insights about the disorder. The remainder of the first part of the book is designed to address the most common questions I am asked when I counsel stutterers and parents. The answers to these questions are basic to an understanding of the nature of stuttering, but the reader should be forewarned. The answers are not neat and tidy. I want to reiterate that there is much we simply do not know about stuttering. It is a communication problem that does not conform to simple answers. There is very little we can say by way of description or explanation that will be true for all stutterers because the disorder is extremely variable and because individual stutterers who might share many of the same symptoms, will react to those symptoms differently. With this disorder, the reactions of the stutterer are often far more critical in determining the impact of the disorder on that person's life than the symptoms to which he is reacting. The reader should also be aware that some of the answers I will provide might make some stutterers uncomfortable because I will repeatedly restate my view that the stutterer is ultimately responsible for his problem. No matter how much he eventually understands the problem, no matter how competent a clinician is in providing treatment and counsel, the stutterer must decide if he is a person who sometimes stutters, or if he is a stutterer, first, last, and always. The answer to that question will ultimately determine the stutterer's fate, at least that part of his fate that will be affected by his speech.

The second major part of the book is concerned with the treatment of stutterers. It deals specifically with the treatment of adult stutterers, young beginning stutterers, and young advanced stutterers. It includes advice about environmental therapy, interviewing techniques, and about how to counsel the parents of young stutterers. The final chapter describes some of the problems involved in evaluating stuttering, and while recognizing that there are as many ways to evaluate stuttering as there are to treat it, I suggest an evaluation protocol with which I am comfortable.

It will not escape the attention of careful readers that a number of general themes will be visited and revisited in this book. Even some basic facts about stuttering will be mentioned more than once. Any repetition of general themes, such as taking responsibility for one's life, being tough-minded in dealing with difficult problems, and remaining objective even when it seems easy to give in to self-pity and anger, is calculated and purposive. One of the lessons I have learned as a teacher, parent, and coach is that one should never assume that a message sent one time will be received. If the message is important, it should be stated, restated, reviewed, resurrected, and reinforced; so if some of my messages sound familiar, you are correct, and they may actually become so familiar, you will remember them. There are certain theoretical views about stuttering, and pieces of evidence that tend to support or refute these views, that I will mention more than one time. In each case, I will try to re-establish context and extend understanding, but you should be forewarned that you will be exposed to some pieces of the stuttering puzzle more than once. There is, in all of these restatements, what I call *purposive redundancy.*

Because I am writing this book for a wide audience that includes adult stutterers, the parents of children who stutter, teachers and other professionals who interact with stutterers, speech-language pathologists in training, and speech-language pathologists in practice, it is not written in a traditional textbook style. I will not be making reference to a long list of journal articles and scholarly books, for example. I will make these references only when absolutely necessary, but it is proper that I mention several people who have profoundly influenced me as a teacher, clinician, scholar, and stutterer through their writings. They are Charles Van Riper, Oliver Bloodstein, and Wendell Johnson, three men whose insights into stuttering have shaped the collective thinking of my profession about this disorder for many decades. They have facilitated my understanding of my own stuttering. They have inspired me to continue to search for answers to questions that sometimes seem unanswerable. I have used several of their works as references in this book, and their theoretical and clinical views will be heavily represented in the pages that follow.

And Now A Few Words About Political Correctness . . .

We are living in an era of great sensitivity about political correctness. There is serious debate about how far we should go in our efforts to avoid hurting people by using language that some people, or some groups of people, might find offensive. In this debate, I tend to come down on the side that asserts that we should call people what they prefer to be called, that no group can decide for another group what labels or descriptive terms are appropriate. I believe, for example, that only Native Americans can decide if using words referenced to Native Americans to name athletic teams or mascots is offensive. I believe that women have a perfect right to be offended by terms of endearment that are clearly demeaning.

The debate about political correctness has now touched stuttering, and I must confess I am troubled by the arguments in this case. Some in my profession, and many people whose lives have been impacted by stuttering, are insisting that we should no longer use the word, *stutterer,* that we should instead use the phrase, *the person who stutters.* I understand the argument. That is, the phrase, *the person who stutters,* supports the view I have already expressed in this chapter, that stuttering is just one behavior this person produces, that stuttering is not the beginning, middle, and end of this person's identity. I am troubled by the argument, however, because *stutterer* is a perfectly legitimate agentive form. That is, a stutterer, by definition, is a person who stutters. That is what the agentive form of a verb accomplishes. A worker is a person who works. A runner is a person who runs. A singer is a person who sings, and a stutterer is a person who stutters. I have chosen to use the word *stutterer* in this book, therefore, because I do not find it personally offensive. It is not demeaning. It is simply the agentive form of *stutter,* and in that capacity, it works quite well.

The issue of gender language must also be addressed. I am certainly sensitive to this issue because I believe that attitudes about gender are reflected in the words people use to describe women and men, and I believe that children's attitudes about women and men are, to a large extent, shaped by the words they hear in reference to each sex. It is not difficult to understand, for example, that a boy who hears words in reference to women such as *babe, chick, sweetie, honey,* and *darling,* will come to believe that females are people who need to be protected and taken care of, as opposed to people who are strong, capable, and independent. I have no problem with the idea that we should avoid language that is clearly sexist, language that demeans people based on gender. As a writer, I do have a problem with using *he/she,* or with a careful rotation of *he* and *she,* because this unnatural attention to gender words gets in the way of the message. Unfortunately, English does not include the kind of gender-neutral pronouns that would solve this problem.

While I am willing to acknowledge the problem and assert my sensitivity to it, I will not write in a gender-neutral manner because it is simply too awkward. In this book, I will refer to the stutterer as *he* and to the speech-language clinician as *she.* My rationale for this strategy is based on two simple facts: (1) There are many more male stutterers than female stutterers, and (2) There are many more female clinicians than male clinicians. The gender references, therefore, accurately reflect the real world regarding the sexes, at least relative to stutterers and clinicians. More importantly, there are absolutely no value judgments involved in making these gender distinctions.

If any reader is offended by my decisions regarding political correctness in reference to people who stutter or the sex of people who provide therapy to people who stutter, please reread this sentence, and you will have a pretty good idea about why I made the decisions I made.

Chapter 2

STUTTERING: UP CLOSE AND PERSONAL

This chapter contains two messages. The first message is most directly aimed at people who stutter, but it is a message I believe should be heard by the parents and teachers of children who stutter, by speech-language pathologists who treat stutterers, and by anyone else who must interact with people who stutter. The second message is most directly aimed at all people who must interact with stutterers, but its message should be important to stutterers as well because it suggests that people who stutter are remarkably similar to people who do not stutter. Sometimes stutterers seem to believe that people who do not stutter are perfect communicators who have no empathy for the stutterer's communicative fears or failures. Stutterers need to know that all speakers experience communicative failure, that normal speakers are sometimes fearful in speaking situations, that all speakers are familiar with the embarrassment and frustration that are byproducts of speech failure, and that when fear and failure are great enough, all speakers sweat.

The first message is contained in a speech I gave to a group of stutterers, parents, and speech-language clinicians in New Brunswick, Canada. It is a personal account of my own stuttering, my own therapy experiences, and my personal perspective about this disorder that has so affected my life. The second message is contained in an article I wrote that was published in the *Journal of Fluency Disorders*. It describes an exercise that all of my graduate students must complete when they take my advanced course in stuttering. They go out into the community as simulated stutterers to learn for themselves, albeit on a very limited scale, what the stuttering experience is about. I have edited both the speech and the article so they will fit more neatly into the context of this book, but I have carefully preserved the message contained in each.

My Life as a Person Who Stutters

My story as a person who stutters is remarkable because it is remarkably typical. The events of my life are not necessarily typical, but how these events relate, seem to relate, or do not relate, to the development of stuttering are typical, so a short journey through my personal history may help you understand how stutterers get from there to here, and also how some stutterers manage to get back to there, or at least as close to there as is feasible.

I am a male, and that is quite typical for stutterers. Stuttering is much more common among males than among females. My mother's pregnancy with me was full-term and uneventful, and that is also typical for stutterers.

I first became aware that I stuttered at the age of six years when I was in first grade in Lima, Ohio, but according to my parents, I began to stutter when I was about three or four years old. Both of these ages fit what we know about the onset of stuttering. Stuttering is considered a childhood disorder that usually begins between the ages of two and six years. Adult onsets do occur, but they are rare, and there is evidence that many apparent adult onsets are actually recurrences of childhood stuttering.

In order to appreciate the next part of my story, you need to understand some of the basic causality issues surrounding this disorder. Most experts agree that there are three kinds of causes that impact stuttering: (1) There are **etiological** factors, or underlying causes, those factors ultimately responsible for a person's becoming a stutterer. Most theories of stuttering address these causes. They suggest, for example, that stuttering is an organically based problem, caused by a defective larynx or by a central nervous system that is abnormal in some way. Others suggest that stuttering is a symptom of an underlying psychological problem, or that stuttering is strictly learned behavior. (2) There are **precipitating** causes, those factors that trigger the disorder when the right etiological factors are operative. Writers over the years have suggested that stuttering is triggered by shocks, illness, imitation, or by some emotional conflict in the person's life. (3) There are **maintaining** causes, those factors that cause stuttering to persist even when the etiological factors and precipitating factors are no longer operative. My personal story certainly has its share of possible causes. As I look back over my life, I tend to believe that these factors were probably coincidental to my stuttering, but I think you will agree that if one were inclined to want to find reasons for my stuttering, he would not have to look very far.

At the time I became aware of my stuttering, there were a number of dramatic things happening in my life, events that could easily have been blamed for causing me to stutter, or at least blamed for making my stuttering worse. My family was getting ready to move from Ashland, Ohio to Lima. My father had just finished college and was preparing for his first teaching job.

My mother was pregnant with my younger brother, and it had been a difficult pregnancy. My parents were Rh incompatible, a condition easily controlled today, but a condition that threatened the health of neonates at that
time. Because we had to relinquish our house to the people who bought it,
we lived with friends for about a month before the move. School was to
begin after Labor Day. My mother was due about mid-August. She spent
most of the last two months of her pregnancy in bed, and even though my
two sisters and I did not know exactly what the potential medical risks were,
we knew there were problems, and we were worried. The friends who took
us in had a farm just outside of Ashland. It was a great place for kids to be.
They had horses, a wooded area behind the house for exploring, and a creek.
Most of our time there was a grand adventure, but there were two events in
the midst of that adventure I will never forget. One day while riding one of
the horses, I was thrown to the ground and trampled. I was not seriously
hurt, but when you're not quite six years old, the sight of a horse's hooves
taking aim at your head is a bit frightening. On another occasion, I was playing in the hayloft of the barn, and not watching carefully enough, I tumbled
too close to the edge. I fell about ten feet to the ground below and landed on
a pitchfork, the tines of which poked three small holes in my back. Again,
there was no serious damage, but I was a bit shaken. Shortly after these
events, my mother went into labor, and consistent with the last two months
of the pregnancy, the labor was difficult. Because of the Rh incompatibility
problem, the hospital had blood available to do a complete blood transfusion
if the baby were born *blue*. Fortunately, my brother was born with normally
oxygenated blood, but everyone was worried, and we children were caught
up in the anxiety. Within a week, we were all loaded up for the move to
Lima. I rode in an ambulance with my mother and little brother, experiencing a mix of feelings. I was sad about leaving the only home I had ever
known and traveling to a city that seemed a world away. I was excited about
riding in an ambulance, but I was also worried about what this all meant
about my mother's health and about what my father was not telling us. In
another week, it was time for me to start school. I had not gone to kinder-
garten, so this was my first school experience. Apparently, all the anxiety
associated with these changes affected me physically. I developed a severe
rash over my entire body, a rash our physician said was an allergic reaction
to grass. Twice each day I had to take baths in a solution of baking soda. So
here I was, six years old, about to begin school, with a bright red rash from
my head to my toes, three puncture wounds on my back, and several large
bruises on my legs and shoulders courtesy of an obstinate horse. In addition,
I had been traumatized by a move and by my mother's pregnancy struggles.
Were any of these things responsible for my stuttering? I have thought about
this often over the years, and I have decided that none of these events had

anything to do with my stuttering, but there are other aspects of my personal story that I think do provide insight into my own stuttering experience.

For this part of the story, we need to go back to the first year of my life. According to my parents, when I was perhaps nine months old, I sat in my high chair and arranged colored blocks into precise patterns. I separated the blocks by color, all the reds together, all the blues together, etc. I then alternated colors, so that I had blue, red, green, yellow followed by blue, red, green, yellow, etc. In short, at a very early age, there was emerging a Type A, compulsive-obsessive, anal retentive personality, a personality that has flourished in my life ever since.

When I was six years old in Lima, Ohio, facing my first day of class, my mother wanted to take me to school, but I refused her assistance. I told her that I wanted to go to school by myself because, in essence, "There are certain things a man must do on his own." I remember that day like it was yesterday. It was sunny and moderately warm. I was wearing a shirt my mother made for me and blue jeans that were so new they were still noisy when I walked. I clutched my pencils and crayons and my tablets and walked straight ahead, my eyes firmly fixed on my destination. As I walked, I had one recurring thought, one recurring worry. Will I do well enough in first grade that I will be able to get into college? From the earliest days of my life, I could not tolerate disorder, and I could not accept failure. These attitudes provide far more insight into my own stuttering problem than any event or person outside my own thoughts and perceptions.

There is no debate about what happened over the next few years of my life after I began school. The severity of my stuttering escalated. On a scale of 1–7, on which seven represents *very severe stuttering,* I was at least a six by the time I was 10 years old and in the fifth grade. We know that once stuttering begins, it rarely remains the same. The research evidence suggests that about half of all children who begin to stutter will spontaneously recover, and most who recover will do so by the age of six years. Recovery did not occur in my case. Those who do not spontaneously recover almost always become worse, and I did. By the time I was in the fifth grade, I could not, would not respond in class, and as is often the case, I was the recipient of teasing and mocking from my more insensitive peers. The greatest pain for me, however, was not the teasing which I dismissed as the product of ignorance. The greatest pain was not being able to participate in class. You see, I was one of those *geeky* kids who loved school, but when I knew the answer, I would not offer it. Even when I was called upon and knew the answer, I would seldom give it because I was afraid to talk, afraid to stutter, afraid to fail.

I began therapy at the age of eight years, and in retrospect, I believe the therapy I received had a great deal to do with the progressive severity of my disorder. From the perspective of today's therapies, the therapies I received were primitive and generally awful. My first therapist discovered that I loved automobiles. Seizing upon this interest, she cut pictures of automobiles out of magazines, pasted them onto large cards, and instructed me to name the automobiles as she showed me the cards, one by one. This is what we did every Tuesday and Thursday morning for an entire semester. As long as I was saying only a word or two at a time, my speech was pretty fluent, and my therapist thought she was doing wonderful work. She decided at this point that I needed to practice speech in longer units, so she had me recite tongue twisters like "Peter Piper picked a peck of pickled peppers. . . ." I began slowly, and then she required me to speak more rapidly. My speech deteriorated . . . rapidly! The worst part of this therapy was that there was a home version of the torture. My poor mother was required to do the same thing to me at home. In order to appreciate how difficult and painful this was for her, you must understand that her reaction to my stuttering was utter pity laced with guilt about her possible responsibility for my problem. We sat at our kitchen table, she in her hard chair and I in mine. She said, "Let's try the first one," and I would begin, "Peter Piper picked a peck of pickled peppers. . . ." Following the therapist's orders, she then required me to say it faster, and faster, and faster. As my stuttering became worse and worse, the tears flowed down her cheeks, but we continued nonetheless because we were obedient to the therapist's instructions. By the end of that year, my stuttering had progressed from moderate to severe, and it had become a heavy emotional burden in my life. At this point, I viewed myself primarily as a stutterer. I escaped this self-concept only in my school work and in my beloved sports. When I took tests and wrote reports, I was a straight "A" student. When I played baseball, football, and basketball, I was an athlete. In virtually every other part of my life, I was a stutterer.

Over the next two years, I had therapists who tried to teach me how to breathe and how to use my tongue properly. In the breathing therapy, I spent 20 minutes at a time ". . . breathing out the bad air and breathing in the good." The teachers at my school always knew when I had just finished with therapy because I would walk down the corridors clutching the walls, fighting the light-headedness associated with hyperventilation. Passing me in the hallway, a teacher would say, "How did speech go today, Lloyd?" I would mumble, "Oh, just fine, thank you. By the way, what day is it, and would you mind pushing me in the general direction of my classroom?" This therapist also wanted me to learn how to play the clarinet, reasoning that this would help me build up the breath support I needed to speak fluently. My father rejected this suggestion, not only because of the expense, but because he did not want the noise of instrumental practice in his house. The tongue therapy involved exercises in which I would move my tongue rapidly from side to side, thrust it out forcefully and pull it back in, and try to touch my nose and chin. What I remember most about that therapy is being amazed at how tired a tongue can get. I also remember the chapped lips.

All of the therapies I experienced during my elementary school years were typical of the interventions used from about 1920–1960. They were based on three basic assumptions about stuttering: (1) The person who stutters does so because of underlying weakness in the muscles of the speech mechanism, (2) stuttering is the consequence of neurological spasms, and (3) stuttering is a bad habit that can be broken by practicing normal speech. The research evidence supports none of these assumptions as valid explanations for stuttering, even if there are aspects of the assumptions that may be true for some individuals who stutter. They did have an impact on me, however. Because my stuttering worsened over these years, my public school therapists decided I was better off without therapy, and they were probably right. I was better off without these therapies, but they did make me think about my stuttering, and that was good.

The turning point in my stuttering life came when I was 15 years and preparing to enter my sophomore year in high school. I was old enough at this point that I no longer harbored hopes that this nightmare would suddenly and magically end. I was looking ahead to beginning college, and I was giving serious thought to what I wanted to do with my adult life. I considered the impact my stuttering might have on that life. I made a conscious decision that I would not allow stuttering to affect my vocational life, and I would not permit stuttering to influence my personal life. Although it's difficult to briefly summarize the thought process, I can share with you some of the critical pieces of my mental journey from helplessness to hope and eventually to self-discipline and fluency control.

I first tried to determine exactly what the stuttering experience was for me. I knew, for example, that I did not stutter all the time. There were times, when I was playing sports and when I was angry, when I did not stutter at all. I did not stutter to the same degree when I talked to certain people. I was fairly fluent in conversations with my friends, but I stuttered frequently and severely when I talked to my father and to other adult male authority figures. There were certain words that gave me more trouble than others, but I could say even the most difficult words when I was talking to myself. As I began to put the pieces of this puzzle together, I concluded that stuttering was not something that happened to me, but something I did. This was an incredible insight, an insight that allowed me, for the first time, to understand some aspects of my problem and allowed me to begin to find reasonable solutions to my problem. I realized, for example, that certain words were *hard* only because I thought they were hard. I understood that when I thought a word would be hard to say, I prepared for speech failure by creating too much muscular tension and by struggling. I reasoned that if I could create the excessive tension, I could also reduce the tension. Over the course of that year, I practiced reducing tension whenever I felt tension build. I concentrated on producing potentially difficult words with light, loose contacts. True to my personality, I confronted feared words and situations rather than running away from them. I also had help, even though he never knew it, from Mr. Smith, my sophomore English teacher. Mr. Smith was the most demanding teacher I ever had. He required his students to read a novel each week and to give a report, either orally or in writing, each Friday. While it would have been easy for me prior to this time in my life to simply turn in written reports, I chose the oral report every week because I wanted to fight my speech battles under the toughest possible conditions. The first few weeks were awful, for me, my classmates, and I'm sure for Mr. Smith, but his reactions to my reports were perfect. He never commented on my speech. He criticized and occasionally praised my analyses and my conclusions, but he never mentioned my stuttering. By mid-year, my oral reports were delivered with greater fluency than most of my nonstuttering peers could manage. I looked for an even greater challenge, and found it in the annual high school speech contest. In this contest, each speaker memorized and delivered a speech composed by a famous person from any era of history. I chose Abraham Lincoln's second inaugural address. I practiced every night in my room, relishing the difficult words and the unusual phrasing. When the night of the contest arrived, I was terribly nervous but also terribly excited by the challenge. My parents were in the audience that night. My performance was flawless, and I won. My teachers and my friends were astounded. I was ecstatic. When I tried to find my parents, they were gone. I was crushed. This had been the most triumphant moment of my life. In September, I had been a severe stutterer. In May, I won a speech contest, and my parents were not there to share my victory. When I went home that night, they were waiting for me. They told me that they left the auditorium because they were too overwhelmed by what they had heard. They did not want to try to explain their tears to people who could not possibly understand the transformation they had witnessed.

I wish I could tell you that this was a *happy for evermore* stuttering story, but it was not. I continued to work hard on my speech every day for the next 18 months, but sometime during my senior year, I came to a terribly erroneous, and equally dangerous, conclusion. I concluded that I was cured, that I was no longer a stutterer, that I could communicate as well as other people, with no more attention to the process of speaking than that exercised by other people. It was a mistake in judgment that put me in the company of most stutterers because the rule in stuttering is relapse, precipitated by the belief that a problem under control is a problem solved. From the second half of my senior year in high school and throughout most of my freshman year in college, I went backwards, back to my old motor habits, back to my old perceptions of difficulty, back especially to my old coping strategies of avoidance and postponement. Like so many other stutterers in this situation, I rationalized my failures away, and I blamed other circumstances in my life, but because I had been down this road before, I eventually recognized where I was going, and I remembered where I had been, and I knew what I needed to do to get back to where I wanted to be. I made speech a priority once again. I refused to give in to the fear. I practiced the motor modifications that allow me to prepare for fluency when I anticipate fluency failure.

I have not experienced a relapse of that magnitude in all the years since that time, but I still have bad days, bad weeks, even bad months. I have learned to expect them, and when they come, for whatever reason they come, I know I am prepared to confront them. While I do not always understand why some days are tougher than others, I know that my will to be in control is stronger than my fear of failure. I know that my understanding of my disorder is greater than my ignorance, and I know that my ability to manipulate the physiological adjustments that make speech fluent is facile enough to overcome mere habits of motor failure.

Over the course of a university teaching career that has spanned four decades, I have been asked countless times by speech-language pathologists in training if my own stuttering has been an asset or a liability in my career as a teacher and a clinician. I always give the same answer: "Yes!" This might not be the answer students expect to hear, or want to hear, but it is a truthful answer. In truth, I was drawn to this profession, in large part, because of my own stuttering experiences. As is true of most people who stutter, I wanted to know why I stuttered. I wanted to understand this communication disorder that had so affected my life. What I have learned over the years, of course, is that there are no clear answers to thousands of fuzzy questions about stuttering. I have learned that no communication disorder has been studied by so many people from so many different disciplines who have collectively reached so many conclusions that are refuted by so many others. Stuttering has been described as a mystery, an enigma, a riddle, and even an enigma wrapped in a riddle. This is not to say that we do not know more about the disorder today than we did 100 years ago. We certainly do, but we have yet to define stuttering in a manner that is acceptable to a majority of experts, and we have yet to answer some of the most basic questions about it. What causes stuttering? Is there one cause, or are there many causes? Is it one disorder, or are there many disorders covered by a single label? Why does it affect males more often than females? Why do some who stutter spontaneously recover and others do not? Why do most stutterers sing fluently when they cannot speak fluently? Why can most stutterers speak to trees and small furry animals without stuttering? I think you can see that if this were a vote, the "whys" would have it!

Now, I am sure you have noticed that I have seemed to drift away from my original observation that my own stuttering has been both an asset and a liability. All of this mystery and enigma business is related to what I perceive to be one of the assets of being a speech-language pathologist who stutters. Although my personal experiences with the disorder have not provided definitive answers to the great questions about stuttering, they have provided me insights I would not otherwise have. More importantly, my own experiences and my own unanswered questions keep my level of curiosity high. As long as I have a powerful personal vested interest in this disorder, which I do, I think I can bring a commitment to the teaching and therapy processes that nonstuttering teachers and clinicians will have difficulty matching. When a nonstuttering clinician tells a client she *understands* what he is experiencing, she may have some idea about what he is going through, but she cannot know the experience exactly. I know the experience, from the inside out, and on balance, this up close and personal familiarity with stuttering has been an asset.

In what sense is my own stuttering a liability? You have all heard that there is no more impassioned antismoking advocate than a former smoker. The same can be said for recovering alcoholics, recovering drug addicts, and people who have had long-term success in dealing with weight control. For many of the same reasons, a recovering or controlled stutterer can be a real pain in the neck for people who are fighting the stuttering battle with less success. I have been a severe and uncontrolled stutterer. I experienced the classic developmental patterns. I have used every category of stuttering behavior described by the experts. When I tell a client that I understand what he is experiencing, I mean it, and in most respects, as I have already noted, this understanding is a good thing, but there is a down side. I also understand what is required to wage a successful battle against this disorder. I understand the absolute necessity of self-discipline and will in dealing with powerfully entrenched misperceptions, fears, and motor habits. I know the levels of motivation and commitment that are necessary for success, and sadly, I know the levels of motivation and commitment most people who stutter are willing to give. I know how deadly the *I can't* attitude is that dooms therapy effectiveness. I know how easy it is to blame other people for causing the problem, or for not solving the problem, and I know how easy it is to say, "The program didn't work," when, in fact, I know that people solve this problem, not programs. The bottom line on the liability issue is this. As a person who stutters, I have very high expectations for what must happen in therapy, and when clients demonstrate an unwillingness to meet those expectations, I am disappointed. Although it may not be true in my personal life, I am a fairly patient person in my professional life, but when it becomes apparent that I care more about dealing with the problem than the person who owns the problem, my patience wears thin, and that can be a liability for someone who treats people who stutter.

If you are a stutterer or a stutterer's caregiver, I want you to pay close attention to the ending of this section of this chapter. In preparation for a recent visit to Wheaton College, a small liberal arts college in the Chicago area, I asked students to write out some questions they would like me to address about stuttering. One of the questions I received I will never forget: "Have you derived any benefits from stuttering?" I later learned that this question was posed by a stutterer, but knowing that would not have changed my answer. I want to share with you just a portion of my response to this question.

I believe I have derived enormous benefits from my stuttering experiences, some of which relate directly and specifically to my stuttering and some of which relate to my life in general. Stuttering has helped me understand the necessity of assuming responsibility for one's own life. No matter what or who may have been responsible for my stuttering in the beginning, there is nothing I can do about that now. I can only deal with my stuttering as it exists today. If I expect to deal with it successfully, I must assume ownership of the problem and its solution. My stuttering has taught me invaluable lessons about self-discipline, motivation, the power of will, and the necessity of practice. Stuttering has taught me that fear, and especially the fear of failure, is a paralyzing force that must be controlled if one is to live meaningfully. Stuttering has taught me that the most influential person in my life, the person who will affect me most powerfully for good or ill, is me. You might recognize that these lessons sound somewhat like the lessons learned, and then taught by, the child I mentioned in the first chapter, the little girl who was dying of cancer. This is not mere coincidence. The underlying lesson I have learned from dealing with my stuttering, and the underlying lesson the little girl learned from confronting her cancer is that every person, no matter what obstacles may intrude, is in charge of his or her life. There is a certain comfort in that knowledge, but there is also an enormous challenge. The challenge in being the master of one's fate is to stop laying blame, stop making excuses, stop whining and complaining, and get on with the business of solving problems to ensure the most satisfying fate one can achieve.

A Stutterer Like Me

"Unless you have walked in my shoes . . ." is the common lament of someone who feels misunderstood. We have all been on both sides of the empathy problem. There are times when we feel others cannot relate to what we are feeling or experiencing, and there are times when we stand accused of not being sensitive to the feelings, attitudes, or experiences of someone else.

One of the more courageous attempts to understand the experience of others was made by John Howard Griffin during the fall of 1959. Griffin, a Caucasian, lived for five weeks as an African-American. With the assistance of a physician in New Orleans, he used drug and sun lamp treatments to darken his skin. He traveled across Louisiana, Mississippi, Alabama, and Georgia. In his book, *Black Like Me,* Griffin chronicles his experiences, most of which were as distressing as they were enlightening. For those five weeks, he came as close as possible to true empathy for the African-American experience.

I have often thought about John Howard Griffin and his quest for understanding when I have tried to explain to my students what it is like to be a stutterer. As a teacher and clinician in the area of fluency disorders, I have become increasingly convinced that understanding the person who stutters and the nature of stuttering is essential to success in the clinical process. Toward that end, I require my graduate students to live as stutterers for a brief time in order to gain some insight into what the stutterer experiences during communicative failure.

The assignment has been gradually modified over the years to optimize the educational value. The students go out into the community in pairs. Each takes a turn as the stutterer while the other observes from close distance. They must go to retail stores, talk to people they do not know, and they must stutter as severely as possible. The assignment is preceded by a comprehensive in-class discussion and demonstration of stuttering behaviors. At no time may the student reveal that she or he is a normal speaker. Following the exercise, each student writes a report on the experience, detailing what happened during the communicative situation and identifying her or his physical and emotional reactions to the simulated stuttering and to the responses of the listener(s). We also devote class time to an open discussion of the students' experiences. The following is a summary of the reactions of one class of twenty-nine female graduate students. The summary is divided into four sections: Physical Reactions, Emotional Reactions, Listener Reactions, and Insights Gained.

Physical Reactions

The physical reactions were predictable and not unlike those experienced by stutterers themselves. Eight students said that their faces "turned red," "flushed," or "burned." Another six reported that their "stomachs were upset" or "tied in knots." Almost all indicated that they felt muscular tension when they stuttered. Nearly half wrote about their hands shaking, their voices quavering, their faces or mouths twitching. Three students felt their pulses quicken. Two mentioned an increase in perspiration. One student said she felt "dizzy," while another said that she was "in a daze." Several indicated a feeling of "no control." One student said that she felt like she could not stop being nonfluent once she started. Four students said that, without thinking about it, they looked away from their listeners when they simulated stuttering. One student reported that she "played nervously" with the buttons on her coat. Another student felt the pitch of her voice increase. Another said that her legs were weak. One student wrote, "I felt like my lips were glued together." In a variety of ways, these students frequently mentioned feeling physically fatigued when the experience was over. One student wrote, "When I got out of the store, my adrenaline was really going. It was like finishing a tough exam but still not being relieved."

Emotional Reactions

There was considerable uniformity in the emotional reactions of these students. Almost all reported that they were "nervous," and several indicated that this sense of anxiety existed before, during, and after the simulation. Other common reactions included feeling "embarrassed," "uncomfortable," "self-conscious," and "frustrated." In one way or another, every student wrote about "fear." One student used the word "panic" to describe how she felt. Several used the word, "paranoia." Others felt "angry," "vulnerable," "confused." Still others wrote that they felt "inadequate," ". . . like a failure," "intimidated," "stupid." One student said that she was afraid she would faint because her emotions were so high. Several mentioned that they could not remember what they were talking about. One student wrote, "My concept of time was distorted because I felt like I had been there forever." Almost half of these students described attempts to avoid or flee. One wrote that she ". . . wanted to stop and walk far away." Another wrote, "The whole thing was very isolating. It was just me and those words trying to get out. I hated it." In summary, these students experienced the entire range of negative emotions commonly experienced by adult stutterers. Many of them reported that they felt "emotionally drained" at the end of the simulation.

Listener Reactions

There was a wide range of perceived listener reactions, but on balance these students perceived more negative reactions than positive. Six students wrote about listeners "staring" or "gawking." Others reported that listeners were "embarrassed," "uncomfortable," "rude," "impatient," "annoyed," "disgusted," "condescending." Several indicated that listeners were "compassionate," but several others used the word, "pity." Some students wrote about listeners moving away or looking away. Four students encountered listeners who finished their sentences. One reported that the listener's "eyes widened," another that the listener "rolled her eyes." Two students wrote that they were treated like children, and three others said that they were treated as though they were mentally retarded. In all of these cases, the students reported that the listeners spoke slowly, loudly, and in simple sentences.

There were, according to these students, some listeners who responded in more appropriate ways. Students wrote about listeners who were "patient," "concerned," and "calm and relaxed." Two students wrote about listeners who were not rude but who were "startled" or "astonished." One reported that the listener "laughed nervously," and another that the listener was "as nervous as I was."

Insights Gained

The goal of this task is to teach students something about the nature of stuttering and how it impacts the individual who stutters. However limited and flawed the experience of simulated stuttering may be, there are lessons learned. Although students are nearly unanimous in dreading this assignment, they are also nearly unanimous in asserting that it is worthwhile, educational, and enlightening. Two students in this class observed that it made them more aware that the stutterer's experience extends from prior to the actual stuttering to a period of time after the moment is complete. Several students noted that they learned how perception plays a role in the stuttering experience. They indicated that they selected female listeners, for example, because they thought it would be more difficult to talk to males. One student learned something about the nature of speech-related fears: "Needless to say, I was relieved when we left Wendy's, and I will probably never set foot in that place again even though I love it. Now I understand how a stutterer can develop situation fears and how this fear could generalize to McDonald's, Burger King, etc." Another student learned something about the power of communicative failure to live beyond the moment: "My heart started pounding and I could feel my cheeks get red just writing about the experience." Yet another student learned that the end of a moment comes with mixed feelings: "I felt relief when I finished the sentence but not a sense of accomplished communication." Several students wrote about the overwhelming sense of frustration one experiences before and during fluency failure, but one student captured this thought particularly well: "The tension of only thinking about talking is incredible. A simple question I've asked to so many people with no conscious effort had become a task of enormous difficulty."

The Simulated Stuttering Experience in Context

So many of our research efforts over the past half-century have focused on potential differences between stutterers and nonstutterers, and that focus is understandable. If we can identify differences, we can perhaps uncover the cause or causes of stuttering, and if we can discover the causes, we can devise more effective treatment and prevention strategies. Unfortunately, this preoccupation with differences obscures the fact that people who stutter are remarkably similar to people who do not stutter.

As a clinician and teacher, I have tried to impress upon clients and students that the stutterer is, in almost every important respect, a normal person, or at least as normal as the majority of human beings are allowed to be. Virtually every physiological and psychological difference that has been noted can be more easily explained as an effect of stuttering than as a causative factor. There are also those annoying exceptions that make potential explanations of stuttering troublesome. It is true, for example, that stuttering is much more common among males than among females, but there are females who stutter. Stuttering usually begins during childhood, but there are cases of adult onset. Fluency problems are more common in individuals who are mentally retarded, but there are also intellectually gifted stutterers. Too many people who try to explain stuttering assume that stuttering is a single disorder with a single cause. If our research and clinical efforts have taught us anything over the past 50 years, it is that this is an unrealistically simplistic view of a very complex problem, a problem we increasingly understand is not limited to the speech apparatus.

Perhaps the most important lesson to be learned by normal speakers in the simulated stuttering exercise is that perception plays a major role in stuttering. A stutterer has difficulty with certain words, certain situations, and certain listeners, not because there is anything inherently difficult or justifiably frightening about these cues, but because he believes they are difficult or frightening. One of the cruel twists in this disorder, a cruelty bound up in perception and fear, is that the stutterer stutters most when he is convinced it is most important to be fluent. Stuttering then is more than repetitions, prolongations, facial grimaces, and disordered breathing. It is also fear, ranging from vague doubt about the ability to speak fluently to uncontrollable panic, that precipitates the physiological reactions that result in the inappropriate articulatory adjustments that make nonfluencies inevitable. More importantly, this chain reaction is not unique to stutterers. Any speaker, given enough fear, will experience the same physiological reactions, the same articulatory maladjustments, and at least similar fluency failures. This is the lesson to be learned in simulated stuttering, and it is a lesson that has the potential to make a clinician more understanding and more empathic when working with the *real thing*.

Despite my efforts to minimize the differences, there is one crucial difference between stutterers and nonstutterers that cannot and should not be ignored. Two students in this class alluded to this difference. One wrote, "This assignment was a tough one, but it was a good learning experience. We thought about the difference between just pretending to stutter and not having a choice." Another student made reference to a scene from the film, *Soul Man*. In this film, a young Caucasian man passes as African-American in order to win a scholarship to the Harvard Law School, a scholarship reserved for African-Americans. The ruse becomes complicated when he falls in love with the young woman who should have been awarded the scholarship he received. Eventually, his identify is revealed, and he faces his mentor with the truth. His mentor, a distinguished law professor who, not coincidentally, is African-American, tells the young man that he has learned some valuable lessons about what it is like to be African-American. The young man admits that this was not really true because he always knew he could choose to be white again.

The analogy is clear. Students who submit themselves to the assignment of simulated stuttering experience, to some degree, the physical and emotional reactions the stutterer must endure every day, but these students know that when they wake up the next day, they will be normal speakers. For the stutterer, the communicative failures continue, and the normal speaker should not be deceived about what this means. Just as an African-American never accepts bigotry and discrimination in their obvious and subtle forms, the stutterer never adjusts to the physical discomfort and the emotional pain that mark his disorder. Walking in his shoes is the beginning of the journey to understanding, but a short walk is just that–a short walk. It is not the same as the complete, uninterrupted trip.

Chapter 3

IN SEARCH OF A DEFINITION

Having established some personal perspective on this disorder, I want to go back to what would seem a logical beginning point. What is this disorder we call *stuttering?* Obviously, what we need here is a good definition. What we do NOT have here or anywhere else is a good definition of stuttering. In fact, we do not even have a mediocre definition that would be acceptable to a sizable majority of experts. The reasons for this problem are not simple, but I will try to provide a reasonable explanation.

To *define,* according to my edition of Webster's dictionary, is "to determine or set down the boundaries of; set down or show the precise outlines of; to determine and state the limits and nature of; describe exactly; to give the distinguishing characteristics of" whatever it is one is trying to define. Stuttering presents some serious, although not unique, problems when it comes to establishing a definition. All experts would agree, for example, that the word *stuttering* is properly used to describe a speech disorder characterized by disrupted rhythm or fluency, but if we apply this definition, we must conclude that all speakers stutter since all speakers, at one time or another, experience disrupted fluency. In fact, many people we would all agree are nonstutterers are more nonfluent than some people who are accurately diagnosed as stutterers. The mere fact that someone occasionally repeats sounds, syllables, or words does not make that person a stutterer. Stuttering goes beyond normal fluency failures, and therein lays the rub. If we had a solid handle on what constitutes normal speech, we would be in a better position to define stuttering, or other communication disorders for that matter, but we do not.

There are wide ranges of normal along every dimension of speech, including fluency. There are individuals who do not make all the sounds of speech according to standard form who are paid obscene sums of money to be television journalists. We might agree that their speech is not perfect, but it would be difficult to argue that their speech is *defective* since they are employed as professional speakers. In truth, some of these people seem to be more appealing because they do not have perfect speech. Their communicative imperfections are part of their charm in much the same way that sports fans came to view butchering the English language entertaining and charming in the baseball legends, Dizzy Dean and Casey Stengel. Fluency is an even more troublesome aspect of speech than the production of speech sounds because *every* speaker experiences fluency errors. Speech-language pathologists make a distinction between *normal nonfluencies* and *stuttering*, and any relatively intelligent, insightful stutterer knows the difference. I can readily discern the difference between normal and abnormal nonfluencies in my own speech, but it might be difficult to make the difference clear to someone else, especially to someone who does not stutter, and the differentiation is made even more difficult when we add the age and developmental factors. I could tell you, for example, that my stutterings are anticipated and that they involve struggle and that my normal nonfluencies are not anticipated and do not involve struggle, but I also know that most young stutterers produce behaviors I would consider stuttering that seem not to be anticipated and are not characterized by struggle, so where and how does one draw the line between normal mistakes in fluency and stuttering? Whatever lines might be drawn are largely arbitrary. Consider that when experts, listening to tapes of normal and stuttered speech, have tried to agree on what is stuttering and what is not, their agreement has been very poor, not appreciably better than when laypersons have attempted the same task.

Wendell Johnson, a man whose views about stuttering shaped our understanding of the disorder for much of the 20th century, was particularly sensitive to the problem I have been addressing. He believed that the only real difference between stutterers and nonstutterers, at the onset of stuttering, is that stutterers are labeled *stutterers*. He contended that all of the other problems we associate with stuttering are caused by the child's reactions to the label, reactions that are considerably aided and abetted by his parents' evaluations, attitudes, and perceptions related to the child's speech failures. Johnson believed and preached that there is nothing the stutterer does that the nonstutterer does not also do at some times to some extent. In other words, Johnson saw no line between stutterers and nonstutterers, PRIOR TO DIAGNOSIS, except the one arbitrarily drawn by those who overreact to the normal nonfluencies in children they identify as stutterers. The struggle and facial contortions and disordered breathing and the substitution of words we associate with severe stuttering, according to Johnson, are the result of reactions to the line, the diagnosis, the label *stuttering*. This view of the problem results in what might be called a Johnsonian definition of stuttering: "Stuttering is what the stutterer does in order not to stutter." That is, the child is normally nonfluent. An adult, usually a parent, responds to these natural mistakes by calling them *stuttering* and by calling the child a *stutterer.* The child, believing that adults and especially his parents are infallible in their judgments, accepts this evaluation as valid. In an effort to correct this problem, to eliminate this flaw, the child struggles to make his speech perfect. In valiantly trying to shed the label and repudiate the diagnosis, he becomes the very thing he was trying to escape. He becomes a stutterer.

I will hasten to point out that not all experts agree with Johnson's views on stuttering, but they do provide an opportunity for the reader to consider some of the problems involved in defining stuttering, not the least of which is distinguishing between normal nonfluency and stuttering.

If you are feeling a bit frustrated at this point, do not despair. I hope to convince you that a definition of stuttering is probably an overrated commodity. By its very nature, a definition limits, and the process of limiting may not be what we need in this case. I would suggest that we are better served by seeking an understanding of stuttering that does not set rigid limits because it is a disorder that does not lend itself to rigid limits. It is a highly complex and multi-faceted problem that cannot even be limited to speech. By the time we reach the end of this chapter, you will not have a definition of stuttering, but you should have a much better understanding of its primary, and widely varied, features.

One Disorder or Many?

In order to understand what stuttering is, we must distinguish it from normal nonfluency, but we must also separate stuttering from other fluency disorders. This has long been a problem in the stuttering literature and has added fuel to the debates concerning the cause or causes of stuttering. We know, for example, that fluency problems are more common among mentally retarded individuals than among normally intelligent individuals, and we know that fluency problems are even more common among Down's syndrome people than among mentally retarded people who do not have Down's syndrome. Fluency problems more frequently occur in the cerebral palsied and epileptic populations than among people who are neurologically normal. We also know that some victims of stroke develop fluency problems, along with language and articulation problems. Many writers over the years have called all of these fluency problems, *stuttering,* and have made little attempt to distinguish between fluency problems associated with brain damage and fluency problems that develop in children and adults who show no evidence of neurological damage. Common sense would suggest that there have to be some differences, and common sense is correct. The neurologically normal stutterer, for example, is significantly affected by speaking situations, by the listeners to whom he is speaking, by the words he is trying to say. When there is little stress, when he feels comfortable with his listeners, when he is confident in his ability to say the words he wants to say, he is likely to be quite fluent. When there is a great deal of stress, when he is talking to people he finds intimidating or threatening, when he is trying to say words he believes are inherently difficult, he will almost certainly stutter, and he might stutter badly. While the severely cerebral palsied individual will also be affected by stress, he is more likely to be nonfluent in all speaking situations. At the risk of making a differentiation that is too simplistic, the neurologically normal stutterer's problem is heavily perceptual and the neurologically damaged individual's problem is heavily motoric. Although both of these individuals have fluency problems that combine perceptual and motoric components, the neurologically normal stutterer is likely to do well when he **thinks** speaking will be easy, and he is likely to struggle when he **thinks** speaking will be difficult.

One of the great unanswered questions concerning stuttering, therefore, is whether we are dealing with one disorder, several, or many. There are several possibilities. Stuttering might be one disorder with one cause. Although a number of theorists have approached it this way, the one disorder/one cause view seems a highly unlikely possibility. Stuttering might be a single disorder with several causes. It might be several disorders with one cause, although this seems even more unlikely than the one disorder/one cause view. The view most plausible to me is that *stuttering* is a term traditionally applied to several disorders, each of which probably has more than a single cause. The only common denominator in all of these disorders is nonfluency, and the nature of the nonfluency will vary to some extent with each disorder. We must guard against thinking of nonfluency as the disorder because nonfluency is only a characteristic of speech, disordered or not. The stutterer, the spastic cerebral palsied speaker, and the normal speaker all produce nonfluencies, but they are not necessarily, or even plausibly, the same behaviors, and it is difficult to imagine that they have precisely the same origins.

Having expressed an opinion about this issue, I want to caution the reader that my comments should not be interpreted as an answer to the question about how many disorders and how many causes we are addressing. I am comfortable with the multiple disorders/multiple causes view because it fits my interpretation of the research data and because it fits my sense of most reasonable understanding, but reason, understanding, and data are not enough to make this view *the truth*.

Although I cannot prove, beyond a shadow of doubt, that my view is correct, I ask that you consider the following. Over the past several decades, our understanding of cancer and its causes and our understanding of depression and its causes have changed dramatically. At one time, we viewed both of these conditions as limited disorders/limited causes problems, but the more we learn about these disorders and most disorders with which human beings are afflicted, the more we understand that the disorders themselves are very complex and that they can have widely varied origins. We now understand that cancer can have genetic connections, that it can be caused by improper diet, by smoking, and even by stress. We know that all cancers are not the same, except that they all involve abnormal cell growth. At one time, we believed that depression was a strictly psychological problem, but we now have evidence that depression is often the result of biochemical imbalances, and we believe that some individuals are genetically predisposed to depression. These changes in our understandings of cancer and depression have significant implications relative to the diagnosis, treatment, and prevention of these conditions, and I have only used these two conditions to make a point about causality and human problems, including stuttering. If you had the opportunity to observe the speech behaviors of a severe spastic cerebral palsied individual, a severely mentally retarded Down's syndrome individual, and a stutterer who is otherwise normal, I suspect you would agree with me that not all people who are labeled *stutterers* are experiencing the same condition. I suspect you would become convinced that the term, *stuttering,* is used to identify different disorders with somewhat different symptoms that require different treatments.

You may feel that I have belabored this point somewhat. I will confess that I have, but I have done so for good reason. I want to make it clear that this book is not concerned with all fluency disorders. It is not concerned with *cluttering,* a disorder characterized by rapid rate, fluency breakdown, and slurred articulation. It is specifically concerned with the fluency problem that develops in the absence of severe neurological or psychological problems. When nonfluent speech develops suddenly in a child or adult who has experienced a serious emotional trauma, the nonfluency is probably symptomatic of a psychological problem. Treating the speech in this case is something like putting a bandage on your forehead when you have a migraine headache. You are doing something to be sure, but it is not likely to have a medical impact because you are reacting to pain, a symptom, and not to the cause of the pain. On the other hand, the person who has neurologically-based fluency problems needs speech therapy, but the therapy appropriate for this client would differ significantly from the therapy designed for a neurologically normal stutterer. What is written beyond this point, therefore, pertains to neurologically and psychologically normal stutterers, with the understanding that *normal* does not mean *without problems* since no one would fit that definition. *Normal* in this context means *without serious, debilitating problems.*

I want to add a personal observation about *normal* before we move forward. The longer I deal with people professionally and personally, the more convinced I am that there are no really *normal* people, and we should be grateful for this fact of life. We all have our little problems and idiosyncrasies, and they make us more interesting and more acceptable to all the world's other imperfect people. I would argue that only when imperfections begin to interfere with a person's ability to function in healthy ways, should we use the word *abnormal,* and even then we should all confess that we are more tolerant of imperfections in our friends than in strangers. I will allow you to determine if you fit this rather vague and liberal definition of *normal.* After a brief period of introspection, please rejoin me as we continue to try to answer the question, "What is stuttering?"

The Confusing and Incomplete Facts about Stuttering

We have considered a few of the difficult and disturbing questions about stuttering. Let us now consider what we actually know about stuttering–the sometimes confusing and almost always incomplete facts about stuttering. When I was a student in a graduate seminar on stuttering, the professor began the term by distributing a handout, the title of which was *Everything We Know About Stuttering.* The handout consisted of one page, and that one page was not completely covered with information. Furthermore, almost every bit of information included was qualified in some way. What follows is my version of that handout, considerably elaborated. You will notice that much of what we know is quite superficial. I will tell you what we know, and then I will tell you what we do not know about what we think we know. Confused? If so, join the legions of confused and frustrated people who have tried to understand this mysterious disorder. I will try to make clear what can be made clear, but some confusion is inevitable because we just do not have many answers to the big stuttering questions, and those answers do not seem to be lurking over the horizon.

We know that stuttering is primarily a childhood disorder. That is, it most often begins during childhood, typically between the ages of two and six years. Adult onset cases are rare. There is, in fact, some evidence that many cases of stuttering that seem to begin during adulthood are actually recurrences of childhood stuttering. Nevertheless, there are people who begin to stutter as adults, usually following a psychological trauma or as a consequence of a neurological trauma. Fortunately, many adults who begin to stutter as adults stop stuttering when, or if, they recover from the trauma.

We also know that many children who begin to stutter stop stuttering, without therapy, before they reach adolescence. There is considerable disagreement about how many children spontaneously recover. The estimates range from about 40 percent to 80 percent. Some experts reject the high number because, they argue, many children who are considered *recovered from stuttering* were probably not stutterers in the first place. You may recall the earlier discussion about how problematic it is to separate normal nonfluencies from stuttering. The question about how many children spontaneously recover from stuttering is directly related to this problem. Writers who are skeptical about high spontaneous recovery rates point out that some children who are considered *recovered* are diagnosed as stutterers when they are two and three years old and are declared *recovered* six months or a year later. There is no question that this is a difficult judgment to make, and one can readily see the potential for false positive identifications, but we should be certain that we do not lose sight of several points to be made here. Many children, perhaps 50 percent, who have what speech-language pathologists perceive as more than normal difficulty achieving fluent speech, recover from this difficulty without direct intervention. In addition, speech-language clinicians would agree that the younger the client, the more favorable the prognosis when a stutterer is enrolled in therapy. Conversely, the longer a person stutters, the poorer the prognosis is for a complete recovery.

We know that the *prevalence* of stuttering worldwide is approximately 1 percent. Prevalence tells us how many people in a given population are stutterers at this moment. Assuming there are 300 million people living in the United States today, there are about 3 million stutterers. The *incidence* of stuttering is about 4 percent. The incidence figure tells us how many people in a given population were, are now, or will become stutterers in their lifetimes. There are, therefore, about 12 million people in the United States who are stutterers today, were stutterers at one time, or will become stutterers in the future. Since stuttering usually begins at an early age, the difference between the prevalence figure and the incidence figure can be mostly explained by the rate of spontaneous recovery. These are fairly hopeful numbers in a couple of ways. First, there are relatively few people who become stutterers. This is of little comfort, of course, to those of us who are stutterers, but the numbers should help us maintain reasonable perspective about how widespread the problem really is. Many people I talk to have never personally known a stutterer because it is such a rare disorder. I always tell these folks that their lives would be much richer and fulfilling if they did know some stutterers because we are infinitely more interesting than the smooth talkers of the world, but having gauged the true value of my opinions, they ignore me. The prevalence and incidence figures are also hopeful in that they suggest that stuttering is not necessarily, or even usually, a permanent condition. I should also point out that many experts today believe that the incidence of stuttering is declining, although it is difficult to prove this apparent tendency for a number of reasons, not the least of which is our inability to agree on a definition of stuttering. It could be that what seems to be a decline in incidence is really just a shift in the general perception of what stuttering is. I believe, for example, that we are much more tolerant of all kinds of differences among people today than we were a generation or two ago, even though we have miles to go before we are as tolerant as we should be. Nevertheless, it may be that we think there are fewer stutterers because we accept children today as normally nonfluent who would have been diagnosed as stutterers 30 or 40 years ago. I want to emphasize, however, that even if the decline in incidence is only due to more tolerant attitudes, that is still very good news because many clinicians, including this one, believe that intolerant and critical attitudes about the imperfections in children's speech can contribute to the onset and/or development of stuttering.

If stuttering is a constitutional predisposition problem, as many theorists have suggested, there may be a decline in incidence because people are healthier and stronger today than they have ever been. One needs to be extremely cautious about this connection, however, because the declines noted have occurred over a period of only 40 to 50 years, which seems hardly enough time to account for genetic improvements in human beings that would make them less vulnerable to constitutional predisposition problems. If the decline in incidence over just two or three generations is real, it is more likely to be explained as an environmental phenomenon than as a genetic or biological phenomenon.

One of the more interesting, although unexplained, things we know about stuttering is that it is much more common among males than among females. The ratio of males to females ranges from about 2:1 to 5:1, increasing with age. This ratio increase could mean that females are more likely to recover from stuttering than males, but we have no evidence to support that explanation. Instead, the evidence suggests that as children grow older, boys remain vulnerable to the onset of stuttering for a longer period of time than girls. As you might imagine, there are many arguments about why males are more likely to become stutterers than females. Some writers suggest that boys are more likely to become stutterers simply because they are members of the biologically *weaker* sex. Males are weaker in the sense that they have more difficulty surviving childbirth and the first year of life than females. In adulthood, males die younger, and they are more susceptible to a wide range of disorders and diseases than females. It is not surprising, these pundits assert, that males are more likely to stutter than females because they are victims of their own sex. Another point of view suggests that males are more prone to stuttering because there is more environmental pressure on males than on females to compete and succeed. If this is true, we should see different sex ratios in societies that treat males and females more equally than our own or less equally than our own, but we do not find different ratios. Cultures that promote apparent equality between the sexes in terms of opportunity, expectation, and competitive stress, produce stuttering sex ratios that are virtually identical to those produced by cultures that promote or allow differences in the treatment of the sexes. A third explanation that strikes a balance between these views suggests that more males than females stutter because boys mature physically and emotionally more slowly than girls, and therefore, cannot tolerate the ordinary pressures all children experience to talk early and talk well. Some writers point to data that seem to suggest a sex-modified genetic transmission of a greater constitutional predisposition to stuttering among males, and still others theorize that the sex ratio can be explained by the higher levels of testosterone in the male fetus in comparison to the female fetus. According to this view, testosterone retards the development of the left cerebral hemisphere, making the child more vulnerable to the full range of communication disorders, including stuttering. And where do all these possible explanations leave us? Even though we have added a few new ideas to the speculative mix, we are probably not much closer to knowing the *truth* about the sex ratio today than we were a half century ago, but we might find some solace in knowing that this imperfect closure is not unique to stuttering. There is much we still do not understand about differences between males and females in general, and the debate about whether these differences are largely biological or largely environmental endures. The stuttering sex ratio issue is one very small element of a mystery about the sexes that is not likely to be solved any time soon. I am reminded that it was not many years ago when running experts were convinced that women could not, or perhaps should not, run marathons. Today some of these same experts believe that women, because they may be uniquely suited to this kind of running, may someday complete faster marathons than men. The point is we have much to learn about the capacities, limitations, and differences between males and females before we can deal with issues such as the sex ratio in stuttering with any degree of confidence.

Is stuttering the product of genetics or the environment? The preceding discussion should lead you directly to the answer to this question. We do not know. We do know that stuttering often appears in successive generations of a given family, a fact that has fueled speculation that stuttering is inherited. There are survey data that appear to support a genetic link. When asked if they know anyone in their families who are stutterers, 33 to 66 percent of stutterers report that there are. Only 6 to 18 percent of nonstutterers report that there are stutterers in their families. On the surface, these numbers would seem to suggest a genetic link, but there are at least two nongenetic explanations for these numbers: (1) Stutterers are more likely than nonstutterers to be aware of the existence of other stutterers in their families simply because they are more interested. Any person with any condition that makes him or her unusual becomes immediately interested in possible genetic explanations for the condition. (2) As was pointed out to me years ago, there are many things that are passed from generation to generation that have nothing to do with genetics, including political views, religious beliefs, and money. Stuttering could, therefore, be an environmental problem that is handed down from one generation to the next because the child-rearing environment that gives rise to stuttering is handed down from one generation to the next. I want to carefully note that I am not suggesting there *is* a connection between child-rearing environment and the development of stuttering, but I am suggesting there are plausible environmental explanations for what may appear to be genetic connections.

Genetic research itself has not provided a clear answer to the heredity question. We do know that stuttering among family members cannot be explained on the basis of traditional genetic transmission. That is, it is not a classic recessive or dominant genetic trait. In more recent years, there has been the suggestion that stuttering might be a human trait resulting from the interaction of genetic and environmental factors. If there is a majority opinion among speech-language pathologists on this question, taking into account all the relevant research, it would be that there is probably a fairly strong genetic factor related to a predisposition to stuttering, but this factor does not operate independent of the environment. This would mean that if two people are born with the same genetic predisposition to stuttering, one might become a stutterer and the other might not. If a person with this predisposition is reared by exceptionally loving, accepting parents who exert no pressure on him to talk sooner or more competently than he is capable, and if they are not critical of the child's normal speech failures, and if the child does not apply undue pressure on himself, or develop a perfectionistic attitude about speech, he might very well emerge a normal speaker. The other person, born with the same genetic predisposition to stuttering, if reared in an environment characterized by unrealistic expectations, competition, perfectionistic attitudes, and criticism, might become a stutterer.

You should note here that I have not crawled very far out onto a limb because we can have the same argument about many other behaviors caught up in the never-ending *nature versus nurture* debate. Is a child's intelligence a product of heredity or environment? Is the child's personality a product of heredity or environment? Most reasonable people would agree that a person's genetic makeup certainly contributes to intelligence and personality, but they would also agree that environment plays an important role in developing intellectual capacities and personality profiles. The point is, there are few things about human beings, beyond things like eye and skin color, that are purely genetic, and there are few, if any, behaviors that can be described as purely environmental. Unless a child is born with some innate musical talent, for example, he or she will never be a world-class musician, no matter how many hours are devoted to practice. We should also keep in mind that something as obviously genetic as eye color can be manipulated environmentally. A brown-eyed person can have blue eyes if he or she can afford color-altering contact lenses. Pushed to the wall on this issue, I will say I am confident that future research will verify the popular view today that stuttering is a genetic AND an environmental problem, not one or the other.

One of the more interesting facts about stuttering, and a focal point in the *nature versus nurture* argument, is that stuttering is much more common among twins than among singletons. Furthermore, there is some evidence that when stuttering occurs in one member of a set of identical twins, it is likely to occur in the other member, a phenomenon referred to as *concordance* of stuttering. While the evidence gathered over the past 60 years suggests that there is a fairly high degree of concordance of stuttering in identical twins, the data do not indicate that there is significant concordance in fraternal, or nonidentical, twins. The researchers who first discovered the high concordance among identical twins were quick to conclude that this proved a genetic link. They argued that since identical twins are the products of the cleavage of a single fertilized ovum, we can assume they have the same genetic background, and since identical twins are much more likely to share stuttering than fraternal twins, who do not have identical genetic backgrounds, this must mean that stuttering is genetically transmitted. Reviewers of this research reach a more cautious conclusion. While conceding that these data might support a genetic link, they point out that there is an alternative, nongenetic explanation for this difference in concordance. Identical twins not only share a common genetic background, they also share a common environment. These children, because they are so strikingly similar, are typically treated by their parents and all significant others in identical ways. If stuttering is an environmental problem, we would expect that identical twins reared in the same environment would both likely become stutterers if the conditions for creating stuttering were present. Perhaps the most intriguing aspect of the research on twins is what it could yield in the future. If we could show that identical twins, separated at birth and reared apart in significantly different environments, have a high degree of concordance of stuttering, we would have strong evidence of a genetic link, at least for twins. These data are not yet available, and they may never be available because the separation of identical twins is rare in an era of humanitarian sensitivity and concern for the rights of newborn children.

Have we found any significant environmental differences in prevalence that might help us resolve the nature versus nurture argument? During the period from about 1935 to 1955, there were some researchers who came up with promising leads, but their conclusions probably exceeded the limits of their data. In general, these investigators found that there were fewer stutterers in cultures not characterized by pressure and perfectionistic attitudes, particularly in regard to speech. In other cases, researchers identified cultures characterized by unusual degrees of pressure that produced more stutterers than the worldwide average. Taken together, all of these studies would lead us to conclude that there are probably no stuttering-free cultures, but there are cultures that seem to produce more or fewer stutterers than others. It should also be noted that there are enough questions about research design and biases in the interpretation of these data that we cannot accept the conclusions of these investigators without considerable reservation.

In many cases, the environmental research is inconclusive. In other cases, it is simply contradictory. For example, some research has demonstrated differences in prevalence of stuttering on the basis of families' socioeconomic levels or on the occupational levels of primary income earners, but other studies, considering the same factors, have found no differences.

So what do we conclude? We conclude that the genetic and environmental arguments concerning the origin, or origins, of stuttering are still open issues. It is appropriate to assert, however, that all of the evidence in aggregate increasingly supports the view that stuttering probably has a genetic basis, at least in terms of predisposition, and it is equally appropriate to assert that environment plays a role in the development of stuttering, no matter how strong the genetic link may be.

The title of this section warned that the facts about stuttering are sometimes confusing and almost always incomplete, but they do add to our understanding of the disorder even if they do not provide simple, neat answers to our questions, and even if they do not result in a tidy definition of stuttering.

The *Moment* of Stuttering

There is some debate about who first developed the concept, *moment of stuttering,* but there is no debate about the impact this concept has had on how we have come to think about stuttering, study it, and treat it. The moment concept was developed during the early decades of the twentieth century and has dominated theoretical, research, and clinical thinking ever since. Prior to the understanding that there are moments, or discrete episodes, of fluency failure in otherwise normal speech, writers talked about stuttering as though it were a disease or pervading condition of some kind, in much the same way we think about blindness or deafness. The blind person does not have moments of not seeing. The deaf person does not have discrete episodes of not hearing, but the stutterer DOES have moments of fluency failure. He does not stutter all the time. He does not stutter when he is silent, of course, but neither does he stutter constantly when he talks. Sometimes when he talks, he does not stutter at all, and even when he does stutter, he does not stutter on every word. In analyzing the stutterer's speech, we identify his moments of stuttering, the behavior or behaviors that make up each discrete episode of fluency failure. The moment concept has led researchers to ask some very interesting questions about stuttering. These questions and their answers will lead us to a better and more complete understanding of stuttering.

If the stutterer does not stutter on every word when he talks, are there some words, or types of words, that are more likely to be stuttered than others? We could try to answer this question for an individual stutterer or for stutterers as a group, and given the idiosyncratic nature of the disorder, we would be correct in assuming that what is true for the group will not necessarily be true for the individual. Since we are primarily interested in understanding the disorder in the most general sense, we will focus on group findings, and while we are safe in assuming that what is true for the group will also be true for most individuals, we should always remember that stuttering is a disorder marked by exceptions. More males stutter than females, but there are female stutterers. More twins stutter than singletons, but there are singleton stutterers. There is a higher concordance of stuttering among identical twins than among fraternal twins, but there are concordant fraternal sets and there are discordant identical sets, etcetera into mind-numbing etcetera.

Before we examine the answers to the question about which words are more likely than others to be stuttered, we must consider another concept that underlies the interpretations of most of these answers. That concept is *anticipation*. Many theorists, researchers, and clinicians believe that stutterers anticipate or predict their moments of stuttering. There was considerable research in the 1930s that appeared to support this notion, the findings of which have not been seriously challenged and certainly have not been dismissed. On the basis of these studies, researchers concluded that many adult stutterers can anticipate 90 percent or more of their moments, although some stutterers seem unable to anticipate any of their moments, and there were other inconsistencies. Even those stutterers who were able to predict a high percentage of their moments were not perfect in their anticipations. Not all of their moments were predicted, and not all of their predictions of stuttering were followed by actual moments. Despite the imperfect relationship between anticipation and stuttering, the concept of anticipation has been widely embraced by speech-language pathologists as an explanation for the occurrence of specific moments of stuttering.

The significance of anticipation is that it suggests the stutterer is somehow conscious, not only of the act of speaking, but of the words and sentences he is planning to produce. Wendell Johnson popularized what is called the *Anticipatory Struggle Hypothesis*, which asserts that the stutterer stutters because he anticipates that he will have difficulty saying a particular word, and he tries very hard not to fail, as he believes he will. The struggle not to stutter results in the behaviors we recognize as *stuttering*. In trying to explain why anticipation is not perfect and why some stutterers seem not to antici-pate at all, Johnson and others have suggested that anticipation might some-times operate at a very low level of consciousness. That is, the stutterer might anticipate without being aware that he is anticipating. While this might seem a specious argument to some, I find it convincing. I suspect we have all expe-rienced situations in which we think we are feeling little or no anxiety about something we must do only to find ourselves terribly relieved when the doing is completed. The relief we feel is evidence of the anxiety we felt, anx-iety we did not know we had. I am convinced, based on my own stuttering experiences and on the experiences of my clients, that stutterers often antic-ipate when they are not acutely aware that they are anticipating. One needs only look at the stutterer's face to see signs of anticipation, signs that often appear before words are spoken. Eyes widen. Lips become rigid. Breathing stops. Whether or not the imperfections between anticipation and stuttering can be explained to everyone's satisfaction, the Anticipatory Struggle Hypothesis is widely accepted as an explanation for why certain words are stuttered more often than others.

Factors Influencing the Distribution of Moments

When we analyze the stutterings of adult stutterers, we discover that nouns, verbs, adjectives, and adverbs are more likely to be stuttered than articles, prepositions, and conjunctions. The explanation most often given for this tendency is that nouns, verbs, adjectives, and adverbs, collectively called *content* words, are the meaning carriers of language. Content words are perceived by the stutterer as more important than the smaller parts of speech, typically referred to as *function* words. It is reasonable to assume that if the stutterer is going to anticipate difficulty, he will anticipate difficulty on words that matter most in the context of speech.

It is interesting and important to note that young beginning stutterers do not show the same tendency to stutter on content words. In fact, these chil-dren often stutter on function words, not because they recognize some gram-matical quality in these words that makes them seem difficult, but because function words often appear at the beginning of syntactic units, and the non-fluencies of these children tend to occur at the beginning of syntactic units. One interpretation of this tendency is that the child is using nonfluencies to hold the listener's attention while he formulates the next phrase or sentence. A more plausible explanation focuses on communicative responsibility in the context of speech and language development. That is, the child at the typical age of stuttering onset is still acquiring language, and is struggling to master the nuances of conjoining and embedding phrases and clauses. Even adults, when they are trying to formulate long, complex sentences often pause at syntactic junctures to make sure they are headed in the right language direction. It is easy to understand that the child, with a more restricted vocabulary and less sophisticated language competence will hesitate and stumble when he comes to all those syntactic forks in the road. These nonfluencies, therefore, do not reflect concerns about how difficult it might be to produce a particular word or perceptions about the relative importance of some words in comparison to others. They do reflect, or at least seem to reflect, the child's uncertainty about how to apply the rules of syntax so that complete, correct sentences are produced.

It has been noted by many researchers that adult stutterers tend to produce more moments on the first words and other early words of sentences. The general explanation for this tendency is that the beginning of a sentence is especially conspicuous. From a communication point of view, the beginning is also particularly important. If the opening portion of any communicative attempt–a play, movie, letter, essay, speech, or a simple utterance–fails to gain the listener's attention and fails to set the communicative agenda, the efficacy of the entire communication is in jeopardy. The stutterer recognizes the importance of the beginning of his utterance. If he is going to anticipate difficulty, it is reasonable to assume he will anticipate difficulty on the most conspicuous and important part of the utterance, the beginning.

If other variables are held constant, the stutterer is more likely to stutter on longer words than on shorter ones. That is, this tendency holds if we compare nouns with nouns, verbs with verbs, if we compare words in the same positions of sentences, and if we keep all other important variables constant. I doubt that anyone is surprised by this tendency because all speakers are more likely to be nonfluent on longer words than on short words. We all find longer words more challenging to produce. We perceive them as difficult to pronounce and articulate, even when there is no legitimate reason to view them as difficult.

The stutterer's perception of difficulty and subsequent anticipation of stuttering are also affected by how frequently a word occurs in his normal expressive language. That is, he is more likely to have trouble with a word he does not use very often. The infrequency of usage makes such words stand out in the stutterer's perception. The more familiar he is with a word, regardless of its grammatical class or its length, the less likely he will perceive it as difficult, at least in contrast to a comparable word he seldom uses.

Factors Influencing the Frequency of Stuttering

Are there factors that affect how frequently a stutterer will stutter? Will there be a higher frequency of moments of stuttering under some conditions than others? Yes, there do seem to be some conditions that cause stuttering to occur more or less often than usual.

I have used the word *stress,* and synonyms for *stress* a number of times in this chapter. The typical stutterer, regardless of age, is noticeably affected by the degree of communicative stress or pressure he feels at any given time when he is talking. The truth is, we are all affected by communicative stress. At one time in my life, I was a high school speech teacher. In this position, I saw students every day who were affected by the stress they experienced when they were delivering simple speeches to their peers, and there was not a stutterer among them. Some students perspired and shook when they were frightened. Others became quite nonfluent, and one young woman fainted into the chalkboard in response to the overwhelming stress she felt. It would be quite surprising then if stutterers were not affected by the stresses of communication.

One of the most common ways communicative stress is created is by heightened responsibility. That is, frequency of stuttering is related to the degree of responsibility the stutterer ascribes to his role as a speaker, and to the importance of what he is saying. If he feels that his role as a speaker gives him considerable communicative responsibility and/or that what he is saying is important, he is likely to stutter more frequently than usual. On the other hand, if he believes what he is saying is relatively meaningless, or if he feels little personal responsibility for communicating a message, he will probably speak more fluently than usual. For example, the typical stutterer has little difficulty talking to trees, small children, animals, or to himself because in these situations, he has little communicative responsibility, and he does not see his messages as particularly important. It really does not matter what he says to his oak tree or to his Doberman, and there is not much pressure in a self-to-self conversation. Because he is not afraid of failing as a communicator in these situations, he does not anticipate failure. As a result, he does not stutter at all, or he stutters less frequently than he would under normal conditions. Furthermore, if he does fail, he does not care because he is not concerned about critical reactions he might receive from himself, his tree, or his dog. If, however, he must pick up the telephone to report a fire, he feels very responsible. He knows he must communicate the message accurately, and he is concerned about the consequences of failing as a communicator. This is a classic example of communicative stress created by significant communicative responsibility. Under this circumstance, he is likely to stutter often and severely. He might struggle so much that he is unable to say anything at all.

Communicative responsibility might be related to the words the stutterer is going to say. Many stutterers have little or no trouble with social gesture talk, counting, profanity, or anything that is memorized, such as a nursery rhyme or a pledge. What do all these things have in common? They are all relatively devoid of semantic meaning. We say, "Hello," "Hi," "How are you?" without really thinking about what the words mean and often without expecting a response. It is not uncommon, for example, for one person to say, "How are you?" and for the other person to say, "Hi" in response. When we count, we are engaged in an exercise that has little to do with thinking about what each number really means. The profanities people use do not convey semantic messages as much as they convey emotional messages. After all, how many of us would be truly offended if someone called us a "puppy," but we might get terribly bent out of shape if someone used the comparable profane phrase, which roughly translated means "male offspring of a female dog." As far as memorized material is concerned, I can still recite the Boy Scout laws in about 10 seconds, but I would have to pause and think about each one before I could tell you its meaning. Every week in worship services of all kinds, people recite prayers and creeds without giving much thought to what the words mean. Stutterers seldom have difficulty with speech activities such as these, words that are spoken with little or no intentional meaning.

The stutterer feels greater or lesser responsibility, and therefore, greater or lesser communicative pressure depending on the perceived status of his listener(s). If the stutterer feels superior to his listener(s), he usually stutters less than he normally does; but if he feels inferior, intimidated, or threatened by his listener(s), he is likely to stutter more than usual. What the stutterer experiences in this regard is simply a higher degree of what all people experience under comparable circumstances. We are all slightly intimidated by persons we perceive as authority figures or by people who are threatening to us for any reason, and even normally fluent speakers tend to become nonfluent when they talk to these people. This is what causes the admirer of a movie star to say, when meeting the object of his or her adoration, "You're my biggest fan!" We all get a little flustered in the presence of real or perceived greatness or authority. The stutterer may just be more affected than the nonstuttering speaker.

One of the stranger phenomena the stutterer might experience is reduced or no stuttering when he is reading in unison with someone else. The most common explanation for this reduction is that in unison or choral reading, there is shared, and therefore, reduced communicative responsibility. The stutterer who is fluent when he is reading with someone else might have considerable difficulty when he reads the same material by himself. Some people have speculated that the reduction in frequency of stuttering that occurs during unison reading results from distraction. That is, because the stutterer is either concentrating with unusual intensity on his own speech because of the competing voice or because he is attending to the other voice and not to his own speech, he does not think about the *difficulty* of speech, and he does not stutter. The fly in this particular ointment is that when the stutterer reads together with someone who is reading different material, he does not show the same reduction in stuttering as when he and the other person are reading the same material. Surely, two people reading different material at the same time is more potentially distracting than two people reading the same material, but reading the same material has a greater effect on reducing the frequency of stuttering. This certainly seems to suggest that the effect of choral reading is more likely to be the product of shared responsibility than distraction.

The frequency of stuttering is often affected by the time pressure a stutterer feels. If he believes he has all the time he needs to talk, he will tend to speak fairly fluently, but if he senses an urgency to talk, he will be more inclined to experience fluency failures. If he speaks slowly, he will have little difficulty, but if he tries to speak quickly, the stuttering may come in torrents.

Stutterers generally stutter more when they are talking to groups of people than when they are talking to only one person, and they usually do not stutter at all when they are talking to themselves. It should be noted, however, that most normal speakers are more prone to fluency failures when they talk to groups of people than when they are engaged in conversation with one person or with just a few people. According to many polls, more people fear public speaking than fear death. Fear of speaking results in speaking failures, whether the speaker is a stutterer or not.

Although generalizations are always dangerous, they are also sometimes helpful in understanding a point that is larger than the sum of examples of the point to be made. Here come two such generalizations I hope will help the reader understand why stutterers stutter when they do, and why they are likely to stutter more in some situations than in others. (1) In general, the words most likely to be stuttered are those that are the most semantically or personally meaningful and those that because of their length, unfamiliarity, infrequency of occurrence in the speaker's expressive language, position in an utterance, or for any other reason, are conspicuous. (2) In general, the frequency of stuttering increases in relation to the importance or meaningfulness of speaking situations. In other words, when it is most important for the stutterer not to stutter, he is most likely to stutter, and when it does not matter whether he is fluent or not, he does not stutter or he stutters less than usual.

I am sure you have noticed, and I have specifically pointed out in some cases, that none of the factors that affect when and how often stuttering occurs are unique to stutterers. All of these conditions, and similar conditions I have not mentioned, might very well produce nonfluent speech in normal speakers. This is perhaps an appropriate time to recall Wendell Johnson's assertion that there is nothing the stutterer does that the nonstutterer does not also do at some times to some extent. The stutterer is not an unusual person in the sense that he reacts to stimuli differently than others do. He is a normal person who reacts to stimuli and to threatening conditions in very normal ways, even though his reactions might be more severe than the reactions of people who do not stutter. There are some differences between stutterers and nonstutterers, of course, and we will take a look at some of those differences in Chapter 6.

Our goal in this chapter has been to discover what stuttering is. I have certainly not included everything that might be considered in trying to understand the nature of stuttering, but I believe I have included a representative sampling of the information we should consider. I hope at this point that the reader understands why we have not been successful in drafting a definition of stuttering that captures the essence of the disorder and that is embraced by all the experts who view stuttering from many different theoretical perspectives. Stuttering is a complex and multi-faceted problem. Some stuttering can be seen and heard, but much of the disorder cannot be observed, and many people who study stuttering, including this writer, believe that the unseen components of the problem are largely responsible for the components that can be observed. I believe that if we could change the way the stutterer thinks about the act of speaking, if we could change the way he perceives and reacts to the words he speaks, the people to whom he is talking, and even his own self-image, many of the observable behaviors would cease to exist, but this is infinitely more difficult to achieve than to assert.

In the next chapter, I want to explore the behaviors included in what we call *stuttering*. We will take a look at those behaviors that can be seen and/or heard, and we will examine the hidden aspects of the disorder, the portion that lies beneath the surface.

Chapter 4

THE BEHAVIORS OF STUTTERING

When a typical stutterer is asked, following a moment of stuttering, what he did on the fragmented word, he answers, "I stuttered," or "I blocked," or "I got stuck." When he is pressed to describe *exactly* what happened, he is often unable to respond. The listener is sometimes surprised by the stutterer's inability to describe his moment because stuttering behaviors often involve so much struggle and last for such a long time that it is hard to believe the stutterer does not know what he did. We need to keep in mind, however, that because stuttering behaviors are characterized by struggle derived from fear, panic is very much a part of the formula for stuttering. Sometimes the panic is mild, but sometimes the panic is so severe the stutterer feels paralyzed by his stuttering. We also need to remind ourselves that any person in the midst of panic is unable to provide the details of what he was experiencing during the moment of panic. Anyone who has been in an automobile accident can relate to this. Accidents usually happen so quickly, and the panic is so intense the victims cannot remember what happened during the accident even if they can remember what happened before and after the accident. The stutterer's experience with a moment of stuttering is very much like this. He may remember the target word. He may be able to explain why he thought it would be a difficult word to say, and he will probably be able to explain how he felt after he extricated himself from the moment, but the moment itself is a blur, the details lost in struggle and panic.

The reader might conclude that the preceding paragraph lets the stutterer off the responsibility hook. This is certainly not my intention. While I am willing to acknowledge that most stutterers, prior to therapy, have a difficult time identifying what they do when they stutter, I am adamant in asserting that they MUST learn how to analyze their own behaviors if they expect to modify or eliminate them. Furthermore, I believe that any reasonably intelligent and properly motivated stutterer can become an exceptional analyst of his own behaviors. How the clinician teaches the stutterer to identify his behaviors will be a subject for consideration in the second half of this book. The purpose of the present chapter is to describe the behaviors we are likely to find in moments of stuttering. It is highly unlikely that one will find all of these behaviors in a single moment, but it would not be uncommon to find a half dozen or more.

As a clinician and as a teacher of future clinicians, I believe it is absolutely essential that the stutterer be able to differentiate his stuttering behaviors. Stuttering behaviors are not random, accidental, and meaningless. They are predictable, lawful, and purposive. Some behaviors exist only because they are superimposed on others or because they are used to cover up or end other behaviors. It is crucial that the stutterer understands this because as long as he believes that stuttering is random behavior beyond his control, and as long as he believes there is nothing he can do to prevent, eliminate, or change stuttering behaviors, he will continue to be hostage to his disorder. Stuttering is a speech disorder that testifies to the truth of the old maxim that we fear the unknown more than we fear the known. We will all concede that stuttering is a mystery to people who do not stutter, but it is equally true that stuttering is a mystery to people who stutter. Most stutterers have no idea what is happening to them when they experience fluency failure beyond such general and useless insights as, "Well, that word is always hard for me, so when I tried to say it, I stuttered." The understanding inherent in this kind of observation is so minuscule that it tends to be more harmful than helpful. It seems to suggest that stuttering is a kind of general and nondescript behavior, a suggestion that falls far short of fact. Stuttering consists of many behaviors linked by a few critical common denominators. Stuttering does not happen to the stutterer as a kind of random accident. Stuttering is created by the person who stutters. He sets up the perceptual conditions and makes the physiological adjustments that result in stuttering, in a fairly clear and easy to understand cause-effect manner. In this chapter, I will identify categories of stuttering behaviors, define them, explain why they are used, and discuss how our knowledge about stuttering behaviors gives us direction in therapy.

The classification system I will be describing was first introduced by Charles Van Riper. Over the course of my own career, I have added some organizational structure I believe will assist the reader in understanding how these behaviors are linked. I will also take full responsibility for interpretations, assumptions, and conclusions that go beyond Van Riper's original descriptions. I do want to note that this classification system has become central to my own understanding of stuttering, that it drives my approach to therapy, and that it has greatly influenced the way I teach this disorder to my students. If you derive from these preceding sentences that I think this system is basic and important, and that it is a significant part of the total message I want to share with you in the pages of this book, you are correct.

The Seen and the Unseen

As has already been noted, only a portion of the stuttering problem can be observed by listeners. There are many behaviors that can be seen and/or heard, but there are other dimensions of the disorder that are hidden in the stutterer's feelings, perceptions, and attitudes. Joseph Sheehan, a psychologist with a strong professional interest in stuttering, compared stuttering to an iceberg. He observed that only a small part, about 10 percent, of an iceberg is visible, above the surface of the water. The larger portion, the remaining 90 percent, is below the surface. The hidden part of the iceberg is often the most dangerous dimension because one cannot always tell how large the mass of ice is by looking at the portion that is visible. Sheehan argued that stuttering is very much like an iceberg in that a small portion of stuttering contacts the senses, but the greater part of the problem is hidden, below the surface. One would expect a psychologist to view stuttering in this way because psychologists are always probing beneath peoples' surfaces into their emotions and feelings to discover what makes them functional or dysfunctional. What might be surprising to some is that the iceberg view, or at least some modified version of it, is widely accepted among speech-language pathologists. The major arguments between psychologists and speech-language pathologists would center on exactly what is hidden. The psychologist would probably talk about anxieties related to disturbed interpersonal relationships, and somewhere in the explanation we would hear the word *conflict*. The speech-language pathologist would probably argue that the hidden portion of stuttering includes the stutterer's misperceptions about speaking, words, himself, and others. Both professionals would almost certainly agree that as far as stuttering is concerned, what you see and hear is only a small part of what you get.

The Core Behaviors of Stuttering

When most people attempt to imitate stuttering, they produce repetitions of sounds, syllables, or words, and they produce prolonged sounds. There is a general impression among laypersons that these behaviors are the beginning, middle, and end of stuttering behaviors. While it is not true that stuttering can be reduced to just repetitions and prolongations, it is true that these behaviors are the most basic of the stuttering behaviors. They are so basic, in fact, that all other observable behaviors are related, directly or indirectly, to these two categories. This is why repetitions and prolongations—which we will subdivide into two categories—are considered the *core* behaviors of stuttering. They are like the core of an apple. The core is the middle part of the apple, around which the meat of the apple is wrapped. In stuttering, repetitions and the two forms of prolongation constitute the core of the disorder, or at least the core of the disorder's observable behaviors. All other behaviors are *wrapped around* them.

The first of the core behaviors is **repetitions.** All speakers occasionally repeat, so what makes the stutterer's repetitions special? When a nonstutterer repeats, he usually repeats a whole word, although he might repeat a sound or syllable. When the stutterer repeats, he usually repeats a fragment of a word, either a sound or a syllable, although he sometimes repeats whole, single-syllable words, and in some circumstances, he will repeat two or more words. The difference then centers on tendencies. That is, the nonstutterer tends to repeat whole words, and the stutterer tends to repeat fragments of words. A second difference is far more significant in terms of understanding what the stutterer is doing when he repeats. The nonstutterer's repetitions are produced without struggle and without any sense of anticipation of fluency failure. The stutterer often repeats precisely because he anticipates that a target word, or perhaps the first sound of a target word, will be difficult. His repetitions are also produced with excessive force, and because of his belief that the word or sound will be difficult, in combination with the excessive force, he uses inappropriate positioning of the speech structures when he makes his ill-fated attempt.

It is intriguing to think about why the stutterer produces this strange behavior. If he is trying to say "top," for example, why does he repeat the "t"? If he produces "t" the first time, why does he go back and produce it again and again? In this case, if at first he does succeed, why does he try, try again? It may be helpful to think of a series of repetitions as a search for articulatory correctness. The first repetition of "t" might be recognizable to the listener as a "t," but it does not *feel* like a "t" to the stutterer. This attention to feeling is important because speakers, whether they stutter or not, depend as much, if not more, on what they feel as on what they hear to determine if motor speech is correct. If the "t" does not feel right to the stutterer, therefore, he tries again in order to get the feeling that suggests *articulatory correctness.* Each repetition in a series of repetitions moves him a step closer to the target sound in terms of placement of the articulators and in terms of degree of muscular tension. When the placement and muscular tension feel right, the stutterer finishes the word. Within this understanding of what happens during repetitions, the problem is not simply that the stutterer is repeating. There are actually two problems: (1) finding the appropriate placement for the speech structures, and (2) finding the proper degree of pressure or muscular tension for the production of the target sound, syllable, or word. The repetitions are actually attempts to *solve* these problems. That is, the stutterer adjusts and adjusts until the targeted segment feels right. He then moves on to the next segment. Simplistically speaking, therefore, the stutterer can eliminate repetitions from his speech by always articulating as he should. Prior to therapy, many stutterers know what repetitions are, but very few understand that repetitions are the products of inappropriate physiological adjustments, and even fewer understand that they are produced for the purpose of readjusting toward articulatory correctness.

Repetitions are often the first behaviors to develop in young stutterers, and in the beginning, they tend to be produced with little struggle or tension. As the disorder progresses, repetitions become increasingly effortful, distorting the sounds or syllables on which they occur. As the severity of stuttering increases, we see the emergence of the other two core behaviors: **closures** and **postural fixations.** These two categories are often subsumed in the more commonly used term, *prolongations,* but it is important to differentiate them because each category is more closely associated with a particular group of speech sounds than the other, and because there are real and significant physiological differences between them. Even as I write these words, I am aware that I am inching out onto a branch that may not bear the full weight of my message. The reader should keep in mind that virtually everything I write about stuttering behaviors will be in the form of generalizations. The truth is there is probably no statement I can make about any stuttering behavior that will be valid for every stutterer or for every moment produced by a given stutterer. The reader must consider that the purposes of this discussion are to identify and describe stuttering behaviors in a generic sense and to offer the most plausible explanation for why these behaviors are produced and how they are interconnected.

One of the most uncomfortable of stuttering behaviors is the second core behavior, **closure,** also referred to as *blockage* or *block.* When the stutterer produces a closure, he feels as though he cannot get the sound out at all, as though the air is stuck in his mouth or throat. Actually, this is exactly what happens during a closure. There is a brief, very real blockage, at some point in the vocal tract, a blockage that occurs as a direct result of the stutterer's trying too hard to produce the sound. It usually happens something like this: The stutterer approaches a word he thinks will be difficult for him to say. He concludes that if the word is going to be hard to produce, he should prepare himself for a serious articulatory battle. Now, let's fade to a different scene for just a moment. Actually, it's a split-screen scene. On one side we have a boy preparing to swing a baseball bat at a pitched ball. He concludes that this is going to be nearly impossible, using a round bat to contact a round ball being thrown at tremendous speed. Because he thinks this task will be extremely difficult, he tenses the muscles in his hands, wrists, arms, and shoulders, and as a consequence of all this muscular tension, he produces a swing that is stiff and awkward, and he misses the ball as it flies into the catcher's glove. On the other side of the screen, we have a girl who is preparing to shoot a basketball. She concludes that this is a very difficult feat, throwing a ball from a distance of 15 feet into a hoop that is barely two times the ball's width and that stands 10 feet off the floor. Caught up in her conviction that this simply cannot be done, she tenses the muscles in her hands and wrists, she does not bend her knees, and when she shoots the ball, it misses the front edge of the rim by two feet. On both sides of the screen, we have observed athletes *choking*. They have failed to perform basic athletic skills because they perceived difficulty and made inappropriate physiological adjustments that made success impossible. As we turn our attention back to the stutterer, we see exactly the same thing happening. He thinks the word will be hard. He prepares for it to be hard. The preparation makes a normal production impossible, and he *chokes*. If he is trying to say the word "boy," for example, he might press his lips together so tightly when he tries to produce the "b" sound that he traps air inside his mouth and nothing comes out. This is a *bilabial closure,* which means that the air is blocked by locking the two lips together. If the stutterer continues to struggle, he will eventually break through the closure and complete the word.

Closures can occur at several places in the speech mechanism. They can occur, as in the example above, when the stutterer presses his lips together to close off the airflow. They can also occur when he pushes his tongue so hard against some part of the roof of his mouth that he cuts off the air flow, or when he strains so hard to set his vocal folds into vibration that he actually forces them closed so tightly that air cannot pass through. Some readers who have a good understanding of speech physiology will observe that a stutterer could press his tongue hard against the ridge behind the upper front teeth and still release air flow. This is true. When the stutterer presses his tongue against this ridge, as in producing the "t" sound, the excessive tension he produces flows down into the larynx, resulting in locked vocal folds. What is important to keep in mind is that the struggle and excessive tension result in closure at some point in the vocal tract. From a therapy point of view, we concentrate on what the stutterer *feels*. In this example, he will probably *feel* closure at the point where the tongue contacts the alveolar ridge. If he can produce the "t" without producing excessive force between the tongue and the alveolar ridge, there will be no tension to spread into the larynx, forcing the vocal folds closed, and he will not produce a closure.

Although closures can and do occur on all speech sounds, they are most commonly produced on sounds, which by their nature, involve some degree of closure. These sounds, called *plosives* or *stops,* are "b, p, d, t, g, or k." When we produce any of these sounds in a normal manner, we stop the airflow temporarily and release it. In his struggle and panic, the stutterer exaggerates this normal stoppage, producing a closure. Laypersons often observe stutterers producing this behavior, and they cannot understand why they do it. In addition to the baseball and basketball examples I offered earlier, I want to add two more. My hope is that one or more of these examples will cause the reader to say, "I can relate to that," because what the stutterer does is not extraordinary. It is a very common reaction. The only thing that makes it extraordinary is that the reaction occurs in speech–an act that most people produce easily and naturally. With minimal effort, however, most of us can think of motor acts that might cause problems similar to what the stutterer experiences when he tries to say words he thinks are inherently difficult. For example, when a child is first learning to ride a bicycle, he is so sure he will fall down that he struggles and fights to steer the bicycle properly. The very effort to keep the bicycle on a straight course results in failure to do so. Only when the child learns to relax will he steer properly and avoid falling down. Notice that it is only when the child stops thinking about the impossibility of riding a bicycle that he rides the bicycle successfully. Many people, including many adults, perceive that putting a thread through the eye of a needle is very difficult, so they tense up and struggle to get the thread through the needle's eye, a struggle that invariably results in frustration and failure. The stutterer's problem is remarkably similar to the problems depicted in these examples. If, when trying to say "boy," he approaches the "b" sound with confidence, and if he articulates it in a relaxed manner, he will say it without stuttering. When he perceives *difficulty,* however, his natural reaction is to struggle, an adjustment that guarantees that stuttering, often in the form of a closure, will occur.

The third core behavior, and the second subcategory of *prolongation,* is **postural fixation.** As is true of closures, postural fixations occur only if there is a significant degree of muscular tension when the stutterer is trying to produce the target sound or word. There can be mild, struggle-free repetitions, but it is highly unlikely you will hear a stutterer produce mild, struggle-free closures or postural fixations. These behaviors occur when the stutterer is trying to blast through a word, and blasting through requires more than the usual amount of muscular tension and effort. The difference between closure and postural fixation is simple. Closure occurs when there is complete stoppage of airflow. A postural fixation involves abnormal constriction at some point in the vocal tract, but airflow does continue. This behavior usually occurs on *fricatives,* sounds that involve some degree of constriction, sounds such as "s, z, sh, f, or v." As occurs in the production of a closure, the stutterer produces a postural fixation by exaggerating a natural characteristic of a sound. The panicky tennis player hits his forehand over the back screen because in his struggle, he exaggerates the motion and force of his natural forehand stroke. The golfer, even the excellent golfer, when he is under stress, might hit a putt 10 feet past the hole because he panics and exaggerates the length of his back swing or the force with which he strikes the ball.

In much the same way, the stutterer approaches the word "ship," panics, and exaggerates the natural articulatory constriction of the "sh" sound and produces a postural fixation.

Behaviors Superimposed on the Core Behaviors

The core behaviors form the foundation of observable stuttering. There are a number of other behaviors that are produced on top of this foundation, usually as a result of the stutterer's attempts to fight through the repetitions, postural fixations, and closures. Although these superimposed behaviors comprise the more bizarre aspects of stuttering, they are really not as significant as they may seem to the stutterer or to his listeners because they exist only as additions to the core behaviors. If the stutterer makes the physiological adjustments that are necessary for the elimination or modification of the core behaviors, the superimposed behaviors will quietly go away. Why this is so will be clear when we examine each of the superimposed behaviors in more detail.

It is perhaps easiest to see the superimposition of **vocal fry,** so we will begin with this behavior. Since it is possible you have heard this term or the equivalent term, **glottal fry,** I need to make it clear that there are two kinds of vocal fry, only one of which is of concern here. In a generic sense, vocal fry is produced when the vocal folds vibrate very slowly so you hear a ticking quality in the speaker's voice. The term is most commonly employed to describe the sound made when the vocal folds are very relaxed, giving the impression that the folds are so tired they are barely moving. The other kind of vocal fry, the kind produced by stutterers, is a hypertense version. The vocal folds vibrate slowly, but in this case they vibrate slowly because the stutterer is exerting so much pressure on the folds in the closed position he must strain to get them to vibrate at all. When they do vibrate, you hear the ticking quality of vocal fry, but you hear the fry within a strained voice, not a relaxed voice. Hypertense vocal fry is unpleasant for the listener, and if produced frequently or for long periods of time, it is physically uncomfortable for the stutterer. Furthermore, if this behavior becomes a dominant feature of the stutterer's speech, it might eventually lead to vocal fold pathology such as nodules, polyps, or contact ulcers. The discussion to this point has provided some clues about which core behavior is most commonly associated with vocal fry. Here is another clue. Many stutterers report that they use vocal fry to "loosen" a "tight larynx." Putting the clues together, we conclude that vocal fry is most often superimposed on closures produced at the level of the vocal folds, and it happens as follows. The stutterer produces a laryngeal, or vocal fold, closure. He struggles to break the closure. The struggle against the tightly closed vocal folds causes them to vibrate, but the vibration is under considerable strain, resulting in vocal fry. As the struggle continues, the vocal folds vibrate more rapidly until the stutterer is able to complete the production. The hypertense vocal fry is undoubtedly the most disturbing characteristic of this moment of stuttering, both to the listener and to the stutterer, but it is clearly not the major problem in this moment. The problem is the closure. If the stutterer makes the adjustments necessary to prevent the production of the closure, the vocal fry associated with the closure can never occur. In fact, if he makes the adjustments necessary to end the closure as soon as he feels himself creating it, the vocal fry will not be produced.

A second superimposed behavior is called **complemental air.** Sometimes a core behavior produced on a single sound lasts for an unusually long time, 15 to 20 seconds or longer, and the stutterer uses up the air he would normally exhale for an entire sentence. Sometimes, in his struggle to fight through the core behavior, he releases too much air too quickly. In either case, by the time he gets to his final attempt on the target sound or word, the stutterer does not have enough air left to say the word normally. At this point he has two choices. He can begin again, in which case he risks starting the stuttering all over again, or he can try to finish what he has started in spite of the fact that he has used up too much air. Keeping in mind the nature of panic behavior, the reader should not be surprised that the stutterer often takes the second choice. Panic promotes obsessive reactions. When the stutterer gives in to the panic and makes his final attempt after he has used his normal supply of air, he is speaking on what Charles Van Riper calls *complemental air.* The word is finally spoken, and it is usually fluent, but it is produced with extraordinary effort, not unlike the words spoken by a dying man or by someone who is trying to talk after completing a strenuous workout program. Complemental air probably does not occur with any one of the core behaviors more often than the other two, but it does seem to be produced most often on sounds that naturally involve more rapid release of air. The best example would be the "h" sound because this sound is produced by simply expelling air with no constrictions or closures anywhere in the vocal tract to slow the release. As with vocal fry, words produced on complemental air sound unnatural, and the stutterer looks as though he is about to lapse into unconsciousness when he uses this behavior, but looks and sounds can be deceiving. Complemental air, in itself, is not a serious problem. If the stutterer learns to modify or eliminate the core behaviors, complemental air has no opportunity to occur.

One of the most bizarre of all stuttering behaviors and one of the most unsettling for stutterers is the **tremor.** A tremor is a rhythmic vibration of a muscle or a group of muscles. When a tremor is superimposed on a core behavior, it typically occurs in one of four places in the speech mechanism: the lips, jaw, tongue, or the larynx. According to Van Riper's description of this behavior, three conditions must be present in order for a tremor to develop. First, there must be a *localized area of hypertension*. That is, even though excessive muscular tension is characteristic of most moments of stuttering, there must be comparatively more excessive muscular tension in the structure that tremors than in the surrounding structures. If muscular tension is evenly distributed, no matter how excessive it is, there may be stuttering, but there will be no tremor. Second, there must be an *abnormal positioning of the muscle or muscles involved*. This condition is likely to exist with any core behavior since one of the natural results of speech struggle is distorted positioning of the speech structure that is the primary target of the struggle. For example, if the stutterer is trying to say "mother," and stutters on the "m," his lips may be drawn in too tightly, pushed out in a kind of strained pucker, or perhaps they will be in a open, frozen position. In any case, the position is not normal. Third, there must be a sudden movement, a surge of tension, or a spurt of airflow to *trigger* the tremor. These triggers are not in short supply since they are characteristic of any kind of struggle, speech or nonspeech. The unsettling, even frightening, aspect of the tremor for the stutterer is that it makes him feel like he is out of control. The tremor seems to happen spontaneously, and it seems to have a life of its own. This is not true, of course, since the stutterer creates the physiological conditions that give birth to the core behavior and to the tremor superimposed on the core behavior, but the *feeling* that he is being controlled by the tremor is very real. The tremor usually ends when the stutterer, often by accident, produces a behavior that is not synchronized with the rhythm of the tremor. This behavior might occur in the structure that is being affected by the tremor, or it might occur in a structure adjacent to the tremoring structure. For example, the stutterer who produces a lip tremor might suddenly and forcefully push his lip upward. If this movement is synchronized with the tremor, the tremor will continue, but if it is not in rhythm with the tremor, the tremor will be terminated. The stutterer might end the same tremor by jerking his head forward. It should be made clear that these movements are seldom, if ever, planned and executed consciously and deliberately. They are usually the products of continued struggle.

A tremor might also end simply because the muscles fatigue. A man hanging from the ledge of a window on the tenth floor of a skyscraper will struggle to hang on, but eventually his hands will fatigue, and he will let go. The stutterer who produces a tremor might fight and fight to overcome the tremor, only to discover that if the muscles involved get tired enough, the tremor will fade away. The lesson is obvious. Just don't struggle. Many stutterers know this lesson, and they try not to struggle, but they are usually as successful in trying not to struggle as worriers who try not to worry. The worrier, terrified by medical research that indicates that worry and stress contribute to a wide range of illnesses, worries about not being able to stop worrying. The stutterer understands that struggle is his enemy, not his ally. He struggles not to struggle. Alas, life is not fair, and it is not easy. Incidentally, the man who was hanging from the window ledge was not injured. The fire department was waiting below with a net. I love happy endings.

One of the fascinating things about stuttering behavior we can learn from the tremor is that the more the stutterer struggles, the more behaviors he creates and the more behaviors he must fight through in order to complete a targeted word. It is no wonder that severe stutterers are often physically and emotionally exhausted after long conversations. The severe stutterer may have to battle through moments on 50 percent or more of the words he speaks, and each moment may consist of six or more different behaviors, some of which might be repeated two or more times within a single complex moment. Knowing that it is he who creates all these behaviors is small consolation to the stutterer when he is in the midst of struggling, but this knowledge is crucial to his treatment. Once the stutterer understands and accepts the fact that he produces his stuttering behaviors, that he is truly the master of his own mouth, the long journey to fluency control can begin.

It is also helpful to understand tremor as a microcosm of the stuttering problem. That is, this single behavior includes the common denominators of stuttering that—if not produced or if adjusted during struggle—will prevent stuttering or release moments once they are created. Think about the three conditions for the development of a tremor: (1) localized area of hypertension, (2) abnormal positioning of the structure involved, and (3) a triggering behavior. What three pieces of advice could I give the stutterer that would absolutely guarantee he would never produce a tremor again? (1) Always speak with a *relaxed* speech mechanism. (2) Make sure you use *proper articulatory positioning* when you speak. (3) *Don't make any sudden movements* when you are speaking. If a stutterer is able to follow this advice, he will not produce tremors, and . . . he will not stutter. Why then does he not follow this sage advice? To answer this question we need only retreat to the comparative conditions I have mentioned before: weight loss, alcoholism, and drug addiction. I will not suggest that these three conditions are *directly* comparable to stuttering, of course, but in this regard, they are. If a person is trying to lose weight, what does he or she need to do? He needs to consume fewer calories than he burns. If a person is trying to win the battle against alcoholism or drug addiction, what does he or she need to do? He needs to stop drinking or stop taking drugs. Wow! These are such simple problems to solve, but they are NOT simple problems to solve because in each case—weight loss, alcoholism, drug addiction, and stuttering—there are many factors contributing to the problem, factors that take the solution beyond will and beyond intellectual understanding. Knowing what needs to be done in problems such as these is not enough. Knowledge is necessary. Discipline is essential. Having the will to overcome is critical, but attitudes and perceptions must be changed. In many cases, a person's entire self-concept must be transformed. Old habits must be broken and new habits established. All this takes time and patience. These problems CAN be solved, but the journey is not easy, and it is not swift.

The final and most often produced superimposed behavior is the **interrupter,** or **escape.** An interrupter is any behavior the stutterer uses to end, break, or overcome a core behavior and any other behavior that might already be superimposed on the core behavior. An interrupter can be verbal, but it is usually nonverbal. It is a quick, forceful behavior that clearly reflects the stutterer's attempt to impose rhythm on his obviously disrupted speech. Why does the stutterer react as he does to this disruption in rhythm? Human beings like and are soothed by rhythm. Our physiological functions, especially our respiratory and cardiovascular functions, are rhythmic, and when they are out of rhythm, we do not feel well. The expression, "out of sorts," is one way of saying that a person's natural rhythms have been disrupted in some way. Speech too is a rhythmic function. Every spoken language has its own "music," its own rhythm. Even if we do not know how to speak French or Japanese, we will immediately recognize the rhythms of these languages. The stutterer, like all human beings, wants and needs the natural rhythms of his life. When they are disrupted, he tries to restore them. When his speech is arrhythmic, he is uncomfortable. As a speaker, he is out of sorts. He does whatever he needs to do to regain the rhythm he has lost. He uses an interrupter to open a closure, release a postural fixation, or to halt a series of repetitions. The interrupter might be a physical behavior such as a jerk of the head, a stomp of the foot, or a quick intake of breath. It might be a verbal behavior such as "uh" or "well" produced quickly in the midst of his struggle with a moment of stuttering. Depending on the magnitude of the struggle, he might produce the interrupter once or several times, but it is almost a certainty that if a moment of stuttering persists to the point of arrhythmic discomfiture, the stutterer will try to end it with some form of interrupter. Interrupters can be strange and attention grabbing. The listener might actually pay more attention to the head jerks, facial grimaces, unusual and misplaced interjections, and finger snaps the stutterer uses to get out of his moments than to the core behaviors themselves, but I will emphasize again that these behaviors are merely hangers-on. They are the bit players in the stuttering drama. The main players, the real culprits, are the core behaviors. If the stutterer learns to prevent the physiological conditions that give rise to the core behaviors, and if he learns how to extricate himself from these conditions if he does create them, he will no longer need interrupters because there will be nothing to interrupt.

Anticipatory Behaviors

In the preceding chapter, I discussed the idea that stutterers anticipate that certain sounds, words, or situations will be difficult and that this anticipation determines whether stuttering will occur, and if it occurs, how often it will occur. When the stutterer anticipates that he might stutter, he often tries to do something to prevent the stuttering. Behaviors used by the stutterer when he believes a moment is imminent, and for the purpose of preventing the stuttering from occurring, are called **anticipatory behaviors.** There are two categories of anticipatory behaviors: **avoidance** and **postponement.**

An **avoidance** is any behavior the stutterer uses to prevent saying a certain word or entering a certain situation, and please notice the inclusion of the word, "certain." Avoidance is not a general strategy for coping with the anticipation of fluency failure. It is a behavior focal to specific words and situations. The danger inherent in avoidance is that it causes the stutterer's fear of the target word or situation to increase, and I trust the cruel irony will not go unnoticed. He uses avoidance in the first place because he is afraid he will not be able to say the word or enter the situation without stuttering. In the process of avoiding the word or situation, his fear increases. Although the circumstances I am describing here may be unique to stuttering, the human reaction is not. It is very normal for people to avoid what they fear, but any time a person avoids something because he fears it, his fear of that thing will increase. The old maxim about falling off a horse is about fear and the consequences of avoiding what we fear. *If you fall off a horse, get right back on.* The idea is that if you do not get right back on the horse, it will be much more difficult to get on the next day or the next week because the moment you do not get on the horse, you begin to believe more fervently than ever that getting on the horse is dangerous. Over time, the fear becomes terribly distorted, irrational, completely out of proportion to reality. One of the *facts of life* some people never adequately learn is that human beings conquer their fears by confronting them, not by running away from them.

Charles Van Riper once called avoidance "the pump of fear," a very apt description. By avoiding, the stutterer not only runs away from a word or situation, he runs away from the disorder itself. In a very real sense, avoidance is the stutterer's *denial* behavior. There is no doubt that stuttering can be a painful disorder. The stutterer often feels like a social freak, the object of mockery, ridicule, or pity. Any sensitive person will understand why the stutterer would want to avoid the embarrassment associated with fluency failures, but sympathy for the stutterer, whether it comes from others or from himself, misses the point about the dangers of avoidance and denial, dangers that can be noted in the following scenario.

When the stutterer senses he might stutter, he tries desperately not to stutter by avoiding a word he fears he cannot say fluently. If he successfully avoids this time, it becomes a little easier to avoid the next time. In fact, he may believe he has found a reasonable way to cope with this fears. He reasons that if he avoids all the words and all the situations that might produce stuttering, listeners will not know he is a stutterer—no stuttering, . . . no problem. Unfortunately, the stutterer who avoids does not appreciate the insidious nature of avoidance, and he gets caught in his own vicious web of fear, a web in which fear begets avoidance which begets more fear which begets increased struggle which begets more fear and avoidance, and soon the stutterer finds himself hopelessly mired in an avoidance-fear-struggle quagmire. In the struggle between stutterer and avoidance, assuming the stutterer continues to see avoidance as a solution, there will be only one winner, and that winner will be *fear,* the evil protégé of denial.

As I have often pointed out to my stuttering clients, we see this same pattern in the alcoholic who denies his disease, in the drug addict who insists he is in control of his drug, and in the obese individual who eats salads in public, devours sweets in private, and claims the weight problem is *glandular.* In each case, the individual is avoiding the problem, running away, denying, and in each case, avoidance makes the problem worse, much worse. Avoidance is a strategy that, by definition, cannot solve a problem because when it is used, the problem is not confronted, and any unconfronted problem is an unsolved problem. I may be guilty of verbal overkill here, but it is essential that the stutterer and everyone who interacts with him understand the dangers lurking within this behavior. It is such a seductive behavior because the immediate feeling the stutterer experiences after a successful avoidance is relief. It feels good to not stutter when you are certain you will, but this feeling is short-lived, and the next time the same word or the same situation must be faced, the fear, now elevated, will still be there.

Mild stutterers typically avoid more than severe stutterers because they stutter less often, and are therefore, more likely to avoid successfully. There is a price to be paid for this success, however. Although mild stutterers tend to have fewer word and situation fears than severe stutterers, the fears they do have tend to be more intense. Often, these stutterers are held hostage to their fears. They become hypersensitive to their fear-related cues and are constantly looking for ways out. The strain of constantly avoiding becomes unbearable. For these individuals, the unseen portion of the stuttering iceberg runs very deep indeed. Severe stutterers eventually reduce their attempts at avoidance because no matter what the speaking situation, no matter which words they must say, they are likely to stutter. This does not mean that the severe stutterer has no speech-related fear. It does mean that his fear tends to become more generalized. That is, there is no place to run, no place to hide, no reason to avoid.

There are three general types of avoidance behavior: *refusal, substitution,* and *circumlocution.* The most obvious way to avoid a word or a situation is to simply refuse to say the word or refuse to enter the situation. This is not usually the avoidance strategy of first choice, but when the fear is intense enough, some stutterers would rather be viewed as reticent, stupid, or deaf than to stutter. When asked a question, the stutterer might just glare at the listener, or shake his head and extend his arms in bewilderment. When instructed to speak, he might just fold his arms in defiance, or he might walk away. A more common avoidance strategy than refusal is substitution. If the stutterer is afraid he will stutter on "car," he says "automobile" instead. If he is afraid to call someone on the telephone, he writes a letter or sends a message by FAX or e-mail. Sometimes the stutterer cannot think of a synonym for a feared word, but he still wants to avoid saying it, so he circumlocutes, which literally means "to talk around." When the stutterer uses this strategy, he avoids a feared word by describing it. Instead of saying "sofa," he says "the elongated piece of upholstered furniture." Instead of saying "car," he says "the motorized, four-wheeled vehicle." It is an odd behavior to be sure because the stutterer avoids a single word by saying several words, but no one said fear always makes sense. We all know people who have unreasonable, groundless fears. In truth, fear is rarely as reasonable as it is real. The stutterer's fears are no more or less reasonable than others' fears of height, flying, or water, and they are just as real. Relative to stuttering, the reader should also remember that when the stutterer uses an avoidance behavior, he is reacting to a specific fear, so we should not be stunned that he chooses to say many words rather than one. His fear is of the one word, not of talking. He wants to talk, just as the person who is afraid of flying wants to travel. The stutterer's problem is that one word just as the traveler's problem is that one mode of transportation.

The second category of anticipatory behaviors is **postponement.** Whereas avoidance is used to *prevent* saying a word or entering a speaking situation, postponement is used to *delay* saying a word or entering a situation, but the word is eventually spoken, and the situation is eventually entered. The stutterer delays in the hope that his fear will subside enough that he will be able to say the target word or enter the target situation, and there is some justification for this hope. Fear is not an unwavering phenomenon. It fluctuates considerably from moment to moment. Let's assume that someone is trying to jump off a high platform into a swimming pool for the first time and is somewhat fearful about doing this. He might make several runs toward the end of the platform, stopping short each time, before he makes the last run and leaps into the pool. Each aborted attempt is a postponement. He might postpone the jump three, five, twenty or more times, but the odds are good that if he keeps running across that platform, he will eventually do so when his fear is at a low ebb. During that brief moment of reduced fear, he jumps. The stutterer's postponements work in the same way. He approaches a feared word, postpones its production once, twice, or several times, but if he keeps approaching the word, he will eventually say it when his fear is at a low ebb. The behaviors the stutterer uses when he postpones are the same behaviors all speakers use when they are trying to think of what to say next or when they are trying to hold the listener's attention. These are interjections such as "uh," "um," "well," "ya know," and other equally arcane utterances. Sometimes the stutterer postpones in silence, but this is not a common choice because silence in the midst of conversation is very uncomfortable for both speaker and listener.

Stutterers and people who observe stutterers will notice that postponements change over time. There is good reason for this change. The stutterer postpones because he does not want to stutter. The motive does not change, but the behaviors do. When he begins to postpone, he tries to use behaviors that do not call attention to themselves, and that makes sense too because he is trying to deceive the listener into believing that what is going on is something other than stuttering. As the disorder progresses, however, this deceit becomes more difficult because the articulatory struggle escalates. When the stutterer's struggle exceeds his ability to hide it in a guise of normalcy, postponement behaviors change. Behaviors that began as fairly normal and inconspicuous interjections become bizarre and exaggerated and eventually add to the abnormality they were intended to prevent.

And There Are Still More!

There are three additional behaviors we need to identify that do not fit into the groups above. Two of these are very common behaviors, and the third occurs in some very severe stutterers. Our understanding of the elements that can occur in moments of stuttering will not be complete without their inclusion.

One of these behaviors, usually called a **starter,** is most often associated with postponement, but it can occur even when there is no postponement. A starter is any behavior, verbal or nonverbal, the stutterer uses to end a postponement or to impose timing when he is trying to say a word on which he thinks he might stutter. The name, *starter,* is appropriate because that is precisely what the stutterer is trying to do. He is trying to get started. When he is postponing, he feels something like a motor that just won't turn over on a bitterly cold winter morning. The driver hears that terrible grinding noise, leans forward into the steering wheel, slams down the accelerator, and twists extra hard on the ignition key, as though any of these actions will actually help the old car get going. The postponing stutterer feels the same kind of frustration. He wants to get going, but his speech motor won't turn over, so he jerks his head, closes his jaw hard, or slaps his hand against his thigh in an effort to get started. Even when he does not postpone, he might sense that saying a certain word will be difficult, so he tries to establish a little rhythm to get a running start at the word.

If the stutterer uses a jerk of the head as a starter, he probably uses a jerk of the head as an interrupter as well. This is not surprising since both interrupters and starters are used to impose timing on arrhythmic speech. The difference between an interrupter and a starter rests in when and why each is used. An interrupter is used *after* a core behavior has been produced, and it is used to get out of the core behavior. A starter is used before the stutterer even gets to the target word, *before* any core behavior has been initiated, and it is used to make the production of the target word mandatory. It is quite possible, of course, for a starter and an interrupter to be used in the same moment of stuttering. The stutterer might approach a feared word, postpone, use a starter to get past the postponement, attempt to say the target word, stutter on the word, and then use an interrupter to end the moment. Such is the complex nature of moments of stuttering.

Disguise is one of my favorite stuttering behaviors because it reflects the extent to which stutterers will go to convince people they are not stutterers after all. A disguise is a behavior the stutterer uses to hide or cover up a moment of stuttering after it has begun. Typical disguises include coughing, laughing, throat clearing, turning away, and pretending to think. The stutterer tries to say a word, produces a core behavior, stops himself quickly, coughs to cover up the moment, and then says something like, "Boy, I don't know what's wrong with me today!" He then tries to say the word again. He might try the same disguise two or three times in a row, but there is a point of diminishing returns with this behavior. If a moment is too obvious, there is no point in trying to cover it up. It logically follows that this behavior is not used by the severe stutterer who stutters badly on many words in all situations. Disguises are most often used by mild stutterers who stutter only occasionally in some situations and who produce brief and simple moments. Disguises are used by moderate and severe stutterers only when they find themselves in situations they believe are not likely to produce much stuttering.

One of my favorite personal experiences from my severe stuttering days involves a disguise behavior. As is true of many severe stutterers, I was very selective in my use of disguises. In difficult situations, I did not consider hiding my moments because my moments were so frequent and so involved I would have coughed or laughed myself into a coma. In situations I thought were relatively nonthreatening, however, I used disguises when I thought they might help me pass as a normal speaker. As I look back on that time in my stuttering life, I realize I probably fooled no one, with the possible exception of my cocker spaniel who was pretty naive, but I thought I was a pretty slick stutterer when I was 13 years old. Anyway, in one of those nonstressful situations when my communicative confidence was high, someone asked me my name. As usual, I anticipated I would have trouble saying my name, but I made what I thought was a good attempt. As soon as I felt the beginning of a closure, I stopped and used my favorite disguise—pretending to think. After looking very pensive for a few seconds, I was suddenly struck by my error. One does not ordinarily have to spend time retrieving his own name from the memory vault. My listener was curious about this person who seemed not to know his own name. I was embarrassed, but as you can deduce, I survived to share my story with you.

Finally, we have the strangest of all observable behaviors of stuttering, **abulia.** Abulia occurs only in very severe stutterers and typically only in those who produce silent postponements or prolonged closures. Abulia has been described as the *ultimate of articulatory procrastination,* as a *complete loss of articulatory will power,* or as a kind of *psychosomatic dyspraxia.* If we piece all of these descriptions together, we get a pretty good picture of this behavior. When he is in an abulic state, the stutterer feels as though he cannot move his articulators at all, and in a certain sense, he may feel no inclination to do so. This is the stuttering equivalent of the deer who freezes in the headlamps of the oncoming car, or the guy who walks onto the railroad tracks in front of a train and becomes paralyzed with fear. During an episode of abulia, the stutterer experiences extreme sensory deprivation, especially auditory and visual. We can all relate to this aspect of abulia because we have all been so deep in concentration that someone says something to us, and we do not hear him or her. We have all been so engrossed in thought we have stared at something without really seeing it, and as we stare, our eyes defocus or we feel as though we are peering through a tunnel. This is what happens during an episode of abulia. To the external observer, it looks like the stutterer is having a small seizure. Abulic episodes typically last for a second or two, but sometimes when the stutterer comes back to sensory awareness, he has forgotten what he was saying. This consequence of abulia contributes to the perception by some that what is really happening is some kind of seizure. Abulia disappears, however, as soon as the stutterer learns to control the severity of his moments and when he stops postponing.

The Unseen Dimension of Stuttering

As I have already mentioned several times, not all of the stuttering problem can be observed. Many clinicians believe that the greater part of the problem is invisible to those who live and interact with the stutterer.

Although it is admittedly difficult to deal with factors we cannot see, hear, or touch, we must deal with the unseen dimension of stuttering if we are to successfully treat it, whether we believe it is the greater or the lesser part of the total problem. The unseen dimension includes the stutterer's feelings, attitudes, and perceptions as they relate to himself, to the act of speaking, to stuttering, and to his listeners. There is no question that these invisible aspects of the disorder will affect the stutterer's success or failure as a speaker. Even the severe stutterer is likely to be more fluent when he feels confident about his role as a speaker, when he feels that his status is superior to those around him, and when he perceives that speaking will be easy. This is all part of the *self-fulfilling prophesy* aspect of the disorder we have already addressed.

One of the primary purposes of therapy with the adult stutterer is to correct his misperceptions about stuttering and to adjust his feelings and attitudes about himself, others, and speech. If the speech-language clinician can accomplish these changes, therapy will probably be successful. If the stutterer's feelings, attitudes, and perceptions remain negative, the prognosis for improvement is poor, no matter what the clinician does.

One of the things we must accept as fact about stuttering is that what comes out of the stutterer's mouth is significantly affected by what he thinks and feels, for good or ill. For the umpteenth time, I need to point out that this connection between behavior and attitudes is not unique to stutterers. The connection exists in every human being. A person who thinks negative, destructive thoughts will behave in negative, destructive ways. A person who is truly happy, who believes in himself and in others will behave in ways that will positively impact his own life and the lives of others. That there is a connection between what we feel and believe and what we do is a simple fact of life. If the adult stutterer is to conquer his speech disorder, he must believe he has the ability to conquer it. He must come to understand that he produces the behaviors of stuttering, and he is capable of producing fluent speech. He must understand that there are no inherently difficult sounds, words, or situations, that he creates his own sense of *difficulty,* and he can also decide that any sound, word, or situation can be handled successfully. He must believe that most listeners are positive, supportive, compassionate people because they are. He must understand and accept that normal speech is not perfect speech, that all speakers produce fluency failures, and that relatively fluent speech is an attainable goal. He must find personal satisfaction in coming to grips with his problem, attacking it aggressively, and moving forward with his life in total control of his speech mechanism. He must stop dreading speech and start enjoying it, even loving it. If he accomplishes these attitudinal and perceptual changes, he has a better than fighting chance to be successful in dealing with the total stuttering problem.

For obvious reasons, speech-language clinicians try hard to prevent the young stutterer from ever developing negative feelings and attitudes about speech and nonfluencies. It is far easier to prevent these attitudes from developing than it is to change inappropriate, destructive attitudes later. Caregivers should remember that speech is naturally pleasurable for children. Children do not have to learn to love talking. They are genetically programmed to talk and to enjoy the exercise. Even when the youngster begins to produce behaviors that are worrisome for caregivers, the child is not concerned, and he will continue to rattle on, oblivious to his hesitations, false starts, retrials, and repetitions. The task shared by caregivers, teachers, and the speech-language clinician is to help the child retain this positive attitude about talking. If they can prevent the misperceptions and prevent the bad attitudes and feelings, the odds are very good that the child will emerge from his period of potential stuttering unscathed, ready to move forward as a well-adjusted, albeit occasionally nonfluent, communicator.

There are many feelings commonly associated with stuttering including embarrassment, frustration, shame, guilt, and hostility, but the one feeling that is directly or indirectly related to all others is *fear.* Fear is, by far, the most common feeling experienced by the advanced stutterer. He fears words, specific sounds, certain people, types of people, certain situations, and in some cases, even the act of speaking regardless of the conditions. The fear the stutterer feels needs to be carefully defined, however, because it is not *terror,* and it is not *phobia.* It is the expectation of unpleasantness in a speaking situation. In its mildest form, it is a nagging doubt about the ability to speak fluently. In its most severe form, it is absolute certainty that fluency failure will occur.

What is the origin of these fears? Certainly the stutterer is not born with these fears, and they do not come to him in mystical dreams. They are fears born in real, although usually quite innocent, life experiences. Stuttering fears begin in experiences of speech failure, the kind of speech failures ALL people experience. Perhaps the young stutterer is called into the principal's office to face charges of wrongdoing. This is a threatening experience for all children. The typical child will find it difficult to communicate smoothly when confronted by a huge adult with tremendous status who has the authority to administer frightening punishments. The accused child speaks in his own defense, stumbles on his words, and walks away a shaken person. The average child will feel the intimidation, experience the fear, and speak haltingly, but he will quickly forget the incident and go about his business. The young stutterer, however, reacts in a somewhat different manner. He is more sensitive to the speech failure, and he does not forget so quickly. He remembers specific details about what happened in that experience. He might remember a particular word on which he stuttered, or he might remember certain physical characteristics of the principal, or he might remember the feeling of confrontation. In the future, if he meets with the principal again, even if the meeting is not confrontational, he might remember the details of the first experience. These details have now become cues for his fear, and once again, he stutters.

One aspect of the development of stuttering fears that needs to be emphasized is that these fears tend to generalize. If the stutterer has a bad experience with the principal—an authority figure—he may have problems with other authority figures, such as police officers, judges, and bosses. If he has trouble with the word "soup," he might have trouble with other words that begin with "s." Once fears begin, they usually escalate until they become dominant features of the stuttering problem. Fortunately, these fears dissipate quickly when the stutterer gains confidence and when he gains control over the physiological portion of the disorder. Most adult stutterers who have gained control over their speech still have speech-related fears, but they tend to be relatively few in number, and more importantly, successful clients know how to deal with these fears.

Putting the Pieces Together

By way of summary, I want to build a sample moment of stuttering so the reader can see how the parts of a moment relate to one another and to the whole. Keep in mind that each behavior, no matter how strange it seems, serves a purpose and that each part of a moment of stuttering has a relationship with one or more other parts of the same moment.

Let us assume that a stutterer is trying to say "key." A plausible moment might develop as follows. The stutterer anticipates that this word will be difficult, so he *postpones* its production by saying "uh, uh, uh." Feeling uneasy about the length of the postponement and the lack of rhythm in his speech, he pulls his elbow to his side (*starter*). He then tries to produce the first sound of the word, but in doing so, he presses the back of his tongue so firmly against the back portion of the roof of his mouth that he blocks the flow of air (*closure*). After struggling for several seconds to force his way through the closure, he lifts his head and throws it down toward his chest (*interrupter*). This action breaks the closure, and he completes the word.

This was actually a fairly simple moment, but it is sufficient to make the point that stuttering is not one behavior but many. The stutterer must be able to recognize each part of the moment, and he must understand the purpose each part serves. Only then will he be able to focus on the parts that matter most. The inevitable bottom line relative to stuttering behaviors is this. If the stutterer can successfully attack the anticipatory behaviors that feed fear into stuttering, and if he can successfully eliminate or modify the core behaviors of stuttering, he WILL indirectly address all the other behaviors. This means that if the stutterer successfully manages avoidances, postponements, repetitions, closures, and postural fixations, he will achieve control over his speech. As is often true, it is easier to say this than it is to achieve it, but control is achievable. The first critical steps toward accomplishing this control are recognizing the behaviors that comprise stuttering, understanding why they occur, and understanding which of these behaviors need to be directly attacked in treatment.

Chapter 5

WHAT CAUSES STUTTERING?

There is no doubt that the question I am most often asked by stutterers and by their caregivers is the one that heads this chapter, "What causes stuttering?" Whenever the question is posed, I am reminded of the phase all young children go through when they ask all those wonderful questions for which there never seem to be easy answers, even if someone somewhere has the right answers. My daughters never asked me, "IS the grass green?" I could have answered that one. They asked, "WHY is the grass green?" Even if I could have answered the question with confidence, I am not sure I could have answered it in a way that would have been meaningful to them at the time. Some questions, unfortunately most of the really important questions in life, cannot be answered as simply as they are asked. I have come to the conclusion that philosophy exists to fill a portion of that vast void between obvious questions and unattainable answers. Philosophers can write and talk for hours about the great questions of life and not come close to encroaching on an answer. If you are beginning to sense that the question, "What causes stuttering?" is one of those questions, a question that has no simple answer, you are absolutely correct, but I wanted to break the news to you as gently as I could.

Splitting the Difference Between Honesty and Responsibility

Actually, there is a simple answer to the question. *We do not know what causes stuttering.* There it is, a simple answer and an honest answer, but it does not address the essence of the question, and it does not do justice to the evolution of thinking about the causality of stuttering that has occurred over the centuries since the question was first posed. It is true that we do not know what causes stuttering, but we have some pretty good ideas about some of the possibilities, and if nothing else, we have eliminated some guesses. When

I counsel people about stuttering, I try to split the difference between the simplistic honesty of "We don't know," and the responsibility I have as a speech-language pathologist to provide as much information as I can. I say, "split the difference," only because not all the theories about the causality of stuttering are useful. There are, for example, people who have speculated that stuttering is caused by demons that must be exorcised. I would certainly not present this as a viable explanation for the origin of stuttering to any of my clients. Most clients are afraid of the causality question anyway. Even though they ask, they are somewhat reluctant to hear the answer for fear they will learn something awful about themselves. I refuse to add to their anxiety by sharing with them every wild and crazy idea that has been put forth by marginally sane, semi-intelligent, and entertainingly ignorant human beings who claim to know the secret to the origin of stuttering. I suspect that many of these same people are responsible for Elvis sightings, claim to know where Jimmy Hoffa is buried, and have had close encounters with aliens from another galaxy.

On the other hand, I do not feel comfortable as a counselor, providing only my own opinion about the cause or causes of stuttering. I try to present an honest, but responsible, edited summary of the major theoretical notions that have been developed over the years, most of which have been in and out of favor several times during the last few centuries. Only after I make this presentation do I present my own personal views about what causes stuttering, and I am very careful to label these views as *my views,* not the *truth.* I am convinced that the swell of music in the background and the laser light show that accompany the expression of my opinions have little effect on the client's accepting my views as *the truth.* In any case, sans light show and with the music turned down so low you may not be able to hear it at all, I intend to address this important question as if I were talking directly to you. I will try to provide a broad and responsible perspective on what may cause stuttering, but please remember that despite what some experts might claim, no one knows for sure what causes stuttering, and though I risk revealing some uncharacteristic pessimism, we are probably only inches closer to an answer today than we were a century ago.

Cataloging the Causes

We must first address an issue that usually does not enter the thought processes of people when they ask about the cause of stuttering. What all is included in the concept, "cause," as it relates to stuttering? Most people use the word "cause" in a very narrow sense to mean "origin" or "genesis," at least when they use the word in reference to stuttering, other communication disorders, and a wide range of other conditions afflicting human beings.

Before we proceed, we need to differentiate among kinds of causes that might impact stuttering. We are, of course, primarily interested in discovering the origin of the disorder. This kind of cause is best expressed in the word, **etiology.** Most theories of stuttering concern themselves with the etiology of stuttering. Some theorists believe, however, that two children can be born with the same potential to become stutterers because both have been exposed to, or affected by, the same etiological factor, but one becomes a stutterer and the other does not. Why? This question leads us to another category of causes that can play a role in a disorder such as stuttering, **precipitating causes.** A precipitating cause is a factor that does not account for the origin of the disorder, but it does *trigger* the disorder if the proper etiological factor is operative. Looking ahead a few months or years, what happens if the etiological factor ceases to be operative, if the condition that originally caused stuttering to develop no longer exists? It is possible, of course, that the stuttering will stop if the etiological factor is no longer operative, but assuming the stuttering continues, why does it continue? Yet another category of causes comes into play, **maintaining causes.** The suggestion here is that the stutterer might continue to stutter even if the reason he began to stutter is no longer present and even if the factor that triggered the disorder is nowhere to be found because other factors emerge that cause the disorder to persist. Is this confusing or what? Are we making stuttering more complex than it needs to be? Having lived with the disorder all my life, and based on what I have learned about the disorder in my career as a teacher and clinician, I believe that stuttering is complex enough that it absolutely cannot be explained by etiological factors alone. I believe that if we are to truly understand this disorder and the people who own it, we must also try to identify precipitating and maintaining causes, but I offer a word of warning. It is no easier to identify precipitating and maintaining causes than to identify etiological factors.

In the event that you are just about ready to slam this book shut in frustration, I want you to know that this tangle of causes is not as confusing as it may first seem, and the tangle is certainly not unique to stuttering, but when the disorder itself is so misunderstood, a discussion about different kinds, or categories, of causes can be particularly bewildering. Perhaps a familiar nonstuttering example will help clarify how etiological, precipitating, and maintaining factors are related to one another and how each category explains a dimension of a complex problem, even if it cannot explain the whole problem.

Consider alcoholism, a common and serious problem. There is considerable evidence today that alcoholism is a disease and that this disease often has a genetic basis. To assert that a given person's alcoholism is genetically based is to identify the etiology of his disease, but a genetic connection alone is not sufficient to make a person an alcoholic. If an individual with a genetic predisposition to alcoholism never takes a drink of alcohol, he will not become an alcoholic. Taking that first drink or those first drinks for the person who is genetically predisposed to alcoholism is the precipitating factor that triggers the disease. The disease can then be maintained for all the reasons we have heard from alcoholics. "I drink because all my business associates drink, and I can't afford to not drink." "I drink because it tastes good and because it relaxes me." In the case of alcoholism, the maintaining factors can be emotional or learned, or the disease might be maintained by physical addiction, but if one is to understand alcoholism and the alcoholic, one must understand that the maintaining factors are just as important as the etiological factors. In terms of treating alcoholism, maintaining factors are actually more important than etiological factors because there is precious little we can do about the etiological factors which are almost certainly inoperative or, in the case of a genetic predisposition, therapeutically untouchable. If we are to treat the alcoholic, we must address the factors that are operative and available to us, the maintaining factors.

The reader should carefully note that what I have written about treating the alcoholic, relative to causality, is relevant to the adult stutterer. That is, whatever the etiological factors may have been for a particular stutterer, they are probably gone by the time the adult stutterer is in therapy. While it may be possible to address etiological and precipitating factors in the treatment of the young stutterer, we are usually limited to addressing maintaining factors when we treat the adult stutterer.

Now that I have made an issue about the kinds of causes that might account for the development and persistence of stuttering, I must tell you that the remainder of this chapter will deal only with etiological factors. We will consider possible precipitating factors in Chapter 7. Maintaining factors will be discussed in greater detail in the chapter concerned with preventing stuttering and in the second part of the book that focuses on treatment. It is important, however, that you begin now to think about causality in the manner I have outlined in the preceding section. Otherwise you become vulnerable to the notion that stuttering is a simple problem with a single cause that can be easily identified, isolated, rooted out and destroyed. I wish it were this simple, but it is not. As people who stutter and people who interact with those who stutter, we must accept the possibility that there is nothing we can do about the origin of stuttering in any given case. We may, however, be able to successfully address precipitating and maintaining factors. If we can control or eliminate these factors, we may be able to effectively prevent stuttering in some cases, and successfully treat it in others.

Theories that try to explain the origin of stuttering are traditionally divided into three categories: (1) theories that explain stuttering as an *organic* or *physical* disorder, (2) theories that argue that stuttering is a symptom of an underlying *psychological* problem, and (3) theories that describe stuttering as *learned* behavior.

One of the most intriguing things I have discovered in studying these theories is that they all make sense, in some ways, in reference to some stutterers, and that, in itself, is an important consideration. Perhaps instead of trying to decide which theory is *correct,* we should consider how each theory might explain certain aspects of the disorder, and how each theory might explain the development of stuttering in certain individuals. You would not have to interact with very many stutterers before you would agree with those who have observed that no two stutterers are alike. Having interacted with many stutterers of all ages, both sexes, and from widely varying cultural and economic backgrounds, I am absolutely convinced that we will never find a single theory that explains all cases, but I will hasten to point out that this is a personal bias, not the revelation of *truth.* I am expressing this much of my own view about the causality of stuttering now, however, because I want you to be encouraged to consider all the theoretical ideas I am about to present with an open mind. Consider, as I have, that each of these views has the potential to shed some light, however dimly and narrowly focused the beam, on the question, "What causes stuttering?"

A Defective Speech Machine?

Most of the oldest theories of stuttering make the claim that stuttering is an organic or physical problem. That early theorists would take this view is not surprising when we consider that prior to Sigmund Freud and psychological explanations of deviant human behaviors, and prior to learning interpretations of these behaviors that became popular in the 20th century, virtually everything that could go wrong with a human being was traced to some physical origin or was blamed on evil, either in a general sense or personified in demons. It must also be admitted that stuttering often *looks* like a physical problem. During prolonged and effortful moments, the stutterer often looks as though he cannot breathe or he cannot move his articulators. In the last chapter, I mentioned that abulia looks like a seizure reaction. It is not difficult to imagine that people watching a severe stutterer might conclude that he is epileptic or cerebral palsied. Stuttering is, in many ways, a physical disorder, so it would be reasonable to conclude that it has a physical origin. *Reasonable* is not necessarily correct, of course, just . . . reasonable.

It should also come as no surprise that the physical structure most often blamed in the oldest organic theories was the tongue. If one were to poll a large sample of people from around the world and ask them which structure inside the mouth is most important in the production of speech, the overwhelming majority would name the tongue. In fact, it is hard to imagine what structure would be the runner-up in such a poll. In any case, if the tongue is the main character in speech production, it seems reasonable that it would be the main character, or at the least one of the leading characters, in a speech failure problem such as stuttering. Whether or not the tongue is as important to speech as most people believe it is, it has been a favorite target of those who have looked for the cause of stuttering.

I seriously doubt that he was the first person to blame the tongue, but Aristotle was one of the first historical figures most of us would recognize to blame the tongue for causing stuttering. Aristotle, as you probably know, was an ancient Greek philosopher. Actually, he was not *ancient* at the time he was a philosopher, but he was Greek, and he was a philosopher so long ago that we feel a need to differentiate between ancient Greece and modern Greece, but I digress. Being a philosopher in ancient Greece was something like being a professional know-it-all. If Aristotle were alive today, he would probably work in a think tank. He was a thinker, an idea man, and he offered his thoughts and opinions on a wide range of political, social, ethical, and moral issues of his day. He also had something to say about stuttering. In about 384 B.C., Aristotle offered an opinion about stuttering, concluding that it is caused by a tongue that is weak and/or immobile. He further reasoned that because of this condition, the stutterer's tongue is too *sluggish* to keep up with his thoughts. Wow! I wonder if you have ever heard this idea before. It is usually expressed as follows: "He stutters because he thinks faster than he can talk." There is good news and bad news about this observation. The good news is that it puts the observer in pretty good intellectual company, right there with old Aristotle himself. The bad news is that the observation makes absolutely no sense. We can perhaps forgive Aristotle for not understanding the neurological connections between thinking and speaking, but there are really no excuses for modern day high school graduates to reach the same erroneous conclusion. OF COURSE, the stutterer thinks faster than he speaks. We all think faster than we speak. We all think faster than we can perform any voluntary movement, considerably faster, incredibly faster. In fact, if we could not think faster than we could perform a voluntary motor act, we could not perform the voluntary motor act. Think about it! What is truly amazing about this Aristotelian observation is that it has survived the centuries despite overwhelming knowledge that makes its logic sound childish. Every year I hear people, including many people who should know better, offer this ancient explanation for stuttering. It was not valid in 384 B.C., and it is not valid today. There is an upside-down version of this observation that is even more ludicrous: "He stutters because he talks faster than he can think." Now that's tricky. I'm going to guess that any person who can do this is either an extremely effective salesperson or an inordinately slick politician.

It's for certain that such a person does not know whether he believes what he says until he's had a chance to think about it after he's said it. The point is, of course, that it is absolutely, positively impossible to talk faster than one can think because the motor acts involved in speaking are the results of neural impulses sent from the brain, impulses intended to translate thought into the words by which those thoughts can be expressed. Thinking MUST precede talking. Now . . . one could legitimately point out that some people do not spend enough time in thought before they speak, but that's an entirely different problem.

If we leave the ancient Greek era behind and move forward in history to the time of the Roman Empire, we find another prominent person putting forth a similar explanation about stuttering. A highly respected Roman physician named Celsus, who would have been listed in the Yellow Pages about 4 B.C., agreed with Aristotle that stuttering is caused by a tongue that is too weak, but Celsus was a physician and not just an idea man, so he devised a treatment for stuttering. He believed that gargling and massaging the tongue would increase its strength, and that with a revitalized tongue, the stutterer would be able to speak normally. Whenever I think about Celsus, which I usually do only on odd Tuesdays, I imagine him administering this tongue massage treatment. "Just lay your tongue on the table, Brutus, and we'll work out the kinks." In fairness to Celsus, his treatment was no more bizarre, or groundless, than countless others that have been forced onto stutterers over the centuries and even with the past 50 years.

If you think that things probably got better for stutterers when the calendar turned to A.D., you would be wrong. About 200 A.D., Galen, a famous Greek physician, concluded that stuttering is caused by a tongue that does not function well because it is too short, too thick, or too wet and cold. In the late 1500s, Mercurialis concluded that people stutter because their tongues are either too moist or too dry. In 1627, Francis Bacon offered an opinion about stuttering that will excite vintners everywhere. Most people know that Francis Bacon was a famous person, but they are often not sure exactly what he did. In some ways, he was an Aristotle of his day. He was also similar to Benjamin Franklin in that he was a person of many talents and interests. He is probably best known, however, as an author and a British statesman. Like Aristotle and Franklin, Bacon was not shy about offering his views and opinions on a wide range of matters, and eventually he decided to shed his light on stuttering. He concluded that stuttering is caused by a *frozen* or *stiff* tongue. He suggested that drinking hot wine would thaw or loosen the tongue, thereby relieving the stuttering.

I included Francis Bacon's speculation in this little summary of tongue interpretations of stuttering, not only because it is interesting, but because it allows me to make an important point about the origin of many theories and treatments of stuttering. I am not sure that Bacon formulated his theory of stuttering in the manner I am about to describe, but I suspect he did. I envision that Bacon drew his conclusion after observing the "town stutterer." I figure that every British village in the 1600s had a town crier, a town drunk, and a town stutterer, and wouldn't it be something if one person held all three jobs? Anyway, I am guessing that Bacon observed that when the town stutterer when to the local pub and threw down a few tankards, he became more fluent. Bacon might then have reasoned backwards. That is, if the stutterer is fluent when his tongue has been loosened by hot wine, he probably stutters in the first place because his tongue is too stiff. This would not be an illogical conclusion, I suppose, but it would not be supported by research data. Some stutterers and most nonstutterers become more nonfluent under the influence of alcohol. Some stutterers may *feel* more fluent when they are intoxicated even though they are not, and some observers may believe they are more fluent because they struggle less, even if the frequency of stuttering does not change.

The point to be emphasized here is not what happens to stutterers under the influence of alcohol. The point is that many ideas about what causes stuttering and how stuttering should be treated are based on casual observations of conditions that seem to increase or decrease the frequency of stuttering. Since stuttering is, by its very nature, an extremely variable disorder, it is fairly easy to find conditions that influence its frequency and severity, but to conclude that these conditions hold the secrets to understanding the origins of stuttering or how to treat it are risky at best. The problem in almost every instance is that a condition that causes more stuttering in some stutterers is likely to result in reduced stuttering in other stutterers.

A well-meaning Prussian surgeon, Johannes Dieffenbach, opened one of the most infamous periods in the treatment of stuttering in 1841. Dieffenbach believed that stuttering was caused by neurological spasms of the tongue. The necessary treatment, he reasoned, was to sever the nerves that were causing the spasms. The procedure he devised involved cutting into the base of the tongue and removing a wedge of tissue. Other surgeons in Europe and in the United States joined Dieffenbach in performing this surgery on scores of stutterers. The immediate results were promising. Following surgery, the patients did stop stuttering, but it soon became apparent that Dieffenbach, and the surgeons who followed his lead, had miscalculated. When their patients' tongues healed, the stuttering returned, but now these poor souls stuttered with permanently mutilated tongues. Even more tragically, there were deaths, the result of the primitive conditions under which surgeries were performed at that time. By any measure, this was a tragic chapter in the stuttering story. If nothing else, it illustrates how desperate stutterers can be to rid themselves of their disorder.

Beginning in the twentieth century, there was an increasing tendency to associate stuttering with problems in the central nervous system. Some writers continued to point their fingers at the tongue. They argued that the tongue itself is normal, and the peripheral nerves that innervate the tongue are normal, but there are problems in the motor centers of the stutterer's brain that send incorrect messages to the muscles of the tongue. The problem, they argued, is not a weak tongue but an uncoordinated tongue. Other writers suggested that the stutterer's apparent respiratory problems are not the result of defective respiratory muscles but are produced by inappropriate messages from the higher motor centers of the brain that control breathing.

In a sense, it may seem a fine line between blaming the tongue or the respiratory system and blaming the motor centers that control the musculature of these structures, but it was an important step forward in our understanding of stuttering. We at least recognized that when we compare the stutterer's peripheral speech structures to those of nonstutterers, we find no significant differences. This does not alter the fact, however, that the stutterer does struggle with speech. The obvious explanation for that struggle, according to these writers, is that the brain is defective in ways that cause the speech structures to malfunction.

Some theorists took a broader view of the brain's role in causing stuttering. Instead of attributing the problem to incorrect information being sent to specific speech structures, they argued that the problem is more global. For example, some writers in the 1920s and 1930s argued that the stutterer does not have sufficient cerebral dominance. To appreciate this theoretical view, we need some supportive background. There are two hemispheres in the brain. With few exceptions, the muscles of speech are paired and receive information from opposite hemispheres. That is, the muscles on the right side of the speech mechanism receive innervations from the left hemisphere, and the muscles on the left receive innervations from the right hemisphere. Information from the two hemispheres must arrive at the same time in order for the movements of the speech mechanism to be synchronized, and the movements must be synchronized in order for speech to be fluent. In order for this synchronization to occur, one hemisphere must become dominant over the other, in order to impose its timing on the other. The stutterer, some theorists contended, lacks this cerebral dominance, which means that the signals from the hemispheres are not properly and precisely coordinated. The end result is that the right side and the left side of the speech mechanism are out of synch, and the product is *stuttering*. This particular theory of stuttering generated volumes of research, some of which seemed to support it, but as is true of so many theories of stuttering, it fell from favor because there were some critical pieces of the stuttering puzzle that did not fit the theory. Since the theory was first postulated, we have found motor tracts that descend from the brain to the muscles of speech homolaterally. That is, right side muscles receive right brain innervations and left side muscles receive left brain innervations. These theorists speculated that stutterers' lack of cerebral dominance would show up in differences in handedness, but the research data did not support this speculation. Nevertheless, the cerebral dominance theory has not died. In revised forms, prompted by new research evidence, it is finding some acceptance in some quarters today.

Some writers, no doubt taking into account the fact that stuttering occurs more often in males than in females, and the fact that males mature more slowly than females in nearly every respect, concluded that stuttering is caused by a central nervous system that matures too slowly to keep pace with social demands for communication development. They reasoned that girls who become stutterers must have central nervous systems that mature at a rate similar to the maturation rate of boys who become stutterers, a rate that is slower than that of boys who do not become stutterers. I realize that I have overstated the case here, but I have done so deliberately to reinforce a point I made earlier. That is, a theory of stuttering is often based on perceptions, perceptions that are based on observations. The theorist puts *two* and *two* together and comes up with *stuttering,* which might be *four,* but which might also be *five* or *107.* The point is, we have no proof that stutterers as a group experience central nervous system maturation more slowly than nonstutterers as a group, but the logic, in the face of some of the things we know about stuttering, is almost irresistible. These theorists cover themselves somewhat by contending that it may not be the slow maturation itself that causes the stuttering, but an immature central nervous system might be more vulnerable to fluency breakdown triggered by environmental pressures.

Some organic theories suggest that stuttering may not be a disorder unto itself, but is a form of some other central nervous system problem. That is, stuttering might be a form of aphasia, epilepsy, cerebral palsy, or apraxia. In general, these theories assert that the stutterer probably has a *subclinical* form of one of these conditions, which basically means that he has the condition, but it does not show up when standard diagnostic procedures are applied, although an autopsy might reveal it. It should come as no surprise that there are not long lines of stutterers standing outside coroners' offices to find out if these theories are correct. We stutterers may be curious about our disorder, and we may at times be a little desperate for answers and for viable treatments, but most of us are not unusually stupid or suicidal.

So far I have mentioned the roads most often taken by organic theorists, but there have been other less traveled and equally interesting roads. Some writers, for example, have blamed the tonsils or the uvula for causing stuttering. No doubt these people observed that stutterers, after having their tonsils removed or their uvulae trimmed, did not stutter as much as they did before the surgery. This is probably true, but it is definitely not surprising. Any surgery in or around the mouth will cause the stutterer to speak slowly, carefully, and gently in order to avoid the pain that comes with hard, careless contacts. If the stutterer speaks slowly and gently, he will not produce the struggle that characterizes stuttering. Struggle, after all, is the product of excessive muscular tension and semi-violent movements and contacts. Struggle hurts! When the surgical wounds heal, however, the stuttering returns because the pain is gone. The tonsils and the uvula were innocent victims, at least insofar as stuttering is concerned.

There were a number of theorists during the 1950s and 1960s who thought that stuttering is a problem that originates, not in the speech mechanism or in those parts of the central nervous system that control motor speech, but in the auditory feedback system. They pointed to evidence that normal speakers experience speech breakdowns that, in some ways, resemble stuttering when they hear their own speech after a very short delay. This phenomenon is sometimes experienced by speakers or singers in football stadiums or by people when they talk to radio disk jockeys while trying to listen to their radios at the same time. It is called *delayed auditory feedback,* or *DAF* for short. DAF can be easily created in the speech laboratory. There is no question that delayed auditory feedback can negatively affect the speech of some people. They may hesitate, block, repeat, and experience wild fluctuations in loudness and pitch. Those interested in finding the cause of stuttering could not resist the application of delayed auditory feedback to stuttering. The stutterer, they surmised, must have a built-in delay in his auditory feedback system. This theory was enthusiastically embraced by a few people for a short time, but it has been largely rejected because the research data simply do not support it.

Although many theorists and researchers continue to look for organic clues to the origin of stuttering in the central nervous system, others have invested their energies looking closely at the *larynx* or what is commonly called the *voice box.* The larynx is the structure in the anterior neck that contains the vocal folds. When air is moved up through the larynx by the forces of exhalation, the vocal folds are set into vibratory motion, producing the *voice.* Some theorists have suggested that the stutterer has a difficult time controlling the airflow, and it is this lack of control that causes stuttering. Others have suggested that the stutterer cannot turn vocal fold vibration on and off quickly enough to accommodate fluent speech. Presumably, this inability to control laryngeal function causes stuttering, but evidence to support this explanation is contradictory and inconclusive. It should be noted that no one disputes that these laryngeal malfunctions are characteristic of stuttering. That is, it is easy to accept that these malfunctions are effects of stuttering. There is just no definitive proof that they are evidence of causation.

Stuttering as a Symptom of an Underlying Psychological Problem

Many stutterers and caregivers with whom I talk express the opinion that stuttering is a psychological problem. Although this view is not as widely held in professional circles today as it was 40 or 50 years ago, there are still people, including many lay people, who remain convinced that stuttering is a symptom of an underlying psychological problem. Because so many people are inclined to look for psychological answers to the origin of stuttering question, we should take some time to examine this theoretical perspective, but the reader should be aware that this is something like looking through an historical home. Walking through an historical home is interesting and educational, but it is no longer a real home because real people do not live there. Considering most psychological theories of stuttering, especially those grounded in Freudian concepts, is interesting and educational, but these theories have been largely abandoned by real experts in both psychology and speech-language pathology. Come with me then as we explore what was, in days gone by, a viable view of stuttering.

In the preceding section on organic theories, I made the point that organic theories have emerged, in part, because stuttering looks like an organic disorder. It would also be fair to say that stuttering looks like a psychological problem. The stutterer appears to be frightened and distressed when he stutters, and the fact that he does not stutter all the time, but mostly when he is under stress, would be consistent with the perception that it is a psychological disorder. Furthermore, there is a certain sense in which moments of stuttering look *symbolic*. That is, one could argue, and some have argued that the stutterer's speech struggles symbolize his internal struggles and turmoil. I am not trying to make a case for the psychological view of stuttering, but I do think we should understand and accept that it is not unreasonable for someone to assume a psychological origin, given some of the features of the disorder. In order to appreciate this view, we need some additional background.

Most of the oldest and most influential psychological theories of stuttering were based on the classic Freudian explanation of psychosexual fixations, this despite evidence that Sigmund Freud himself did not believe that stuttering is a psychological problem. I have found that relatively few people outside of psychology and related fields understand *psychosexual fixation* conceptually, even though they think they understand what it is. This is not a psychology textbook to be sure, and I do not claim to be a psychologist, but if we are to understand this view of stuttering, we must at least get the basic facts straight concerning psychosexual fixations, oral eroticism, anal eroticism, etc., and I think I am armed with enough information in this area to provide an adequate introduction.

According to the Freudian view, a psychosexual fixation occurs when an individual is arrested at an early stage of psychosexual development. A fixation can have many symptoms. One of the possible symptoms is stuttering. Within this context, therefore, stuttering is caused by any condition that is likely to result in a psychosexual fixation. It should be noted that within this theoretical perspective, stuttering is really secondary in importance to the psychosexual fixation itself. Certainly the treatments derived from the Freudian view do not concentrate on the stuttering. They are designed to get at the problem for which the stuttering is merely a symptom. Presumably, if this problem can be identified and remedied, the stuttering will disappear, or at the very least, it will cease to be a major concern to the client. As we work our way through this wing of the museum of stuttering theories, therefore, we must first discover what causes psychosexual fixations. Only then can we begin to understand how these theories attempt to explain stuttering.

A psychosexual fixation develops when conflicts occur over the satisfaction of certain psychological needs during childhood. Please note that these are *needs,* according to Freud, not *desires.* If the child is to develop normally, these needs must be met in ways that do not create traumatizing conflicts. These psychological needs include oral and anal eroticism, dependence, aggressiveness, and self-assertion. If, for example, the child is allowed or encouraged to be dependent normally, there will be no problem, but if the child is forced into unnatural dependence, there is potential for conflict over the satisfaction of this need. The conflicts that give rise to psychosexual fixations are usually associated with disturbed child-parent relationships, and are often related to problems such as abnormal nursing behaviors on the part of the mother, excessively harsh or early weaning or toilet training, parental domination, or overprotection. If the mother, for example, nurses her child only because she feels it is the proper thing to do, she might feel guilty about her reluctance. The child senses the mother's reluctance and her uneasiness about what should be a natural, warm, mutually bonding experience. Even though the child is being nursed, the conflict makes it impossible for his oral erotic needs to be satisfactorily met, and he becomes arrested at the oral erotic level of psychosexual development. Please keep in mind as I trudge forward that I am greatly oversimplifying in an attempt to show how a psychosexual fixation might develop. If we follow this example beyond childhood, we might find a person who sucks his thumb, bites his fingernails, smokes cigarettes, chews the ends off of pens and pencils, or we might find a person who stutters. The Freudian psychologist might look at any of these behaviors and conclude that the behavior is symptomatic of an oral erotic psychosexual fixation, assuming that what is learned about the person's background is consistent with that conclusion. Biting one's fingernails, it could be argued, allows the individual to symbolically continue the nursing behavior that was focal to the origin of the fixation. The adult nailbiter is trying to satisfy an oral erotic need that was not satisfactorily met when he was a nursing infant. This all might sound a little strange to most of us, but this kind of explanation of human behavior was very popular at one time, and there are still psychotherapists who maintain this general orientation to many human behavioral problems.

In order to appreciate this view of stuttering, you must understand that stuttering, or whatever the symptom might be, serves a purpose. The symptom–stuttering–is not a behavior of failure. Rather, it is a purposive behavior the stutterer produces because he needs to produce it even if he is not consciously aware of his need to do so. The stuttering helps him satisfy one or more psychological needs that were not met in normal ways during his psychosexual development. As you might expect, not all theorists who march to the Freudian drummer agree about the need or needs that are being met by stuttering, and they are not in agreement about how these needs are met. Examining all the possibilities would go far beyond the scope of this book, but we will consider the most common interpretations of what happens in the stutterer's quest for psychosexual satisfaction.

As already hinted, some theorists contend that stuttering meets an unsatisfied need for oral erotic gratification. That is, stuttering allows the individual to continue the pleasure he enjoyed as a child when he put things into his mouth and nursed at his mother's breast. The stuttering allows him to continue the pleasure he felt when he identified, in an extraordinarily intimate way with the nursing object, his mother.

Somewhat more disturbing to some of us is the view that stuttering satisfies an infantile need for anal erotic gratification. Lest you think these theorists need a basic lesson in human anatomy, I will quickly explain how we get there from here. They argue that the function of the anal sphincter is symbolically moved upward to the oral sphincter so that when the stutterer speaks and stutters, he is *soiling* his listeners. Got that? One of the nice things about psychological theories is that there are few limits on the imagination. This is certainly one of the more creative interpretations of stuttering I have ever studied, and I will admit that as a stutterer, I find it personally offensive, but I have always avoided saying so in public for fear that my being offended would reveal something sinister about my own psychological health. Anyway, you can take or leave this particular interpretation, but if you leave it, make sure you leave it at the right end, and I will not risk trying to tell you which end is right or up.

Another general point of view suggests that stuttering allows the stutterer to express hostile or aggressive feelings in a manner that camouflages them so they are not recognized as hostile or aggressive by listeners. In what sense is stuttering hostile or aggressive? Consider how listeners feel when they listen to a severe stutterer. They feel uncomfortable, sometimes extremely uncomfortable. The idea then is that the stutterer, consciously or not, strikes out at his listeners by making them squirm when his stuttering makes them feel uneasy. I am not suggesting he was a psychologically disturbed stutterer, but I did know a young man when I was in graduate school who used his stuttering as a kind of weapon. It would have been an easy stretch for a psychotherapist to conclude that he was expressing hostile and aggressive feelings. He was a very severe stutterer, about "11" on a seven-point scale. When he said, "Hello" to someone he did not like, he would look for signs of discomfort. If he saw them, he would stretch that "Hello" into an agonizingly long greeting, and he never lifted his gaze from his listener's suffering. After his victim would leave our office, he would turn to me and say in a hauntingly gleeful manner, "Wasn't that fun?" Well, the truth is it was not fun for his listener, and it was not fun for me as a witness, but I definitely think he was having fun. You may be relieved to know that he did not complete a graduate degree in speech-language pathology. Whew! There are some writers who hold this general *hostile and aggressive* point of view who march out into the weeds a little bit. They suggest that by mangling his words when he stutters, the stutterer is symbolically cannibalizing his listeners, making him a kind of "Big Bad Wolf" in pursuit of "Little Red Riding Hoods." It's just too gruesome to ponder.

A final common explanation found in psychological theories of stuttering is that the individual stutters because he has an unconscious desire to not talk. Stuttering results, these theorists contend, from a conflict between the person's conscious and social need to talk and his unconscious desire to be silent. As I have mentioned and will mention again in this book, there is no question about the fact that all human beings have a natural desire and need to talk. Speech is instinctive in humans, and there is a very real need to include speech in the process of establishing and maintaining relationships with other human beings. It is possible, of course, to establish interpersonal relationships without speech, but few would argue with the idea that it is much easier and more convenient to be a social creature with speech than without it. If this is so, why would there be an unconscious desire to not talk? Writers who subscribe to this interpretation of stuttering have provided many reasons. They speculate that the stutterer is afraid to talk because if he talks, he might reveal hidden and forbidden desires, or he might say words he knows he should not say, including profane words. Does the term, *Freudian slip,* ring a bell here? Other writers suggest that the stutterer wants to be quiet because, at some deep level of his psyche somewhere in the general vicinity of the basement, he believes his stuttering is a form of oral or anal gratification. He cannot do anything about his need for gratification, but he can prevent others from knowing he has this need by simply not saying anything. It may or may not occur to him that his silence could be inter-preted as an indication of some kind of emotional pathology or perversion.

In closing this section, I must make it clear that not all psychological the-ories of stuttering have Freudian foundations, but it would be fair to say they all share the same general emphases, on *conflicts, needs,* and *disturbed personal relationships.* And for the most part, all of these theories assert that stuttering is not *the problem,* that stuttering is a symptom of a problem that lies deeper. Some non-Freudian theorists would concede that stuttering sometimes per-sists because it becomes habitual, but they would remain firm in their belief that the origin of the problem lies somewhere in the stutterer's psyche.

Stuttering as the Product of Learning

Over the last several decades of the twentieth century, one of the most widely embraced views about stuttering was that it is learned behavior, although even this generalization is safe only if carefully qualified. Most experts, in the field of speech-language pathology at least, would agree—even in the early years of the twenty-first century—that learning plays some role in the development and/or maintenance of stuttering. Beyond this relatively narrow common ground, there would be much disagreement. Some theorists believe that stuttering can be wholly explained as a learned disorder. Others argue that there is a genetic predisposition to stutter, but that the disorder is triggered by environmental influences, and that the specific behaviors of stut-tering are learned. Other theorists, with backgrounds in psychology, who believe that stuttering is symptomatic of an underlying psychological prob-lem, argue that the primary treatment should focus on the psychological dis-order. They allow, however, that stuttering may persist even after the psy-chological problem is resolved because the speech patterns have become learned and are habitual. The point to be made here is that the learning view is not completely incompatible with the organic and psychological views of stuttering. In addition, there are certain characteristics of the disorder that seem inexplicable except by learning, which also accounts for the wide acceptance of learning interpretations of the disorder, or at least some aspects of the disorder.

Along our journey through this chapter, I have tried to show that stut-tering has the appearance of an organic problem and the appearance of a psychological problem, which helps explain why people have looked in these directions for possible causes of the disorder. Not surprisingly, stutter-ing also looks and sounds like a learned disorder. One of the characteristics of stuttering mentioned by nearly everyone who writes about it is its extreme variability. To say that no two stutterers are alike does not begin to capture the range of variability that exists among stutterers. I can honestly say that I have observed more differences among stutterers than among any other category of communicatively disordered individuals. In fact, I never cease to be amazed that stutterers are so unique, not only in terms of severity, but in terms of the words and situations they perceive as *difficult,* and in terms of the way they produce stuttering behaviors. There are some obvious commonalities among stuttering behaviors, and I tried to identify those commonalities in the preceding chapter, but if one is not cognizant of these common characteristics, it would be easy to conclude that each stutterer creates his own disorder. In a very important sense, this is exactly correct, and this is one of the reasons stuttering appears to be a learned disorder. The experience of *being* blind does not vary widely even though the experiences of blind persons are surely different, but the experience of stuttering is very different for each stutterer. The individual differences stutterers experience strongly suggest a learning influence. Perhaps the most compelling argument in favor of stuttering as a learned disorder is the fact that each stutterer fears certain sounds, words, and situations that can be explained only on the basis of his individual life experiences.

When I was a youngster, for example, I had trouble with the "h" sound, probably because it was the first sound in my last name, and like most stutterers, I had a fear of saying my name. This fear then generalized to other "h" words such as "hello," "hi," and "here." Could my problems with "h" have occurred because "h" is a difficult sound to produce? Hardly. The "h" sound is probably the easiest of all sounds in our language to articulate because it involves only a controlled release of air. Why then was it a *hard* sound for me? It was hard only because I perceived it to be hard. I literally learned it to be a hard sound. As the years have gone by, most of them whizzing by at speeds that substantially exceed posted limits, my word fears and my situation fears have changed in ways that directly reflect changes in my personal life and in my professional life. For example, my word fears today are mostly confined to words I use professionally, including "physiology," "phonology," "phonation," and "diadochokinesis." Because they are words I frequently use when I talk to students and clients about stuttering, I have added "decision" and "deliberate," but I rarely, if ever, have a problem with "Hulit," "hi," "hello," or "here." These changes in word fears and similar changes in situation fears cannot be easily explained by organic or psychological theories of stuttering, but they fit perfectly into a learning interpretation of the disorder.

Although we may think of learning interpretations of human behavior as beginning with classical conditioning and operant conditioning learning theories, there have actually been learning views of human behavior in general, and stuttering specifically, for centuries. Prior to the twentieth century, however, learning explanations were primitive and simple. In fact, learning was most often understood in the context of the familiar maxim that *practice makes perfect*. The oldest and most primitive learning interpretations of stuttering suggest that the deviant speech behaviors of the disorder are *bad habits* that develop because the stutterer repeats nonfluencies over and over again until they become established patterns in his communication system. The nonstutterer might produce the same nonfluencies, but because he does not practice or repeat them, his nonfluencies remain occasional speech mistakes and do not become habitual speech behaviors.

Classical conditioning was popularized at the beginning of the twentieth century by Anton Pavlov and his famous dog experiment. A bell was rung as a dog was given food. The food produced salivation, a reflexive or unlearned response. After pairing the bell and the food over many trials, the bell alone was capable of eliciting salivation, which was now a *learned,* or *conditioned* response since dogs do not naturally salivate when they hear ringing bells. We are all unknowing subjects of classical conditioning. How many of us, for example, feel a little uneasy when we sense an odor that reminds us of the dentist's office? The odor itself is not likely to generate anxiety, but because it has been paired on a number of occasions with the pain or discomfort of dental treatment, we feel anxiety when we encounter the odor. Obviously, classical conditioning has been applied in the quest to find the origin of stuttering or I would not have included it in this discussion, but how has it been applied? In general, theories of stuttering based on classical conditioning contend that all people become nonfluent when they experience a great deal of speech-related anxiety. In other words, normal nonfluency is not learned. It is a normal, natural response to speech-related anxiety. Stuttering develops when a person becomes sensitized to stimuli that are not directly related to the anxiety but are present when the anxiety and the speech failure are experienced. In other words, these are neutral stimuli. The individual might notice a word, for example, or a certain characteristic of the listener, or some other aspect of the situation. After a number of pairings of this neutral stimulus with speech-related anxiety and fluency failure, the stimulus itself is enough to trigger the anxiety, which then triggers the *learned* or *conditioned* nonfluency we call *stuttering*.

B.F. Skinner popularized operant conditioning during the latter half of the 20th century. Throughout the 1960s and the early 1970s, operant conditioning seemed to be THE explanation for human behavior. It was only a matter of time before this learning theory was applied to stuttering in attempts to discover the cause of the disorder and to find a viable treatment for it. Although there are variations among operant theories of stuttering, there is one consistent thread that ties them together. They begin with the idea that all children produce nonfluencies, a normal phenomenon in speech development. If a given child produces nonfluencies, no matter how many he produces, and they are not reinforced, the child will remain a normal speaker. If, however, the child produces even a few nonfluencies that are reinforced, usually by gaining parental attention, they will increase in frequency and will eventually become major features of the child's speech. At this point, according to these theories, we are likely to attach the label, *stuttering*, to the nonfluencies because they are no longer natural speech failures but learned behaviors. They have been positively reinforced in that a positive consequence–increased attention–consistently followed their production. That is, whenever the child's speech became nonfluent, he received extra time and attention from one or both of his primary caregivers.

You may recognize that this is the same explanation used to account for the development of temper tantrums in young children. If a child throws a temper tantrum and he gets the attention he wants, he will throw more temper tantrums in the future. This might seem puzzling in cases in which tantrums are apparently punished, by spanking for example, but the operant theorist would ask us to look beyond the spanking to see a more important consequence, a positive consequence. If a child truly craves attention, it may make no difference to him if the attention comes in the form of a hug or a spanking. The attention, regardless of its form, is the desired consequence.

The same explanation can be applied to stuttering. A caregiver might react to a child's nonfluencies by correcting him, mocking him, pitying him or even spanking him, but if the child wants attention badly enough, he may not particularly care how the attention is packaged. Attention in any form from a caregiver as a reaction to the nonfluencies, therefore, could serve to reinforce them.

So What Do You Think Causes Stuttering?

I was afraid you would ask me that. I could say that I have already answered this question, but that would not really be true. I have tried to outline the major possibilities as they have been formulated in the minds of expert and quasi-expert theorists over the centuries, but I have so far not told you what I think causes stuttering, and since you have been kind enough to read to this point, I think I owe you my opinion. Before I take this risk, however, I need to tell you that my view is just as shaky as all the rest, and I should tell you that my view is not mine alone but is shared by others. I have no data to prove that my view is correct. I have only a perspective gained by my own study of the theoretical and research literature, my own clinical experiences, and last and certainly least, my own experiences as a person who stutters.

I will begin my answer by repeating an opinion I expressed earlier. I do not believe that stuttering is a single disorder. The term, *stuttering*, has traditionally been applied to a range of fluency problems that have a variety of causes, and I am distressed that we have made little effort to differentiate these fluency problems. I have seen cases of *stuttering* that were, in my opinion and in the opinions of psychotherapists with whom I consulted, clearly caused by psychological factors. These were late onset cases linked to specific traumatic events. The fluency problems did not persist but faded away when the psychological problems were resolved or forgotten. I am convinced that the *stuttering* associated with cerebral palsy, or with the kind of brain damage that occurs in cerebral vascular accidents, is not the same as the stuttering that develops in neurologically normal children. The cause in these cases seems fairly obvious, damage to the motor centers of the brain that control speech movements.

The most difficult kind of stuttering to explain is the stuttering produced by most people who are labeled *stutterers*. There is no obvious physical problem in this stutterer, and there is probably no hidden or subtle physical problem. The stutterer is psychologically and intellectually normal. There do not seem to be any unusual factors in the person's environment that could account for the disorder. The stuttering begins under apparently normal circumstances, and becomes progressively worse over the years of childhood and adolescence. What causes this kind of stuttering, the kind we typically call *developmental stuttering?*

I have become increasingly convinced that some cases of developmental stuttering can be explained solely on the basis of learning, probably some combination of the classical and operant views I briefly described in this chapter. I also believe that many developmental stutterers are born with a genetic predisposition to stutter and that environmental conditions trigger the disorder. These conditions need not be obvious or horrible. Given the predisposition to stutter, these individuals have reduced tolerance for the fairly routine communicative stresses that have little or no effect on other people, except perhaps to cause them some annoyance. Although I do not believe it to be a major contributor to the stuttering problem, the influence of parents might be a factor for some developmental stutterers. This type of stutterer might not respond well, in terms of speech at least, to parents who are perfectionistic, demanding, and critical. One could argue that you should not be certified as a parent unless you have these qualities to some extent, and indeed we typically see these characteristics in parents who truly care about their children, who want their children to grow up to be good, productive people. The point is, these are not *bad* qualities, and most children who have parents with these traits grow up happily and normally, but the child with a predisposition to stuttering, who is unusually susceptible to speech-related pressures, might not be able to tolerate the stresses produced by these parental qualities. In fact, he might not be able to handle any kind of speech-related stress no matter how easy-going, tolerant, and accepting his parents might be. This child is not born a stutterer, but he is born to become a stutterer at the first available opportunity.

In the next chapter, we will consider whether stutterers are special people or normal people with a special problem. This is an important distinction because if stutterers differ in significant ways from nonstutterers, these differences might provide clues to the cause or causes of stuttering. If we can establish with certainty the cause or causes of stuttering, we will be in a stronger position to find appropriate ways to treat it and prevent it, but let me give you fair warning. Don't hold your breath!

Chapter 6

STUTTERERS ARE ORDINARY PEOPLE TOO

The Issue of Difference: Clues to Causality

Most of the research designed to determine how stutterers differ from nonstutterers has not been conducted to merely satisfy the curiosity of researchers. It has been conducted in order to uncover clues that might lead us to an answer to the essential question—What causes stuttering? What might be called the *difference strategy* is certainly not unique to stuttering research. It is a strategy employed in the quests to understand the origins of cancer, heart disease, depression, diabetes, and virtually every other human disorder. Cancer researchers, for example, have found that people who develop lung cancer are much more likely to be smokers than people who do not develop lung cancer. Heart researchers have found that people who have diets that are high in fat, who do not exercise, who smoke, and who live under a great deal of stress are more likely to have heart attacks than people who avoid fats, exercise regularly, do not smoke, and who successfully manage the stresses of their lives. These conclusions, and the recommendations for healthier living derived from them, are based on *difference* studies. Those who study stuttering have tried to understand the causality of stuttering using the *difference* strategy. They have attempted to uncover differences between people who stutter and people who do not in order to understand why stuttering develops. So far the results of these research attempts have been inconsistent, confusing, and largely disappointing.

It should be noted, of course, that there are no absolutes when it comes to understanding the causes of lung cancer or heart disease. Some people seem to do all the wrong things and remain disease-free, and others seem to do all the right things and still develop the disease, but the trends cannot be denied. Your odds of remaining disease-free are much greater if you pay attention to the results of the medical research and if you adjust your style of living according to the recommendations based on these findings. Unfortunately, the picture is not so clear when we look at stuttering. No matter how we might turn the picture, it is pretty fuzzy and out of focus. The purpose of this chapter, therefore, is not to startle you with new and amazing findings about how extraordinary stutterers are, but to show that researchers have been conscientious in pursuing every conceivable lead that might shed light on the causality question. Despite their diligence, and I am now about to reveal the last page of the novel, we have found that stutterers are alarmingly ordinary people.

Before we proceed to a brief summary and analysis of the difference research, I want to emphasize that the causality question is not an end unto itself. We want to discover the cause or causes of stuttering for the same reasons we want to find the causes for cancer and heart disease—so we can effectively treat the disorder and ultimately prevent it. While they know there is much more to learn, physicians believe they have enough answers to the cancer and heart disease puzzles to initiate treatment and prevention programs that are much more effective than similar programs a generation ago. Because we know less about the causality of stuttering than we do about the causes of some other human disorders, we tend to operate on a *trial and error* basis when we treat and when we try to prevent, but it would not be accurate to say that our approaches to treatment and prevention are *shots in the dark*. We have enough research and clinical data, generated over many decades of working with thousands of stutterers of all ages and types, that we can make educated guesses about what will work and what will not. Before we try a strategy, we consider the implications of the research conducted so far. As behavioral scientists, we do not attempt treatments that are not as solidly based on theory, empirical data, and rationale as possible, even though we recognize that the evidence in support of a given treatment may be inconclusive. When a given approach does not yield the results we want and expect, we back off, examine the hypothesis upon which the treatment was based, analyze the results of the failed treatment, reconsider the empirical data available to us, develop a new hypothesis, plan a treatment based on that hypothesis, and begin again. Such is the process we must follow in the treatment of a disorder, the cause of which is not known. I would hasten to remind you that medical science proceeds in much the same way. Medical researchers have certainly not closed their explorative books on cancer and heart disease. There is still much they do not know about causality relative to these diseases, but treatments proceed, and efforts to prevent these diseases continue. The responsible physician, like the responsible speech-language clinician, chooses a treatment approach that is judged to be best for a given patient, based on the best diagnostic data available. If the patient responds well, the treatment is continued, but if the treatment does not yield good results, the physician does not simply give up. Instead the physician analyzes what happened, tries to determine why it happened, revisits the original data, searches for new data, develops a new hypothesis, and tries again. The treatment of any human condition is, to some extent, an exercise in educated trial and error. This will continue to be true until our knowledge is complete, and when will our knowledge be complete? Your guess is as good as my ignorance.

The point of all this is that stutterers and those who treat stutterers should not despair. We know more about stuttering today than at any time in human history, and we continue to learn more about the disorder every year. Even though we do not have answers to some of the most basic questions about stuttering, we have clues to the answers, and these clues are sufficient for us to develop reasonable, responsible, professional treatment and prevention approaches. At the same time, the quest for answers continues, and it will continue until our educated guesses and hunches are, one by one, replaced with facts. This is precisely why the issue of differences between those who stutter and those who do not is so important. Common sense screams that there must be explanations for why stuttering develops in some people and not in others, and common sense tells us in a calm voice that the most logical strategy for uncovering these explanations is to continue our efforts to discover how stutterers differ from nonstutterers.

Physical Changes—Causes or Effects?

Much of the research on stutterers completed so far has focused on what happens to the stutterer when he stutters. Are there physical changes that occur during moments of stuttering that might explain why these moments develop? The first part of this question is easy to answer, and you do not have to be an expert to answer it. There ARE physical changes that occur during moments of stuttering. Do these changes explain why the stuttering occurs? Well, that part of the question is much tougher to answer, but it is the more important part of the question, and I will try to address it as this section unfolds.

Even the most unsophisticated observer can detect what appear to be breathing changes during the moments of some stutterers. These are not imagined changes. They are very real deviations from normal breathing patterns. Breathing can become irregular during stuttering. Either inhalation or exhalation might be abnormally prolonged. The stutterer might suddenly stop exhaling during a moment, or he might take a quick inhalation in the middle of an exhalation. He might gulp two or three breaths of air in rapid succession, or he might begin to speak while he is still inhaling before finishing his sentence on exhalation. There is no question that these disruptions are real. Any stutterer who has experienced these respiratory abnormalities can tell you that they are uncomfortable and not just a little unnerving.

Many other physical changes have been observed. For example, a number of studies have shown that heart rate often increases during stuttering, and there are often changes in blood pressure. Even blood chemistry can change after periods of stuttering. Reductions in blood sugar and protein have been noted in some stutterers immediately following periods of non-fluent speech. These same stutterers might have increased adrenaline levels in their urine after particularly severe stuttering experiences. Stutterers often perspire, blush, or pallor when they stutter. Their eyes might twitch up and down, move aimlessly from side to side, or one eye might be fixed while the other moves vertically or horizontally.

Most recently, many researchers have paid special attention to possible brain differences when comparing stutterers to nonstutterers. The results of this research have been interesting, but as has been true of all the research related to possible physical differences, the results have been mixed and inconclusive. Using techniques designed to determine which cerebral hemisphere is dominant for language, some researchers have found that stutterers either have weaker cerebral dominance for processing language than non-stutterers or have right hemispheric dominance in contrast to the left hemisphere dominance shown by nonstuttering speakers. In all of these studies, however, there were stutterers who showed normal left hemispheric dominance for language, and there have been other studies that have shown no differences between groups of stutterers and nonstutterers relative to hemispheric dominance.

Other investigators have looked at brain waves, particularly the alpha wave that fluctuates with a person's level of attention and concentration. When a person is relaxed, asleep, or in a coma, alpha waves are large and slow. When a person is concentrating or is in a state of attentive excitement, alpha waves are suppressed, or reduced, in amplitude and are increased in frequency. Consistent with research on hemispheric dominance for speech and language, when normal speakers concentrate on speech, the alpha waves produced by the left hemisphere are more suppressed than the alpha waves produced by the right hemisphere, indicating left hemispheric dominance for speech. In some studies, a surprising number of stutterers, when concentrating on speech, experienced greater alpha wave suppression in the right hemisphere than in the left. At the risk of sounding like we have been down this road before, other studies have shown no differences, but at least two studies have contributed an amazing twist to this little story. They found that stutterers who showed right hemispheric processing for speech, after being enrolled in a brief, intensive therapy program emphasizing slow and easy speech, showed left hemispheric processing for speech. What in the world is going on here? It's difficult to say, but based on this kind of radical shift over a very short period of time, it would be a strain to conclude that the original right hemispheric processing for speech is substantial proof of a difference between stutterers and nonstutterers that leads us to a definitive neurological cause of stuttering, even if we could show that all stutterers process speech in the right hemisphere. Nevertheless, it is precisely this kind of research, however flawed and inconsistent it may be, that has sparked new interest in the cerebral dominance theory of stuttering specifically and possible neurological differences between stutterers and nonstutterers generally. At the least, the findings are intriguing enough to keep researchers interested and looking for new ways to find a difference that might really matter, a difference that might lead us to a cause.

Another area of research that consumed investigators for several decades at the close of the twentieth century, and still captures the imaginations of some, has been laryngeal function which, of course, cannot be separated from neurophysiology since whatever laryngeal differences we might find would more likely be products of how the larynx is supplied by the brain than how the larynx is constructed. Virtually all of these studies have led us to the same conclusion. As a group, stutterers have slower voice onset and slower voice termination times than nonstutterers. Despite the nearly unanimous agreement on this finding, we should hasten to acknowledge that this does not mean all stutterers have slower voice reaction times than all nonstutterers. Even though there are fewer exceptions in the laryngeal function studies than in most others, there are still exceptions.

It might be tempting to conclude that these findings suggest that for many stutterers, the problem lies in the larynx, but one should take care not to jump this particular chasm. There is evidence, for example, that some stutterers who lose their larynges to cancer and who have to learn to produce voice using artificial devices or other parts of the remaining anatomy, continue to stutter. Others have observed that stutterers engage in stuttering-like behavior when they play musical instruments. Still others have observed stuttering-like behavior in the manual communications of congenitally deaf individuals. If we put all of the laryngeal evidence and related observations together, it probably makes more sense to conclude that stuttering originates in the brain rather than in the larynx, but I need to emphasize that this is still a prematurely formulated speculation, not a confirmed answer.

As we consider all of the physiological evidence, I would suggest that the important question is not *whether* these or similar changes occur during stuttering, but what they mean. There is no doubt that these changes do occur, but they may not mean what some would suggest they mean. At one time, researchers believed that these changes, these differences, were clues pointing to physiological causes of stuttering. Today there is general agreement

among those who are considered experts that these changes are almost certainly the *effects* of stuttering and are not evidence of potential causes. It has
been noted, for example, that these changes usually occur *during* moments of
stuttering or immediately after moments are completed. These conditions do
not exist in stutterers when they are not speaking, and they are not present
when they are speaking fluently. Perhaps of greatest importance, these
changes often occur in normal speakers when they are excited, upset, frightened, or–hold onto your spleens–even when they *simulate stuttering.* If you
review the changes and differences I have mentioned in this chapter, and
even if you search out more exhaustive summaries of these differences, I suspect you will ultimately agree with the conclusion of the experts. These are
not stuttering phenomena. They are the effects any of us might experience
under emotional or stressful conditions, or even when we are exerting ourselves physically. Do not forget that stuttering is *struggle* behavior. The stutterer must work hard to produce the excessive muscular tension and to
achieve the exaggerated and inappropriate articulatory contacts and movements characteristic of stuttering. Should anyone be surprised that in the
throes of this struggle, the stutterer's heart rate increases, his alpha waves are
suppressed, he perspires, he produces increased adrenaline, and he labors to
breathe normally?

Are There Physical Differences that Really Matter?

The total weight of all the physical evidence accumulated so far suggests
that there are no significant physical differences between stutterers and nonstutterers. Taking into account that stuttering has been such an elusive target
for people who have researched it, written about it, and treated it for centuries, it is not surprising that isolated studies seem to suggest differences, and
it is no less surprising that other studies show no differences, and even some
that show differences in directions opposite to other studies. In some cases,
contradictory results reflect unsophisticated or careless research procedures,
but in most cases, they are honest contradictions. How this can be so may be
clearer if we consider how this research is conducted. Understanding how
this research is conducted is relevant to understanding if there are differences
between stutterers and nonstutterers that matter.
    We must first understand that data collected in this kind of research is
subjected to statistical analyses. Numbers may look neat and tidy, but they
can be misleading, and the interpretation of numbers can be even more misleading. When a researcher writes, for example, that he or she has found a
significant difference, that might sound like a *fact* or a *truth,* but this really
stretches the significance of a significant difference. A statistical difference is
based on mathematical odds. A significant difference is a difference we think

we would find again if the experiment were repeated, but our confidence is hedged when we acknowledge that this finding could have occurred by chance, perhaps five times out of 100. The researcher's numbers, therefore, are only as solid as good odds are solid. If my surgeon tells me before my operation that there is one chance out of 100 that I will die on the table, I may be comforted, but I also know there is no guarantee I will survive. In many of the difference studies, the level of confidence is set at the .05 level of confidence, which means that a significant difference could occur by chance five times of 100. I wonder how I would feel if my surgeon told me that there were five chances out of 100 that I would die on the operating table. I think now I am little more uneasy. In the same way, I might be confident that a statistic means what the researcher says it means, but if I understand the odds, I know that there are no guarantees that the numbers are telling the truth, and if the level of confidence is .05, I am more wary than if the level of confidence is .01.

We must also keep in mind that stuttering is a low incidence disorder. This means that most investigations using stutterers as participants draw their participants from a very limited pool, and this means that most of these studies use relatively few participants. Whenever you conduct research on human beings with a limited number of participants, you increase the risk of what is called *sampling error.* Sampling error means that you might find a real difference between your group of stutterers and your group of nonstutterers, but it might not be true for *all* stutterers compared to *all* nonstutterers. It might reflect something unique about the particular people selected for your study, especially the particular stutterers selected for your study. Obviously, researchers are aware of this problem and sensitive to it, and they do all they can to minimize sampling errors, but we can never be sure it is safe to generalize what is found with a group of 20 or 30 stutterers to the approximately 3 million stutterers in the United States.

I mention all this by way of encouraging the reader to be pragmatically and responsibly skeptical, to be cautious about accepting something as *fact,* simply because someone shows you numbers, charts, and graphs. It has been said that statistics can be manipulated to prove almost anything. While that may be a somewhat exaggerated assertion, it is more true than false. The longer I study the stuttering literature, the more skeptical I have become, but it is a healthy skepticism that prevents me from getting too excited or too upset about what someone is touting as a great, new discovery. Too often these *discoveries* are very similar to the improvements we are supposed to see in products on our grocery store shelves. You know the products I am talking about, the ones that are marked, *new and improved.* Some laundry detergents have been *new and improved* so often that by now they should be able to wash, dry, iron, and fold clothes by themselves. Many of the *discoveries* reported in professional journals, and especially in mainstream publications, are rediscoveries, semidiscoveries, nondiscoveries, or fraudulent discoveries. Every year, almost every month, someone shows me a newspaper or magazine article, or a book, or tells me about a television report promising a *new cure* for stuttering, or someone claims to have found *the cause* of stuttering. Believe me when I tell you that when the cause and the cure for stuttering are discovered, the announcement will not be made in the *newspapers* that grace the rack at the grocery store checkout counter or even in respectable news magazines. Such an announcement will almost surely come in small bits in research articles published in professional journals, representing thousands of hours of work and hundreds of years of collaborated insight. In the meantime, try to contain your enthusiasm because there are no indications that any such announcement is imminent.

For all the reasons I hope are now clear, I do not intend to give you any numbers associated with possible anatomical or physiological differences between stutterers and nonstutterers. In fact, I began this section with what amounts to my summary statement. That is, we do not have conclusive evidence that there are any significant physical differences between people who stutter and people who do not stutter. I do believe it is important, however, to take a peek at some of the stones researchers have turned over in their efforts to find differences. They have looked at respiratory function, cardiovascular phenomena, basal metabolic rate, the musculature of the speech mechanism, the action potentials of those muscles, reflexes, general bodily coordination, fine motor coordination, the speed and consistency of speech movements, manual strength and dexterity, hand-eye coordination, brain functions, handedness as a reflection of cerebral dominance, saliva chemistry, blood chemistry, the speed of voice onset and termination, and too many other bodily functions to mention. Let me assure you that it does not matter if you know what all these things mean. It does matter that you appreciate that researchers have looked everywhere, in places that make sense and in places that do not make sense, to find even the smallest difference that might point to a possible cause of stuttering. If you find some of the stones that have been turned over puzzling, welcome to my world. What difference could it possibly make, for example, if the stutterer's grip is stronger or weaker than the grip of a comparable nonstutterer? I honestly do not know, but I do not question the honesty, integrity, or good intentions of the people who looked at this possible difference or any of the others. I respect the perseverance of researchers who continue to look for new questions because the old questions did not yield useful answers, and I respect those who go back to the old questions and turn them over, hoping to find slightly new edges to them, or apply new technologies or use an improved research design in the hope that these modifications will produce more useful data.

Sensory and Perceptual Differences

The research I mentioned in the preceding section focused on possible differences in the speech mechanism itself or in the nervous system that supplies and controls the speech structures. Some writers have suggested that stutterers differ from nonstutterers, not in the structures and functions of speech, but in the way they monitor their own speech signals. This area of stuttering research is based on what is called a *servosystem* view of speech. A servosystem is an automatic or semiautomatic, self-regulating system. Probably the servosystem familiar to most of us is the heating system in our homes. If you set your thermostat at 68 degrees F., and the temperature falls below this setting, the furnace turns on until the temperature reaches 68 degrees, at which point the furnace automatically shuts off. The furnace operates properly and maintains the correct temperature only if its feedback system, the thermostat, is reliable. Speech is also a kind of servosystem. We monitor our own speech by listening to ourselves as we talk, and we also receive information from the speech structures themselves about movements, positions, and contacts. If any aspect of our feedback or monitoring system is seriously disrupted, our speech output will be affected. We know, for example, that if a person becomes deaf as an adult, thereby losing the auditory portion of his feedback system, he is able to maintain good speech for a short period of time, but eventually his speech will suffer. Speech sounds will not be produced as accurately and crisply as they used to be. He may sound a little too nasal. Volume and pitch will not be controlled properly. All of this happens, not because his speech mechanism has changed, but because a significant part of his feedback system has been lost, and the entire system has become less reliable. Naturally, the deaf person tries to compensate for the loss of hearing by paying more attention to what he *feels* when he talks, but as important as the feeling part of the system is, it cannot completely cover the loss of hearing, and speech will deteriorate. The ability to speak will not be lost, and unless there are other interfering factors operating, the person will continue to speak well enough to be understood, but the quality of speech without hearing is definitely not as good as the quality of speech with hearing.

As I mentioned in the preceding chapter, some theorists have suggested that stuttering is the result of a failure in the stutterer's feedback system. That is, when the stutterer monitors his own speech, his internal auditory feedback is delayed or distorted. In order to support this theoretical view, some researchers have tried to find differences between stutterers and nonstutterers in terms of the way their receive and process their own speech signals.

The reception of speech or any other auditory signal actually involves two separate but related processes. We must first get sensory information to the brain. In the case of receiving our own speech signals, auditory signals are sent to the brain, but we also receive sensory information concerning movements, positions, and contacts in the speech mechanism. The term, *tactile,* refers to contact or touch sensations, and the term, *proprioception,* refers to sensations associated with movements and positions. The monitoring of speech then is fairly complicated since it includes reception of auditory, tactile, and proprioceptive sensations, and this is only the first stage of the process. Once sensory information reaches the brain, it must be recognized, organized, integrated, and interpreted. This is the second process involved in receiving auditory signals, *perception.* Perception is just as important to a reliable feedback system as receiving the sensory information. A person can have a perfectly normal hearing mechanism, for example, but if he cannot process the auditory information he is receiving, it is fairly useless information, something akin to my receiving the auditory signals sent out by dolphins. They are interesting noises, but I have no idea what they mean, although I'm just paranoid enough to believe they are saying something nasty about me, but again I digress. Some children with learning disabilities have problems with auditory processing. They have normal hearing and they receive auditory signals as they should, but their perception of auditory data is faulty. The results can be very serious and no less harmful to the communication process than a moderate hearing loss might be.

I have actually used more space trying to make clear the theoretical background and rationale for research in this area than I will use to summarize the results. The results can be stated quickly and easily. In terms of their ability to receive auditory information, stutterers are no more or less likely to have hearing disorders than anyone else. In terms of their perceptual abilities, some researchers believe they have found evidence that stutterers experience some kind of delay or distortion in their auditory monitoring systems, but the evidence is far from conclusive. Other researchers have failed in their efforts to replicate these experiments, and very few experts today believe this is a productive path of inquiry. The research does indicate that stutterers have normal auditory perceptual abilities. Stutterers do not have vision problems that are distinctly different from the vision problems of nonstutterers. Their visual perceptual abilities fall within normal limits, and their tactile and proprioceptive abilities are normal. Although a few studies have shown differences in sensory and perceptual functioning, they have been more than adequately balanced by other studies that have shown no differences. Taking all of this research into account, it is safe to say that stutterers are as normal as humans are allowed to be in terms of sensory and perceptual functions.

Differences in Intelligence

We are a species consumed with an interest in our own intelligence. When something goes wrong in school or in life, we often wonder if the disaster was the product of some deficit in intelligence. It is no wonder then that researchers have investigated possible differences in intelligence when comparing stutterers to nonstutterers.

There is, however, another factor that has influenced this area of research. It has long been observed that fluency problems are much more common among mentally retarded individuals than among normally intelligent individuals. Naturally, this has fueled speculation that stutterers might be somewhat less intelligent as a group than the general population. Before I pursue this issue any further, I want to remind the reader that it is probably a mistake to view the fluency problems of all mentally retarded speakers as equivalent to the fluency problems we see in normally intelligent stutterers. The fluency problems of many mentally retarded speakers can be clearly traced to brain damage. We have already observed, in Chapter 3, that fluency problems are quite common in brain-damaged individuals, including those with epilepsy and cerebral palsy. In order to fairly consider possible differences in intelligence between stutterers and nonstutterers, therefore, we must look at intelligence in the general population without including mentally retarded and other brain-damaged persons.

It must first be noted and duly emphasized that stutterers are found at every level of intelligence, including the very highest levels. We know, for example, that some prominent and highly intelligent historical figures were stutterers, including Charles Darwin, Charles Lamb, and Winston Churchill. Some of the earliest intelligence studies suggested that stutterers, on average, had slightly higher IQs than nonstutterers. There were, however, some basic flaws in that research. Because these investigations were conducted by college professors, and student populations were handy for subject selection, the stutterers in these early studies were college students. We would assume that college students, as a group, would have somewhat higher IQs than the national average. More importantly, it is commonly recognized that stutterers who go to college are probably not *average* stutterers, any more than deaf or blind individuals who go to college are *average* deaf and blind people. They are stuttering, deaf, and blind people who are intelligent enough and motivated enough to carry their conditions into what can be a threatening academic community without being destroyed by the reactions of insensitive and uninformed people. The fact that college stutterers might have slightly higher IQs than college nonstutterers is as surprising as the fact that college football players are bigger and stronger than college students who do not play football.

More recent investigations have selected samples of stutterers and non-stutterers that are more representative of the general population. These studies indicate that stutterers' IQs are within the normal range but are, on average, slightly lower than the IQs of nonstutterers. Since the differences noted were small, and given the present concern about the meaningfulness of intelligence tests, no one has attempted to make much of these findings. The most reasonable and responsible conclusion we can reach is that stutterers, as a group, are normally intelligent.

Personality Differences

Psychologists and others who view stuttering as a psychological disorder have tried to discover personality or adjustment differences between stutterers and nonstutterers that would support their theoretical interpretations of stuttering. Efforts to identify possible differences have relied most often on two types of testing procedures: (1) personality inventories that purport to evaluate psychological adjustment, and (2) projective measures, such as the Rorschach ink blot test and the Thematic Apperception Test, which are designed to examine personality in depth. These tests are called *projective* because the subject looks at a neutral stimulus, like an ink blot or a simple black-and-white line drawing, and tells the examiner what he sees or what he thinks is happening. That is, he *projects* his psychological state of being into his interpretation of what the stimulus is or means.

A review of all the adjustment studies suggests that stutterers are not significantly different from nonstutterers. In general, these tests indicate that stutterers fall within the normal range of adjustment, although on average, they may be *slightly less well adjusted* than their nonstuttering counterparts. I would urge the reader to pay primary attention to the first part of the preceding sentence. That is, stutterers are within the normal range of psychological adjustment. The observation that stutterers may be *slightly less well adjusted* than nonstutterers is not at all surprising, and it is probably irrelevant insofar as identifying a possible cause of stuttering. Most experts today would agree that mild adjustment problems, and that is what these findings suggest, are almost surely *effects* of stuttering, not antecedents. Any person with any condition that makes him stand out in the crowd, that causes others to pay unusual and curious attention to him, that causes personal discomfort, and that interferes with normal social relationships, is likely to produce some degree of maladjustment. It is important to note, however, that many stutterers quickly improve their levels of adjustment when they become fluent. In fact, one of the problems with which the speech-language clinician must sometimes deal in the final stages of therapy is the change that seems to occur in the personalities of some stutterers. Obviously, no stutterer's basic personality changes as a result of speech therapy alone, but when a person who stutters is successful in therapy, his true personality, which has been hidden by the shadow of his stuttering, might emerge in the daylight of fluency. He might appear to be more outgoing, more social, more willing to interact with other people, but he is really only coming out of the shadow. A few stutterers do seem to go too far in their adjustment, but it should not be difficult to understand why this happens. The stutterer who regains fluency is like a prisoner who has been released from his cell after many years of confinement. He might become so outgoing and so talkative when he regains fluency that some listeners might decide they were better off when he stuttered. I am exaggerating a little to make the point that what might appear to be an adjustment problem when the stutterer is severe and uncontrolled can quickly fade when he becomes more fluent, and if he appears to swing some of his personality traits too far in the opposite direction, this is usually only a temporary situation. The released prisoner adjusts to life outside his cell. The recovering stutterer adjusts to his communication freedom.

The results of the studies that employ projective measures, such as the Rorschach and the Thematic Apperception Test, are more difficult to explain because the interpretation of any projective test of personality is extremely subjective. Some researchers have found differences between stutterers and nonstutterers when these techniques are used, but reviewers of these research studies are quick to point out that projective methods are so subjective that two examiners analyzing the very same results might come to opposite conclusions about what they mean. We need only be reminded about the testimonies of psychologists and psychiatrists in some murder trials to understand this point. The prosecution brings in five psychiatrists who all testify that, on the basis of their evaluations, the defendant is a sane and responsible person who understands what he did and that what he did was wrong. The defense team brings in five different psychiatrists who swear that the defendant is insane, that he had no idea what he was doing, and even if he did know what he was doing, he did not understand the difference between right and wrong. The testimonies of these 10 experts are based on evaluative data drawn from the same subject. Which team of psychiatrists is lying? Neither. They are all honest, well-intentioned, competent professionals, but making judgments about a person's sanity or about his basic personality structure is not a science, at least not an exact science. The moral of this story is that we should not get too excited about the fact that a few researchers, using responses generated by projective measures, have concluded that stutterers have personality structures that differ from the personality structures of people who do not stutter. Few responsible authorities in the area of stuttering believe these findings should be taken seriously, especially since they are not consistent with conclusions based on more objective measures of personality and adjustment.

The weight of all the psychological research on stutterers leads us to the comfortable conclusion that stutterers are quite normal in terms of personality, and they are within the normal range in terms of psychological adjustment. This does not mean that stutterers do not have serious psychological problems. It does mean that stutterers are no more or less likely to have serious psychological problems than people who do not stutter. We must concede that *some* stutterers have adjustment problems related to their fluency disorder. They may not feel good about themselves, and they may have some self-esteem issues to confront. They might be reluctant to risk failure, and they might be somewhat more anxious about life than the average nonstutterer, but these are probably effects of the disorder and not clues to causes. These problems tend to be minor, and they tend to drift away in the winds as the stutterer becomes more fluent, more confident in his ability to communicate, and more confident in himself as a person.

Are There Any Other Differences Hiding in the Underbrush?

Some researchers have taken a Sherlock Holmes approach to finding differences between stutterers and nonstutterers. We have all read about detectives, or watched detectives in the movies or on television, investigating crime scenes. They sift through the dirt, cover every square inch of ground or carpet, and examine every tree, bush, and article of clothing looking for something, anything, that might provide a clue to who committed the crimes they are investigating. They consider every possible motive and interview everyone who might know something about what happened or why it happened or when it happened. The Sherlock Holmeses of stuttering research have the same modus operandi. They have interviewed stutterers and the parents of stutterers, asking questions that may seem to have little to do with stuttering. "Was he a full-term baby?" "When was he toilet trained, and did he have any problems with toilet training, in conceptual or practical terms?" "Was he breast-fed or bottle-fed?" "Does he have any brothers or sisters?" "How well does he get along with others, at home, at school, at the circus?" "How do you discipline him?" "Does he have any allergies?" "When did he first learn how to blow milk bubbles out of his nose?" These research detectives read, reread, and read again case histories on stutterers, looking for any clue, any trend, however slight, that might provide a lead. As with all the research I have mentioned so far in this chapter, they are looking primarily for differences between stutterers and nonstutterers. If they should find, for example, that the average stutterer says his first word at about 12 months, that is not particularly interesting because 12 months is the average age at which all children say their first meaningful words, but if stutterers, on average, do not begin to talk until they are 24 months, we have a lead, a clue that might lead us directly to a cause or perhaps to another clue that might lead us to a cause. I should quickly note that this example was fictitious and bears no resemblance to any real clue to the origin of stuttering, living or dead.

Now to the big question related to all this detective work. Have we found any clues to the causation of stuttering in the dirt, bushes, trees, clothing fibers, or DNA samples that cover the pages of thousands of case histories? We have certainly not found anything definitive, and if we are completely honest about this search, we have not found any leads that are rife with promise. We have found that stutterers have medical histories that are virtually identical to the medical histories of nonstutterers who are matched on the basis of important variables such as age, sex, and socioeconomic class. We have found that stutterers develop in most important respects just as nonstutterers do, although stutterers are somewhat more likely to be delayed in speech and language development and are more likely to have phonological problems than nonstutterers. The degrees of difference here are so slight, however, that they barely constitute tendencies. We have found that stutterers come from fairly normal family environments, which is to say they have imperfect parents and imperfect siblings just like every other imperfect person. Of interest, since they are blamed so often for causing their children so many problems, we have found that parents of stutterers are strikingly normal human beings in every respect. Did I hear a sigh of relief from some of you reading this book? We have found that stutterers get along fairly well in school, although some young stutterers do experience some adjustment problems, ranging from academic difficulties to getting along with their peers, and on average, they may be a little behind relative to grade level. I want to stress in the strongest possible terms that all the differences I have noted in this paragraph are very weak. We are not talking about *significant differences* here. We are not even talking about *trends*. We are talking about what might be called the *hint of tendency,* BUT even if these differences were real and substantial, they would almost certainly reflect effects of stuttering and not causes.

After All This, What Can We Conclude?

We can conclude, on the basis of all the research designed to ascertain possible differences between stutterers and nonstutterers conducted to this point, that stutterers are not extraordinary people. They are ordinary people, normal people, who have an unusual problem, and this puts them in the company of millions of ordinary people who have unusual problems that happen not to be stuttering. This is not to say that the books have been closed on possible differences between stutterers and nonstutterers. The results in every area of investigation are so inconclusive that virtually no possible cause of stuttering has been ruled out. Having acknowledged that, I believe that all of us who deal with the problem of stuttering, including stutterers themselves, parents, teachers, and speech-language clinicians, are best served by accepting the only conclusion that is warranted right now. That conclusion is that stutterers are pretty normal folks. This is my position as a teacher of students who will someday work with stutterers. It is my position as a clinician and counselor. I want my clients to accept the fact that they are normal people with normal speech mechanisms, normal personalities, normal intelligence, and normal family backgrounds. I do not want my clients to have anything to blame for their stuttering because blame is deadly. Blame allows stutterers to abdicate their responsibility for their fluency problems and to wallow in self-pity, bitterness, and despair. I want my clients to accept stuttering as their problem, to accept the idea that when stuttering happens, it happens because they create it, to accept the idea that if they create the stuttering, they can make conscious decisions to modify their speech in ways that will promote fluency. I am convinced that only when the stutterer accepts his normalcy, can he take his first healthy steps toward fluency control.

Chapter 7

THE DEVELOPMENT OF STUTTERING

That stuttering *develops* is a relatively recent concept. Prior to the twentieth century, stuttering was considered a condition or disease with which people were born or caught in much the same way one might catch a cold or leprosy. There was a general understanding that stuttering gets worse as time goes by, but not much thought was given to how stuttering changes over time, and even less thought was given to the possibility that there might be consistent patterns of change in stutterers as a group. Beginning early in the twentieth century, writers began to talk about *stages* of stuttering. This was the first recognition that stuttering at onset is not the same as later stuttering, and it was the first recognition that children and adults do not stutter in the same way.

The first *stage views* of stuttering were, by today's standards, simple and only generally descriptive of what happens during the course of development, and they described just two stages. Basically, they recognized that when stuttering first begins, it consists of relatively simple, uninvolved behaviors such as repetitions and prolongations. In its advanced form, stuttering is more complicated and multifaceted. Although these early descriptions of development lacked detail, they were generally on target. As we observed in Chapter 4, a single moment of advanced stuttering can consist of five, six, or more behaviors, some of which are superimposed on others. The early stage views acknowledged this kind of complexity.

The two-stage interpretation was a reasonable beginning to our understanding of the development of stuttering, but as we look back upon these first attempts, we see a rather obvious problem. We could purposely create a nonstuttering version of this problem, this rather serious omission, if we described the construction of a house in two stages. In the first stage, we build the foundation. In the second stage, we finish the house. This is not an inaccurate description of what happens during the construction of a house, but it is definitely incomplete. It fails to capture all the steps and substeps involved in building a house, which quite obviously involves more than just two steps. In the same way, we can agree that stuttering begins simple and ends up complex, but we need more than two stages to show how we get from the simple stuff to the complex stuff because that does not happen in one giant step even if we say, "Mother, may I?"

The next logical progression in our understanding of the development of stuttering occurred when writers began to describe a *transitional* stage of stuttering, a stage that accounts for all the changes that occur as stuttering evolves from relatively simple to complex. This was a definite improvement, but it still left too much to assumption and undisciplined speculation. As the decades have slipped by, researchers have gathered more data concerning the onset and development of stuttering, and clinicians have observed consistent differences among stutterers of varying ages. We have combined the empirical data of researchers and the observations of practicing clinicians to develop a much more complete and sophisticated understanding about what happens from the emergence of beginning stuttering to the entrenchment of advanced stuttering. Some writers have devised development descriptions with as many as eight stages. Some have suggested that we need to identify several types or patterns of stuttering, each of which develops in unique stages. For the purposes of this book, I will describe the development of stuttering as outlined by Oliver Bloodstein. I have chosen Bloodstein's view of development because it is the one I believe most closely fits the research information on development we have so far accumulated, and because it describes major changes in development without getting caught up in reckless and irresponsible speculation about *why* certain things happen when they happen. At this point in time, we can comfortably and responsibly talk about *what* changes occur and *when* they occur, but our knowledge in this area is not sufficient to assert much about *why*.

Before we proceed, I want to add an important caution about the concept underlying this discussion of development. The stage concept of the development of stuttering is useful in helping us understand general changes that occur in the disorder over time, but it is risky to apply this information to an *individual* stutterer as his disorder progresses. Children are not designed to fit into neat and tidy stages of the development of anything. Children do not develop speech and language according to a fixed schedule, although they do follow the same basic developmental map. Children develop motor skills at different ages, although we can expect that all normal children will crawl before they walk and walk before they run. To complicate matters for parents who are anxious for their children to be absolutely, positively normal, but preferably above normal, it is not unusual for children to develop motor skills ahead of schedule while they lag behind in speech and language development, or vice-versa. Stuttering too develops in stages that are meaningful and predictable as long as we are talking about groups of children without names. As soon as we focus on one child, however, these stages are only guidelines. A given child might progress more rapidly or slowly than average through the stages of stuttering development, just as a given child might progress more rapidly or slowly through speech and language development. With stuttering, we have an additional problem we do not typically encounter in communication development. Communication development varies from child to child, but it is at least linear. That is, it moves consistently forward. A child who stutters might appear to be in Stage One today, Stage Three tomorrow, and back in Stage One the next day. Stuttering does not develop in discrete steps, and it does not always develop in a consistently forward moving manner. It is a highly variable process, and for individual children, it is a highly unpredictable process. This is precisely why a caregiver might perceive that the child is *getting better,* but then *gets worse* again. The course of stuttering development is a journey that covers mountains, valleys, and plateaus, and sometimes the trail doubles back before it moves forward again. What follows then is a somewhat artificial description of the development of stuttering because it does not take into account the day-to-day, week-to-week, and month-to-month hikes up and down the uneven terrain of development we would see in a real child

Factors That *Trigger* Stuttering

Writers who describe stages of stuttering do not typically include explanations for what precipitates stuttering in the first place. Since the onset of stuttering is the first step in its development, we should grapple with this issue before we take a closer look at Bloodstein's description of the development of stuttering. One reason that writers might avoid dealing with precipitating factors is that we do not know any more about what sets the development of stuttering into motion than we know about the underlying causes of stuttering. This means that virtually everything we might say about precipitating, or triggering, causes of stuttering is speculative.

Those who wrote about stuttering in the 1800s often blamed the onset of stuttering on events that *frightened* or *shocked* children into stuttering. Most of the events blamed were fairly innocent, but it is not difficult to believe that things most adults perceive as nonthreatening could frighten a young child. One writer, for example, reported that a child began to stutter after been frightened by a dog's sudden barking. Another reported that a child began to stutter after stumbling in a department store. Other events blamed included falling out of a tree, being frightened on an amusement park ride, and being surprised by someone in a ghost costume. Whatever the frightening event may have been, the child would presumably be mute for a time, per-

haps hours, days, even weeks. When the child began to speak again, he stuttered. Few, if any, experts today would cite fright as a likely precipitating factor, although most would concede that it is *possible* for a child to be frightened
into stuttering. The fact is, however, there are very few cases of stuttering in
which this kind of event occurs in the appropriate temporal relationship to
the beginning of stuttering to be considered a viable explanation for its onset.

Over the years, parents and other concerned adults have often blamed
childhood illnesses for triggering stuttering, and it is easy to understand why.
Parents are usually the first people to realize that their child is having problems with his speech. They begin to look for explanations for these problems
with at least two motives. First, they want to understand why their child is
having a problem so they can find a solution. Second, they want to find an
explanation in order to relieve themselves of guilt. Most normal parents
seem programmed for guilt. If something goes wrong with their child, they
are quick to ask others or themselves, "What did we do to cause this problem?" This is a natural reaction, and it reflects genuine love and concern for
their child. We should understand, however, that even though parents are
concerned about their possible responsibility for what is happening to their
child, they do not want to be responsible and they do not want to be guilty,
so they search for other culprits.

The camera fades in on the typical parents of a typical child who is having a typical fluency problem. The parents wonder how this could have happened. They say to themselves, "Well, he was sick a few weeks before we
noticed that he was stuttering. Maybe it was the chicken pox that caused him
to stutter. Whew! And we thought it was something we did. . . ." The camera
fades out as this little mystery is solved, at least to the satisfaction of these
parents, but let's examine what we know about the relationship between illness and stuttering.

Since stuttering nearly always begins during childhood, and since childhood illnesses commonly occur during the ages when stuttering onsets typically occur, it would be easy and convenient to conclude that some childhood illness is to blame for precipitating stuttering. There is a general consensus among the experts, however, that the close proximity of illness to stuttering onset is merely coincidence. After all, there are very few children who
escape the measles, chicken pox, colds, flu, middle ear infections, tonsillitis,
etc. that occur during the childhood years, and only a small percentage of
children become stutterers. If childhood illnesses were significant factors in
the development of stuttering, we would almost certainly see a higher incidence of the disorder. One might speculate that children who stutter have illness and medical histories that differ in significant ways from the illness and
medical histories of children who do not stutter, but this speculation is not
supported by research data. When stutterers are matched with nonstutterers

on important variables such as age, sex, and socioeconomic status, we find that their illness and medical histories are virtually identical in terms of number, type, and timing of illnesses. The experts have concluded that illness, like fright, is not a significant precipitating factor.

Another belief commonly maintained by stutterers and by the parents of stutterers is that stuttering is triggered by *imitation*. At one time, experts considered imitation a plausible precipitating factor as well, but in more recent years, it has been dismissed as a significant factor in the onset of stuttering for good reasons. Although it is not unusual for a young stutterer to have been exposed to another stutterer at the approximate time of onset, the exposure is usually too limited to account for the child's stuttering. More importantly, there are nearly always substantial differences in the behaviors that make up each stutterer's nonfluency patterns. If imitation plays a major role in precipitating stuttering, we should expect to see considerable duplication of behaviors. This is rarely, if ever, the case. Although most experts today regard imitation as a *possible* precipitating factor, either alone or in combination with other factors, they agree it is not a factor in the vast majority of stuttering onsets.

Without question, the factor most often blamed for precipitating stuttering is *emotional conflict*. Many adult stutterers and parents of young stutterers are convinced that some emotional trauma triggers stuttering, even if they are unable to identify the specific traumas they believe precipitated their own stuttering or their children's stuttering. Before we rush to judgment, we should be reminded that many people believe stuttering looks like an emotional or psychological problem. When it becomes apparent that a person's stuttering is causing him emotional distress, this belief is only reinforced. It is not difficult to understand then why so many people naturally assume that stuttering is triggered by some kind of emotional conflict or crisis. An adult stutterer might report, "I began to stutter when I started to have problems getting along with my father." The parent of a young stutterer might conclude, "Johnny began to stutter as soon as we brought his baby sister home from the hospital," or "we noticed he was stuttering when his father and I talked about getting divorced." The conflicts blamed are almost always linked to disturbed interpersonal relationships, usually a child-parent relationship, and because most children, even in an enlightened era of shared parenting, interact more often and more intimately with their mothers than with their fathers, disturbed child-mother relationships are more often blamed for triggering stuttering than disturbed child-father relationships.

Because the subject of child-parent relationships is so delicate, and because I am convinced that an overwhelming majority of parents and other caregivers are making concerted efforts today to make these critical relationships work as well as they can, I want to add some reassuring perspective. We know that disturbed child-parent relationships occur in the homes of nonstutterers as often as they occur in the homes of stutterers, and that is important for the parents of young stutterers to keep in mind. Furthermore, we have no evidence that stutterers are more likely to have problems with their parents than any other group of children. This means that stutterers have normal relationships with their parents, relationships characterized by healthy doses of love and respect, rebellion, cooperation, and inevitable conflict. It should also be noted that it would be extraordinarily easy to find some kind of conflict, and probably a child-parent conflict, occurring near the time of stuttering onset because conflicts of one kind or another are commonplace during the growing up years. Consider the conflicts surrounding weaning, toilet training, learning to share toys, getting along with other children in preschool or school, becoming less dependent on Mom and Dad, and the list goes on as long as the child continues to grow up, become increasingly mature and self-reliant, and interact with other human beings. Conflicts happen! That is a fact of life. No one disputes that conflicts occur in the lives of stutterers, but the occurrence of a conflict at the time of stuttering onset is probably no more than coincidence.

Causes, Causes, Everywhere

So what can we conclude about precipitating or triggering causes of stuttering? We can conclude that even if we could identify *some* possible precipitating factors, it would be very difficult, if not impossible, to identify the factor or factors responsible for triggering the onset of any given case of stuttering. We can also conclude the stuttering typically begins under annoyingly normal circumstances, like a storm that comes up suddenly and without warning on an otherwise sunny and pleasant day. This does not mean that stuttering begins in the absence of illness or conflicts or other possible triggering events. It does mean there are no more or fewer of these events in the lives of stutterers than in the lives of nonstutterers, and it means we have no evidence suggesting meaningful connections between these events and the beginning of stuttering. We can also conclude that if a stutterer, parent, other caregiver, or speech-language clinician really wants to find something to blame for precipitating stuttering, there are plenty of candidates available in the life circumstances of any stutterer. There are at least two problems with pointing fingers at possible triggering events, however. First, it is highly unlikely we can prove we have identified a valid triggering event. Second, there is little or no payoff associated with blaming something or someone for precipitating stuttering even assuming the blame is valid, other than the very transitory satisfaction of having affixed responsibility. The fact is, as I have already noted, the stutterer, his caregivers, and the speech-language clinician can deal with the disorder only as it exists today. Today is too late to reverse the etiology of the disorder, and today is too late to prevent the precipitation of the disorder. It is sufficient that we deal with a stutterer's disorder, as it presently exists. The truth is, of course, that the limitations on moving back to yesterday or ahead to tomorrow preclude us from doing anything else.

And Now Back to Our Regularly Scheduled Program . . .

Let us now return to the major topic of this chapter, the development of stuttering. Once stuttering begins, it rarely remains the same. The stutterer adds new behaviors, drops a few, and embellishes the behaviors he retains. These changes are reflected in a *stage* interpretation of the development of stuttering. Bloodstein uses the term *phase* rather than the more commonly used term, *stage*. In my opinion, *phase* is a much better word in the context of development because it implies *progressive change* and *overlapping of behaviors,* whereas a *stage* is a *discrete step.* One final note is needed before we consider the details of Bloodstein's phases of stuttering. He delineated these four phases and their descriptions based on the case histories of more than 400 stutterers. This is a very large number upon which to base the conclusions he has drawn. It is not large enough to allow us to say, "We now know all there is to know about the development of stuttering," but it is large enough to allow us to be confident that we have a reliable outline of the development picture.

Phase I–When Stuttering Begins

The onset of stuttering typically occurs between two and six years. Onset after adolescence is rare, and there is some evidence that when stuttering begins during adulthood, it is actually a recurrence of childhood stuttering in many cases. Bloodstein describes early stuttering in a manner that does not clearly differentiate it from normal nonfluency. The reader may want to revisit reasons in Chapter 3 for NOT making such distinctions.

In the first phase of development, stuttering is a very inconsistent disorder. It appears for weeks or months at a time and then disappears for variable periods of time. It is during this phase that spontaneous recoveries are most likely to occur. The child goes into a period of fluency and simply never returns to a period of excessive nonfluency. When this happens, parents might conclude that the child was not really a stutterer after all, that they were just imagining there was a problem, or they were overreacting to what was normal behavior, or they might conclude that their child *outgrew* the problem. It may be impossible to determine which of their conclusions is the more correct. The fact remains, however, that what seemed to be a problem is no longer a problem, and that is good news for the child and for his parents. While in this phase of stuttering, the child has the most difficulty when he is excited or upset, when he is trying to do a lot of talking in a short period of time, or when he is subject to any kind of communicative stress, such as interruption or time pressure. The behavior we observe most often is repetition. In fact, repetition may be the only speech symptom. The child repeats the first syllables of words or whole, single-syllable words. He stutters most often on the *small* parts of speech such as conjunctions, prepositions, articles, and pronouns, and he usually has trouble only at the beginning of his utterances. It should be noted that there might be an important connection between these two tendencies. That is, the child might stutter often on the small parts of speech, not because he is influenced by their grammatical functions, but because these words so often occur at the beginning of a basic syntactic unit–a sentence, clause, or phrase. This explanation would be consistent with recent evidence, and interpretations of that evidence, suggesting that young stutterers' moments are reactions, not to the grammatical functions of words, but to the language challenges posed by producing whole sentences or the major parts of whole sentences. Finally and most importantly, the child in this first phase of stuttering does not show much concern about his speech. He continues to talk in spite of his nonfluencies, no matter how many nonfluencies he produces, and he is clearly more interested in conveying messages than he is worried about speaking them fluently.

Phase II–Stuttering Becomes Chronic

Most stutterers in this phase are between six and 12 years of age, although some adult stutterers could also be categorized as Phase II stutterers. Several important changes are emerging as the problem progresses into the second phase. The stuttering no longer comes and goes for long periods of time. It is now chronic. There are specific conditions under which the problem is better or worse, but there are no longer extended stuttering-free periods. Consistent with the chronic nature of the disorder, the individual now thinks of himself as a *stutterer,* even if he is unable to define the term, and even if he does not seem to be particularly concerned about this identity or about his speaking problems. The stuttering now occurs most often on the *major* parts of speech, the words that convey the most meaning: nouns, verbs, adjectives, and adverbs. This stutterer, unlike the Phase I stutterer, does seem to be influenced by the grammatical functions of words, and this tendency will continue through the final two phases of development. Not surprisingly, the Phase II stutterer is most nonfluent when he is excited, upset, or when is trying to speak under time pressure. Despite the chronic nature of his disorder, the stutterer remains a relatively undaunted speaker. He continues to talk even when he stutters, and he does not react emotionally to his fluency failures. He understands he has a speech disorder at this point, but he seems not to view it as a personal liability. Stuttering influences his speech, but it has not yet altered his self-image, nor has it affected his social behaviors. Unfortunately, all of this will begin to change if his stuttering continues into the next phase.

Phase III–Fear Intrudes

The Phase III stutterer is usually between 10 and 14 years in age, but we can find stutterers in this phase who are eight years old, or even younger, and many adult stutterers seem to plateau at this phase. The most significant change occurring in this phase is that stuttering is becoming increasingly tied to specific speech sounds, words, and situations. Which sounds, words, and situations are determined by each stutterer's unique experiences in fluency failure. The stutterer is now likely to identify certain sounds or words as *difficult*. He will contend that talking to a certain kind of person is *easy*, while talking to another kind of person is *hard*. It makes no difference if these perceptions seem accurate to other people. It matters not if they are, in reality, completely groundless. The perceptions are real, and certainly the fears associated with them are real. Although the stutterer's fears are not intense in this phase, they are sufficient to prompt him to use synonyms for feared words, not all the time, but occasionally. As the reader will recall from our discussion of avoidance in Chapter 4, the danger of avoidance is that it creates more fear and leads to more avoidance, so even the occasional use of avoidance is an ominous change. The stutterer has not yet reached the point where he avoids situations. He continues to speak, and he shows few signs of the embarrassment and fear he is feeling. This emotional dam, however, is about to burst.

Phase IV–Fear Becomes Dominant

We can find Phase IV stutterers as young as 10 years old, perhaps even younger, but most of these individuals are adolescents and adults. Bloodstein describes these individuals more in terms of their emotional reactions to their disorder than in terms of specific stuttering behaviors. I believe this is the only way to appropriately describe these stutterers. By the time a stutterer reaches Phase IV, he has been using a wide range of overt stuttering features for some time. It is not observable stuttering that sets this person apart from the Phase III stutterer. What moves the stutterer from Phase III to Phase IV is *fear,* intense fear, vivid fear, speech-altering and life-altering fear.

This stutterer has fearful anticipations of fluency failure, ranging from vague doubt about his ability to speak fluently to panic so complete he is paralyzed by his fear. He has intense fears of speech sounds, words, and situations. He *frequently* avoids words by using substitutions or circumlocutions. He avoids situations he perceives as difficult whenever he thinks he can get away with it, and even sometimes when he knows it is impossible to get away with it. Some Phase IV stutterers are so certain they will fail in their speech attempts they pretend to be stupid, insane, or deaf rather than risk stuttering. It is at this point that stuttering has become a *handicapping* condition. It is no longer just a speech problem. It is a problem that has gripped virtually every aspect of the stutterer's life. His fear and embarrassment are so great, so out of proportion to the reality of the disorder, that he might choose his friends on the basis of how tolerant they are of stuttering. He might choose a job, not because it is the job to which he aspires, but because it does not require talking. Even if he loves people and revels in social interactions, he might choose to be a social loner rather than risk the speech failure he is certain will occur if he makes communicative contact with others. It is in Phase IV that a stutterer's entire identity might be captured in that one label, that one horrible declaration of personal suffering–*stutterer.*

Phase IV is the worst of the bad news, and the good news is that young stutterers are not guaranteed to progress to this last phase. It is possible to choke off the development of stuttering and help the young stutterer return to normal fluency. Of equal importance, Phase IV does not have to represent communicative death for adult stutterers. The Phase IV adult stutterer can learn how to reverse the physiological conditions he creates that make nonfluencies occur. He can correct his misperceptions about speech and speaking. He can become a confident, effective speaker. Beginning with the next chapter, we will consider solutions to the problems of stutterers, young and adult.

Chapter 8

CAN STUTTERING BE PREVENTED?

Having considered the information in the preceding seven chapters, I am confident you will understand that the question heading this chapter is impossible to answer with any degree of certainty. How can we say that stuttering can be prevented if we do not know exactly what stuttering is, and if we do not know what causes it? The truth is we cannot be certain that stuttering is a preventable disorder, and if this is true, we certainly cannot guarantee that there are measures to prevent it. This could then be the shortest chapter in this book because I could truthfully respond, "We don't know if stuttering can be prevented." Because I understand the importance of this question to stutterers and their caregivers, and because I am nauseatingly optimistic about almost everything, I choose to believe that stuttering can be prevented. I also believe there are times when we are faced with problems as perplexing as stuttering that we must take a *chicken soup* approach. You know how the *chicken soup* approach works. The man says to his doctor, "Doc, my head hurts, my muscles ache, and I have a high fever. What should I do?" The doctor says, "Try some chicken soup." The man says, "Will chicken soup really help?" The doctor says, "It wouldn't hurt. . . ." It is my intention to offer a kind of *prescription for preventing stuttering* in this chapter. If you were to ask me if the suggestions I will offer will really work, my immediate answer would be, "They wouldn't hurt." In my heart of hearts, however, I believe the prescription I will offer is valid and useful, based on all we know about stuttering at the present time.

A Question for a Question

We can begin to answer the prevention question by asking another question. Can parents prevent their children from growing up to be bad adults? Most of us who are parents are parents by choice. We love children, and we especially love our own children. We want them to be happy, well adjusted, and secure, and we want them to grow up to be successful, productive adults. We try very hard to do all the things good parents are supposed to do to facilitate the proper development of our children, but the sad truth is there are no guarantees in the child-rearing business. Sometimes loving, caring, responsible parents make all the proper parenting decisions, and the child who has been the recipient of this wonderful parenting turns out all wrong. Why does this happen? At least part of the answer lies in the fact that every child interacts with many people other than his own parents, and sometimes for reasons that may not be clear, the influences of other people are greater than the influence of parents. These other influences can lead a child in a much different direction than the course charted by his parents. Another equally important part of the answer lies in the fact that a child eventually and inevitably becomes his own person, and this may happen sooner rather than later. The child might continue to listener to his parents' counsel and to their opinions, and he might forever respect their values and the standards by which they live, but eventually he will choose his own way, his own values and standards, and these might vary considerably from his parents'. Sadly, some children choose a lower road than the one traveled by their parents, but we all need to keep in mind that the opposite can also be true. Many great men and women have come from less than ideal backgrounds. Many virtuous and productive people have been the children of immoral, unethical, undisciplined, unproductive parents. There are simply no guarantees.

The stuttering prevention question is fraught with many of the same issues involved in the child-rearing question. Many would argue, properly in my judgment, that if stuttering is an environmental problem in any respect, it is probably significantly affected by child-rearing practices, in which case the discussion above is directly relevant to the prevention question. At the very least, the principles are the same.

Many parents who seek my counsel have already burdened themselves with guilt about their responsibility for the development of stuttering in their children. I believe it is safe to acknowledge that parents and other caregivers *can* and *may* contribute to a child's stuttering problem, but I believe it is more important to recognize that the overwhelming majority of parents of young stutterers are responsible, caring people who are doing far more right than wrong in rearing their children. Even the improper things they do are mostly well-intentioned, an issue I will address in greater detail later in this chapter. My immediate objective is to help the reader separate guilt from fact. The fact is we have no evidence that parents *cause* stuttering. The research evidence suggests that parents of young stutterers are as decent, well-adjusted, caring, and responsible as other parents. The fact is there is nothing anyone can tell any parent about rearing children that will guarantee that a given child will not stutter. Why? Read carefully. This should sound familiar. *No matter how positively the parents of a given child influence him, he will, by necessity, interact with other people whose influences are disruptive, who might create conditions that give rise to the beginning of stuttering. In addition, the child himself might set into motion the forces that precipitate stuttering. These forces might include self-imposed communicative pressures, self-created perceptions about the difficulties of speaking, and self-imposed standards of fluency that are beyond the reach of any speaker. No one can guarantee that any child will not become a stutterer because no one is omnipotent enough or omnipresent enough to control all the variables that might contribute to the development of stuttering.*

Before I leave this business of *guaranteed prevention,* I want to point out that what I have asserted about prevention is not limited to behavioral problems and behavioral outcomes. Consider the question, "Can cancer be prevented?" Is there anything a person can do that will absolutely guarantee he or she will not develop cancer during his or her lifetime? Of course not. As I noted in earlier chapter, a person can do all the things the physicians tell him he should do, and he can avoid all the things the physicians tell him to avoid, but there are no guarantees against contracting cancer or heart disease or the common cold, or hundreds of other illnesses. The *big truth* is that there are no guarantees in life! We do the best we can, using the best information available to us, and we count ourselves blessed if things work out more often than they do not. In trying to prevent stuttering, we do the best we can, using the best information available to us, and we count ourselves blessed, and we count our children blessed if they grow up to be cowboys and not stutterers, . . . or something to that effect.

Reducing the Risks

We cannot guarantee the prevention of cancer or heart disease, but there are a number of things we can do to reduce the risks. Based on medical research and recommendations, we can eat foods that are low in fat, low in sodium, low in cholesterol, and high in fiber. We can choose not to smoke, and we can choose not to drink alcohol, or at least drink alcohol in moderation. We can exercise regularly, and we can reduce the stresses in our lives. If we do all of these things, we cannot be assured that we will remain free of cancer and heart disease, but we can be assured that we have reduced the risks. We can put the odds a little more in our favor.

As parents, we cannot be sure that our children will grow up to be the happy, well-adjusted, responsible, moral, ethical, productive people we want them to be, but we can reduce the risks of their failure by trying to be the best parents we can be. We can be good role models. We can provide our children the quality and quantity time the experts believe they need to develop properly. We can provide them proper nutrition and medical care. We can provide them as many educational, cultural, and social opportunities as possible. We can, in short, do all the things the parenting books tell us we should do. After doing all this, if the end results are not what we had hoped they would be, we can mourn the failure but find some comfort in the knowledge that we expended our best effort.

I believe we can also reduce the risks that children will become stutterers, but the reader must keep in mind that the advice I will offer is only that, advice. I cannot offer *rules for preventing stuttering,* and I cannot offer you an *iron-clad warranty against stuttering,* but if you have a child who is showing signs of stuttering, this advice will almost surely help, and remember the chicken soup rallying cry, "It wouldn't hurt!"

Reasonable Expectations

Speech-language pathologists are often surprised that some parents expect their children to be excellent speakers very quickly. Because we are so thoroughly immersed in communication development and disorders, we tend to forget that laypersons, even well educated laypersons, have a limited understanding of speech and language development. Some parents simply accept whatever communications the child offers without wondering or worrying if the child's communication development is *on schedule.* Other parents, however, do wonder and worry. Parents who are concerned about a child's speech and language development might very well have unreasonable expectations about what should happen in this process and when. If these expectations are communicated to the child, and they almost certainly will be whether parents intend it or not, an unnecessary risk will be created. It is beyond the purpose of this book to detail everything there is to know about speech and language development, but I want to provide enough basic information that I might be able to alleviate unreasonable expectations.

It is perhaps most important to understand that a normal child is a communicator from the very beginning of his life. When the infant cries, he is communicating. Some linguists who study the earliest vocalizations of children believe that fairly specific communicative intents can be attached to differentiated cries. This may or may not be true, but there is no doubt that cries convey messages. The child's earliest cries are instinctive and are usually produced in response to varying states of discomfort such as hunger, fatigue, or diaper distress. Parents and other caregivers may learn to associate certain cries with certain problems, or they may simply make educated guesses about what a cry might mean based on the time of day and the child's environmental conditions. In any case, the child's cry does communicate even if the intent is not deliberate and even if the message is not specific. As the child grows older, he acquires learned cries. The messages underlying learned cries are usually more specific and more easily interpreted than the messages underlying instinctive cries. The child might cry to indicate that he wants to be picked up, for example, or he might cry to express anger. Most parents are quick to recognize the meanings of these learned cries. One way then that parents and other caregivers can begin to reduce the risks of communication problems in general, and stuttering specifically, is to recognize the child's communication attempts from the very beginning of his life, and to respond to them appropriately.

When the child is about six to eight weeks old, he will begin to produce his first noncrying vocalizations in the form of *cooing* or *gooing*. Cooing consists of vowel-like sounds and is usually produced when the child is content. The message underlying cooing is probably more general than the messages underlying cries. The infant coos when he is comfortable and when he feels pretty good about the state of his world. Many infants coo most when they are gazing at their caregivers. For this reason, some experts believe that cooing is part of the early bonding that occurs between the infant and his caregivers. It is unfortunate that some parents tend to ignore cooing and respond only to the child's cries of distress. We can begin to reinforce the pleasurable aspects of interpersonal communication by responding in positive ways to the child's coos. Positive responses include smiles and reciprocal coos. We need to keep in mind that speech is instinctive and pleasurable for all human beings. I believe we can reduce the risks of communication problems by reinforcing the pleasures of communication early in the child's life.

By the time the child is about six months old, he will begin to produce vocalizations that contain sounds resembling consonants. This behavior is called *babbling*. Babbling consists of repeated syllables such as *da-da* or *ga-ga*. Some children babble frequently and some seem completely disinterested in babbling, which apparently does not matter since there is little correlation between the amount of babbling in infancy and later speech and language development. At one time, language people believed that babbling was early practice for the acquisition of speech sounds, but the general consensus today is that babbling is probably no more than vocalized play, although it might prepare the child for the intonational patterns he will soon superimpose on speech. If babbling is not critical to speech and language development, should it be ignored? Of course not. We cannot assume that babbling serves no purpose just because we have so far not identified a purpose. I subscribe to the view that since it exists, it must serve some purpose. If we should someday confirm that babbling is no more than vocalized play, that is purpose enough. Parents and other caregivers should not interrupt private babbling because the child will often stop when someone tries to join in. On the other hand, if the child babbles as part of his interactions with other people, the other people should return the babbling. This babbling exchange lays the foundation for interpersonal communication. We can agree that at the very least, babbling is enjoyable for the child, and it can be enjoyable for adults as well. My advice is to listen to private babbling and return social babbling. Some adults may find that they actually prefer babbling to speech. There is less pressure to be profound when you babble, and no one can criticize your grammar or question the veracity of your stories.

The child's first words are usually produced sometime around his first birthday. The normal age range for the production of first words extends from about nine months to about 18 months, but this does not mean that a child who produces his first word at 20 months or 24 months is significantly delayed in speech and language development. Both of my daughters waited until their twenty-first months to say their first meaningful words. By the time they were 36 months old, they were well ahead of speech and language norms. It is vitally important for parents and other caregivers to understand the concept, *range of normal,* because it is usually misunderstanding about this concept that causes unreasonable expectations, and it is often the emergence of first words that causes parents to underestimate or overestimate a child's communication competence. Parents should not get too excited if their child says his first words *early,* and they should not get upset if the child delays the production of his first words. The fact is the emergence of first words is not the big deal many parents think it is. Keep in mind that there is a range of normal, not only for this speech behavior, but for all speech behaviors, and the range of normal for the acquisition of first words is enormous when you consider the ages we are talking about. A range of nine or 12 months is nothing if we are comparing an 80-year-old with an 81-year-old, but an 18-month-old child is *twice* as old as a nine-month-old child, and this is considered the normal range for the acquisition of the child's first meaningful words. The point is, be patient! The child will say his first words when he is ready. As long as he seems to be progressing normally in other areas of development, there is probably no reason to worry about his reluctance to say real words. If the child is slow to develop in other ways, however, or if parents suspect that there might be sensory, perceptual, or cognitive deficits, they should have him examined by his pediatrician. If such an examination reveals that all systems are healthy and working properly, but the child is not talking when his parents think he should be talking, what can they do to help? The answer is almost too simple. They should talk to the child, and they should encourage him to talk, but they should not demand talking.

By the time the child is 18 to 24 months old, he is ready to put words together. His first word combinations are not true sentences because they lack the syntactic structures of true sentences, but these combinations function as whole sentences or whole messages. If the child says, for example, "Daddy work," he might mean, "The big guy with the mustache has grabbed his lunch box and headed for the office," but this same two-word combination could function as a question posed to the child's mother. That is, the child could be asking, "Has Daddy gone to work?" or "Is Daddy at work?" By taking into account the entire nonverbal context, most adults can figure out what these simple utterances mean, and if their interpretations are incorrect, these little humans have ways of letting them know the errors of their guesses.

Over the next two years, the child experiences a virtual language explosion. By the time he is three years old, he has an expressive vocabulary of about 1000 words, with which he can communicate all his basic needs and wants and express his opinions on a wide range of the weighty issues of his day. He will have also discovered how to ask questions, and he will exercise this language form countless times every day. By the time he is four or five years old, he will have mastered most of what he will ever know about the basic structures and rules of his language. The production of speech sounds and the mastery of adult-like fluency will lag behind, and he still has much to learn about how to *use* speech and language effectively within conventional rules of social behavior. The period between two years and five years is another time when parental expectations can become unreasonable. I suspect this happens because the development that had been moving so rapidly now slows down considerably, and many parents do not know that this slowdown is normal. The unreasonable expectations at this time are also derived from the failure of parents and other caregivers to understand that all segments of the communication system are not mastered on the same schedule. Because the three-year-old manages basic language structures fairly well, his parents are sometimes frustrated that he cannot speak clearly and that the flow of his speech is frequently disrupted by hesitations, interjections, false starts, retrials, and repetitions.

Children do not produce all of their speech sounds in all word positions and contexts, and they do not master fluency until they are about seven or eight years old. Skills in both of these areas depend heavily on fine motor coordination, which develops at a relatively slow pace in comparison to other aspects of the child's development, including language and cognition. This means that the child has the intellectual capacity for speech and language, and he has the linguistic knowledge underlying his communication system, before he has the motor skills necessary for producing speech according to adult standards. Even though parents are often impatient with the child's development, he really does amazingly well at an incredibly early age when one considers the complexities of speech and language. Too often parents and other caregivers focus on the few aspects of communication that are not perfect instead of marveling at the many aspects the child has already mastered, and they fail to appreciate how well he compensates for incomplete knowledge and skill in those areas he is still mastering.

Before we leave the normal development segment of this chapter, I want to add two important observations. (1) We need to remember that children develop speech and language differently in every respect. It is tempting to judge one child's development by comparing him to some other child, usually an older brother or sister. I urge all caregivers to resist this temptation. There are real and substantial differences in development between siblings, and parents' memories of what happened with the older child are not always, or even usually, reliable. Many times unreasonable expectations are born in comparisons that are muddied by incomplete knowledge and murky memories. (2) We also need to be reminded that there are differences between boys and girls. Girls tend to develop speech and language a little more quickly than boys, particularly in the area of speech sound production. Boys may master speech sounds a year or more later than girls. The primary admonition here is that comparisons of any kind are not helpful, and they may create serious problems by setting up expectations that simply cannot be met, even by the *superkid* we all want.

A Good Example Is Worth Twice as Much as Good Advice

I saw this statement, nicely framed, on the wall of an insurance office many years ago. I have never forgotten it because its inherent truth is so striking. I must admit that I have never quite figured out what this maxim has to do with the insurance business, but I am perfectly willing to pick up nuggets of truth wherever I might find them. I trust this is a simple truth most of us accept, even if we find the implied advice a little uncomfortable. We all know, for example, that our children are less likely to smoke or abuse alcohol if we avoid these vices ourselves. We know our children are more likely to be honest if they observe their parents obeying all laws and submitting honest and complete tax returns. We know our children are more likely to grow up with good work habits and high moral standards if they see their parents working hard and living according to the moral standards they preach. Too often, however, we hear ourselves saying, "Do as I say, not as I do," or we find ourselves *hoping* our children will hear what we say, ignore what we do, and grow up to be better people than we are. Unfortunately, this hope is seldom realized, and the advice to "Do as I say . . ." is recognized as empty admonition even by young children. The evidence showing a relationship between what parents do and what their children do as adults is overwhelming. Adults who smoke, drink too much, use drugs, commit crimes, abuse children, etc., etc. are much too often the children of parents who engaged in the same or similar behaviors.

Now, let's just wait a minute. Am I suggesting that stuttering should be squeezed into this list of undesirable behaviors that are passed, by example, from one generation to the next? No, of course not, but I am trying to clearly and emphatically make the point that *parental speech models* do affect the speech behaviors of their children. I cannot prove to you that poor fluency models *cause* stuttering, but I can point out some of the dimensions of a child's communication system that are directly affected by the speech models of his parents and other significant caregivers. If a child speaks American English, it is because he learned that language from his speech models, not because he was born to speak English. From his speech models, he learns the speech sounds of his native language, a regional dialect, much of his vocabulary, nearly all of his basic grammar, and even the pronunciations of most of the words he speaks. He learns stress, inflection, rate, and even vocal qualities from his primary speech models. The child's speech is not an exact replica of one of his parent's speech, but it is probably very close, and the chances are excellent that both parents have influenced some aspects of his communication system. Given the powerful influence of the child's primary speech and language models on his own speech and language, one does not have to leap far to conclude that the speech patterns of adults, and especially parents, *can* affect the fluency of a young child's speech.

The point here is painfully simple. I have included the word, *painfully*, because while the point is simple, it is very difficult to practice. The point is, parents can assist their children in normal speech and language development, and they can reduce the risks of communication disorders, including stuttering, by providing their children good speech and language models. When parents talk to their children, they should produce grammatically correct sentences, but their sentences should not be so long and elaborate that the child gets lost in a syntactic maze. Parents should pronounce words properly, and they should articulate all speech sounds clearly and correctly. Parents should not use the child's versions of words or include the child's phonological mistakes, no matter how cute and irresistible those productions might be. When adults speak to children in the language of children, they risk reinforcing the child's incorrect or immature speech patterns. When the child makes a mistake in grammar, pronunciation, or phonology, the adult should not *correct* the error by demanding a second attempt. Instead, the adult should respond to the child's intended message and include a corrected version of the child's error in the response. Consider the communicative difference between these two approaches. In the first approach, the correction says to the child, "I am more interested in the mechanics of your speech than I am in what you have to say." The demand for a corrected attempt also carries the implication, however unintended, that speaking is difficult, and the child needs special tutoring in order to get it right. In the second approach, the adult's response indicates that the child's message was duly received, but the response also provides the child an opportunity to compare his production with a correct model without any pressure to repeat the production at that very moment.

Children learn all dimensions of speech and language through the processes of discovery and experimentation. Adult responses let them know if they are headed in the right direction. Parents need to know that they cannot *teach* speech and language to their child even if they want to. A linguist, using a computer, has estimated that it would take about 10,000 years to *teach* a child all the bits of speech and language he knows by four years if he were taught those bits using the very best of available learning principles and techniques. Remember that speech is *instinctive* in humans. The child is biologically preprogrammed to talk. If parents and other caregivers provide the child proper speech and language models, if they provide him the opportunities he needs to discover, experiment, and practice, and if the child's speech equipment is in proper working order, nature will take care of the rest.

It may be fairly easy to understand how grammar, dialect, pronunciation, and articulation are modeled, but how can parents provide good fluency models? Parents can provide appropriate fluency models by speaking at a slower than normal rate and by speaking in an unhurried, relaxed manner. These models need not be perfectly fluent, but the speech should be relatively smooth, without abnormally long pauses or unnecessary interjections. When adults produce fluency failures, the nonfluencies should be accepted as natural speech occurrences, which they are. Adults should not signal frustration or alarm when they are nonfluent. Rather, they should continue to speak in a manner that suggests the message is more important than the motor speech by which the message is delivered. Good fluency models convey the idea that speech is easy, natural, and pleasant, that mistakes occur, but mistakes are also natural and need not be disastrous. Given speaking examples like these, the child is not likely to conclude that speech is difficult or onerous, and he is not likely to conclude that normal speech is perfect, two conclusions that probably do not *cause* stuttering, but have the potential to pave the way for the beginning of the disorder. Appropriate fluency models like these from adults the child loves and respects are many times more valuable than all the advice and all the criticism the adults might be tempted to heap upon the child when he is nonfluent.

Listen Actively

One of the easiest things parents and other caregivers can do to reduce the risk of stuttering is to learn how to listen to children when they speak. Some parents listen to their children more or less out of a sense of duty, and they typically listen passively. Consider the tale of two fathers to understand the difference between *passive listening* and *active listening*. The first father is sitting in his family room reading his newspaper. His son runs in from outside, yelling excitedly, "Daddy, Daddy, you'll never guess what happened!" The father lowers his newspaper about six inches, peers over the top and says in a flat voice, "What happened?" The second father is sitting in his family room reading his newspaper. His son runs in and yells, "Daddy, Daddy, you'll never guess what happened!" The father folds his newspaper in half, lays it on the floor, reaches out, lifts his son onto his knees, looks him directly in the eyes, and says in a voice as animated as his son's, "Well, what in the world happened? Tell me all about it."

I hope you found the differences between these two scenes as striking as I intended them to be. The message from the first father is pretty clear. Beyond his words, he is saying to his child, "I am listening to you because it is my parental obligation to listen to you, but what I really want to be doing right now is reading my newspaper, so please hurry up and say your piece, and then leave me to my peace." This is a classic example of *passive listening*. If the son has any tendency to be nonfluent, this situation will probably prompt some nonfluency because the child feels pressured to get his message out quickly so his father can get back to more important things. In the second scene, we sense a much different underlying message from the father. As he puts his newspaper down and picks his son up, he is saying to him, "You are more important than anything else I could be doing right now, and I am as excited about hearing your message as you are excited about delivering it." By rearranging the physical dynamics of the situation so the child is on the same visual plane with him and by eliminating all other distractions, he is also saying to his child, "Take your time. There is no rush." In this scene, the child who is vulnerable to fluency breakdown will probably perform well because the attention is on his message, not on his motor speech, and because there is no time pressure. This is a classic example of *active listening*. When the child is speaking to an active listener, he is enjoying communication because he feels important and because he knows that what he is saying is valued.

Obviously, adults cannot and should not always put the child's desire to talk above all else. The child must learn conversational courtesies, including the idea that sometimes we must wait our turn. Unfortunately, some adults rarely, if ever, talk *with* young children, usually because they believe a three-year-old cannot possibly have anything important or interesting to say. These adults are the poorer for not taking the time to have real two-way conversations with preschoolers. These children have marvelous views of the world. They have incredible insights about life and living, and what they say, whatever they say, is important. What the child says is, or should be, important to all his caregivers if only because the child thinks that what he says is important. When adults listen actively to children, they acknowledge the significance of their communications, and they boost their feelings of self-esteem. This is good preventative medicine, another dose of *chicken soup* for communication ills.

Love and Affection

The best preventative measure of all is good, old-fashioned, but never out of fashion, *tender loving care*. I do not mean to suggest here that stutterers are not loved and that the parents of stutterers are not affectionate. We have already established that the parents of stutterers are normal parents in every important respect, which means they are just as loving and caring as other parents. I do mean to suggest, however, that parents should never underestimate the power of love and affection in the processes of healing and in preventing all kinds of pains and problems, including communication disorders. Love is not enough to prevent a child from saying "wabbit" for "rabbit," and it is not enough to prevent a child from developing a fluency problem, but love is just what the doctor ordered to ease the pain of communication problems, and if we ease the pain of the child's first fluency failures, we may be able to prevent the more serious and frequent fluency problems that herald the beginning of stuttering.

When a potential stutterer is experiencing fluency failures, his parents can often help most by simply being supportive, by reminding the child verbally and nonverbally, that he is important, appreciated, and loved. This child is most likely to be nonfluent when he is upset or frightened. Rather than focusing on his speech failures, his parents should try to relieve his emotional pain. This may be best accomplished by holding and hugging the child without saying anything. It may be accomplished by allowing the child to vent his negative feelings, including his fear and anger, no matter how nonfluent his speech is. There is no magic salve quite like love and affection.

Danger Signs

As I stated at the beginning of this chapter, there are no guarantees against the development of stuttering. Sometimes, despite our best preventative efforts, a child will begin to stutter. Since most young stutterers are brought to speech-language pathologists by parents or other significant caregivers, it is important that these people know what changes in behavior might indicate the onset of stuttering, changes that might be called the *danger signs* of stuttering.

One of the most important danger signs is increased awareness of speech difficulty. If the child exhibits obvious signs of frustration *after* periods of nonfluency, if he gets angry or upset with himself because he cannot speak smoothly, parents should be concerned. If the child shows signs of emotional distress *during* nonfluencies, their concern should be somewhat greater. If he shows evidence he is *anticipating* fluency failures *before* they occur, parents should be very concerned. Common anticipatory behaviors we might observe in young stutterers include widening of the eyes, taking a deep breath, or tensing the muscles of the face. If these behaviors are followed by nonfluency, the child is moving toward more serious fluency problems.

When the child's nonfluencies are no longer easy and unforced, but are characterized by struggle and excessive muscular tension, this is evidence that the fluency problem has moved to the next level of development. This is a danger sign that must not be ignored.

If the child begins to avoid words or becomes reluctant to enter certain speaking situations, he is no longer *normally nonfluent*. Remember that we typically do not see any evidence of avoidance until Bloodstein's Phase III, so when parents see any evidence of avoidance in the speech behaviors of a young child, they should be very concerned. The presence of this behavior, even if it is occurring only occasionally, indicates that the disorder is progressing rapidly.

If the child has been an energetic, freewheeling talker, and he becomes unusually reticent for long periods of time, this may indicate that the fun and pleasure of speech are slipping away. This is also a danger sign that must not be ignored.

If parents see any of these signs, or similar changes in behavior that cause them concern, they should consult a speech-language pathologist. It is quite possible that the child is not a stutterer and that the parents are unnecessarily concerned, but there are good reasons for responding to all suspicions. We know, for example, that the younger the stutterer when he begins treatment, the more favorable the prognosis, so if the speech-language pathologist determines that the child is a stutterer, treatment should begin immediately. There is no reason to take a chance that a more serious, life-altering fluency problem will develop later when early fluency problems are usually resolved easily and quickly. If the child is not yet a stutterer, but is a potential stutterer, the speech-language pathologist can help his parents monitor other behavioral changes that might convert the child's status from *potential stutter-*

er to *stutterer,* and she can provide counsel about what might be done to prevent the existing problem from getting worse. If the speech-language pathologist determines that the child is definitely *not* a stutterer, the evaluation will have eased the parents' minds, and that is a valuable outcome. No matter what the outcome of the evaluation, therefore, it is best to have the child examined if there is any doubt about whether or not he is in the early stages of stuttering development.

Chapter 9

HELPING THE STUTTERING CHILD

Do Not Panic!

Nearly all children go through periods of nonfluency while they are acquiring speech and language. Most do not become stutterers, but a few do. Why do some children weather the normal nonfluency storms and others do not? I trust that by now you already know the answer to that question. We simply do not know why some children continue to have fluency problems beyond the speech and language acquisition period. It is tempting to speculate, but there is no way to verify our speculations, so there seems little value in guessing. As a clinician and counselor, I am always particularly concerned about parents' speculations because they inevitably lead to feelings of guilt. I remind these parents repeatedly that sometimes, despite their best and most responsible efforts to prevent stuttering, children do become stutterers, and fault is not an issue. It is also important to recognize that stuttering is not the worst thing that can happen to a human being, although all things considered, we must concede it is better to be a fluent speaker than to be a stutterer. In addition, it is important to remember that when stuttering is treated early, there is an excellent chance for a full recovery. If a child goes beyond normal nonfluency, therefore, his parents should not panic. They will help their child most by not overreacting to his nonfluencies, by remaining calm and collected, by maintaining an objective attitude, by allowing nothing in their verbal or nonverbal behaviors to signal undue worry or anxiety. The young beginning stutterer sounds more disordered than he feels. Even if he is aware of his nonfluencies, he is not terribly concerned about them, but if his parents seem alarmed, he may very well become concerned, and then we have the potential for more serious problems.

The advice parents are sometimes given when their children show signs of stuttering is, "Just ignore it, and it will go away." This is NOT good advice.

Ignore it, and maybe it will go away? It is not enough to pretend that the child's speech difficulties do not exist, and it is not enough to suppress concern. Parents and other caregivers can and must do more. They must become actively involved in trying to solve the problems created by the child's stuttering. The chances for a full recovery will be greatly enhanced if parents and other caregivers learn how to facilitate fluency, and the chances for recovery will be greatly reduced if the child's significant others remain passive observers on the sidelines of his disorder. In this chapter, I will identify some basic strategies parents and other caregivers can employ in their efforts to help the stuttering child.

The Key to Assisting the Stuttering Child Is *Prevention*

The reader will recognize this message from the preceding chapter. There are things we can do to try to prevent normal nonfluency from becoming stuttering and these strategies were identified in Chapter 8, but if the child shows signs of true stuttering, we do not abandon our efforts to prevent. We simply modify our target. Since it is too late to prevent stuttering, we now shift our attention to preventing the existing stuttering from getting worse. The basic rationale for the strategy of prevention is simple. If we can prevent the stuttering from worsening, there is an excellent chance the child will recover without the need for direct intervention. Specifically, we want to prevent any increase in the frequency and severity of the child's existing stuttering behaviors, but we also want to prevent the acquisition of new behaviors. We certainly want to prevent any increase in the child's awareness of speaking difficulty, and we want to prevent the development of any misperceptions about speech, speech difficulties, words, sounds, speaking situations, or listeners because these misperceptions set the stage for the emergence of the fears that characterize the most advanced phases in the development of stuttering.

Perhaps a simple analogy will help to clarify the prevention message. When the child contracts a cold, we do not *cure* the cold because, as we have heard countless times, there is no cure for the common cold. We do, however, put the child to bed, keep him warm, and we make sure he eats well and drinks plenty of fluids. We do these things to prevent the cold from becoming worse. The child's body will cure the cold if we help by preventing needless complications. In the same way, many young beginning stutterers will recover naturally from their fluency problems if we do all we can to prevent needless complications. That is what this chapter is all about, preventing the unnecessary and potentially destructive complications that can convert relatively simple and uninvolved fluency problems into major fluency problems.

Attitudes Are Contagious

Most of what I want to say in this chapter is not arranged in order of priority, but this particular section is included first because its message is of paramount importance. Parental attitudes and the child's attitudes about speech in general, and about fluency failures specifically, will determine, to a large extent, whether stuttering can be arrested in its earliest phase and reversed or progress to more advanced phases.

There is no doubt that how a child feels about himself and about his speech can have a profound influence on the recovery of fluency or the further development of stuttering. There is also no question that caregivers, but especially parents, are largely responsible for how a young child feels about himself and most other things, ideas, and people in his world. As the child advances from birthday to birthday, he will be less and less influenced by what his parents think, but when he is young, their influence is significant, almost overwhelming. If the parents' attitudes toward the child are positive, the child will generally feel pretty good about himself. If the parents' attitudes are critical, unsupportive, and nonaccepting, the child's self-image is likely to suffer. In the context of a chapter devoted to helping the child who stutters, it is most important to understand that how a child feels about himself WILL influence his behavior. It should be fairly easy to see the chain I am linking together. If parents believe their child is incompetent, and if they send this message to him repeatedly, the child will believe he is incompetent. Eventually, this belief will be translated into behavior. That is, the child will demonstrate by his actions that he is incompetent. If the parents of a young stutterer bombard him with messages, verbal and nonverbal, that indicate their lack of confidence in his ability to speak fluently, he will come to believe that he cannot speak fluently, and if he believes he cannot speak fluently, he will not speak fluently. I am convinced that it is impossible to overestimate the importance of parental attitudes on the future course of the child's fluency problem, and, as melodramatic as it may sound, even on the future course of the child's life. The chain from parental attitudes to a child's behavior can be broken, just as any metal chain, no matter how powerful the metal, can be broken, but it will not be broken easily. We must appreciate that even the most powerful metal alloys cannot match the strength of the attitudes that determine behaviors and shape lives.

Parents need to be aware that they can shape positive attitudes in their child as easily as negative attitudes, and when this happens, the chain takes on an altogether different nature. It becomes a chain that promotes healthy attitudes and constructive behaviors. If parents are loving and accepting, their child will feel loved and accepted. He will have a positive, healthy self-image, and his behaviors will reflect that healthy self-image.

Before I advance one more word, I want to make it clear that I am not suggesting all parents of young stutterers have attitude problems that need to be fixed. On the contrary, the research evidence suggests, and my own clinical experiences confirm, that most of these parents are caring, concerned people who want to do what is best for their children. I am suggesting, however, that the parents of a young beginning stutterer should examine their attitudes toward their child to determine if there are any attitudes in the inventory that might negatively impact their child's speech.

Having said that, I want to change the focus of this discussion. Rather than focusing on what might be wrong about parental attitudes, I want to concentrate on the kinds of attitudes that will be most constructive. Much of the advice and encouragement contained in the remainder of this section and in the remainder of this chapter will be revisited in Chapter 23. The difference in the two presentations is that in this chapter I want to address parents and other caregivers directly. In Chapter 23, this material will be discussed within the context of parental counseling and will be addressed primarily to speech-language clinicians.

It is most important that parents *accept* and *appreciate* their child. Depending upon your personal experience, it may sound easy or impossible to accept and appreciate your child. I want to suggest that it is neither easy nor impossible. Acceptance and appreciation of one person by another come only with effort, although some people are naturally more accepting and appreciative than others, and, quite frankly, it is easier to accept and appreciate some folks than others. The point is, with few exceptions, we can learn to accept and appreciate other human beings if we try. Having identified what is possible, I now want to target a common problem in the accepting/appreciating process and then suggest a solution to this problem.

It is universally accepted that parents *should* love, accept, and appreciate their children without reservation or qualification. In reality, even the most loving and conscientious parent does not feel completely positive about any child all the time. Even the best, top-of-the-line child is flawed in ways that make it impossible for parents to accept the child with no reservations whatsoever. I honestly do not think I could love my daughters, now grown and parenting children of their own, any more than I do, but there were times during their formative years when they disappointed me, times when they made me angry, and times when I wanted to send them into exile. There were other times when they made me so proud I cried, times when they filled me with so much joy I thought I had exceeded maximum federal guidelines, and times I just reveled in their company. My experience as a parent was not unusual. It was the norm. It is natural for parents to feel ambivalent about their children, just as it is natural for children to feel ambivalent about their parents. Another of those facts of life I am compelled to point out is that a normal child-parent relationship is neither all good nor all bad. This then is the problem—that what we sometimes think we *should* do or be as parents, we cannot always do or be. We may think we should always be perfect parents and that our children should be perfect children, and that we should all live happily ever after, but that is simply not the way life is scripted. The sooner we understand and accept this fact of life, the sooner we can begin to work on the solution to the acceptance/appreciation problem.

The solution is not complicated, but it does require a little effort for most people. As parents, we must accept our own ambivalence as normal and natural. We cannot truly accept and appreciate our children until we accept this ambivalence. We must then come to terms with what it means to *accept* our children. To *accept* does not mean that we always understand what our children do, and it certainly does not mean that we always condone what they do. It means that we love and appreciate our children *in spite of* their weaknesses, faults, and failures. It may be useful to remind ourselves that our children accept us, usually without reservation, in spite of our flaws. It may also be useful to remind ourselves that a good marriage works, not because it is the union of two perfect people, but because two imperfect people love, accept, and forgive one another in spite of their individual faults and failures.

We need to go at least one more mile in accepting and appreciating the child with a fluency problem. This child needs to hear and feel the acceptance. He needs to know for sure that he is appreciated, but the expressions of acceptance and appreciation must be sincere because children, even very young children, are not fooled by hypocrisy or duplicity. The parents of the young stutterer need to identify their child's strengths and his positive qualities. If these are not readily noticeable, the parents need only talk to other people who know the child to discover that he is appreciated and to discover why he is appreciated. Once parents see appreciation for their child mirrored in other people, they can more easily identify the child's assets and respond to them. Parents need not flood the child with excessive expressions of love and praise. This would not be natural and might lead the child to imagine that his parents are protecting him from something too dreadful to talk about, but the child does need to hear more positive comments than negative. Perhaps for every statement of criticism or rebuke, the parents should provide 10 expressions of praise and support. Such a ratio of negative to positive comments would undoubtedly bolster the child's self-image without conveying the misconception that he is perfect. After all, we adults know that perfect children were no longer conceived after our generation was hatched.

So far I have focused on attitudes in the most general sense, but general parental attitudes do affect the child's speech because his speech is affected by his feelings of self-worth, and his feelings of self-worth are directly affected by the attitudes of his parents. If parents and other caregivers do no more than improve the young stutterer's self image and enhance his self-confidence, they will have taken a giant step toward easing the fluency problem. The remainder of this chapter will be devoted to attitudes and reactions that are more specific to speech, but these speech-directed attitudes are no more important than the general attitudes of *acceptance* and *appreciation*.

No Advice Is Better Than Bad Advice

It is very tempting to give advice to young stutterers because, at face value, the problem seems so simple, and the necessary adjustments seem so obvious. Parents and others who want to help the child freely offer advice such as "Slow down," "Stop and start over again," or "Take a deep breath before you begin." These may all seem like good pieces of advice because they just ooze common sense. In actuality, each of these instructions is bad and potentially harmful advice.

Follow along as we retrace some familiar ground and then hike to a new conclusion. As I have mentioned several times in the preceding pages, speech is instinctive for human beings. It is as natural for children to talk as it is for children to walk, and it is almost as natural as spitting up. When the child is taking his first tentative steps and falls down, we do not typically offer advice. We pick him up and let him try again, believing that given enough opportunities to walk, he will eventually walk. We seem to understand that walking is biologically preprogrammed in humans, but we really struggle with the idea that talking is also biologically preprogrammed. When the child has problems in the process of acquiring speech, we conclude that he does not know how to talk, that talking somehow is a more conscious, cognitive, and learned activity than walking. I will not minimize the connection between cognitive development and speech and language development, and I will be about third in line to agree that learning plays an important role in language acquisition. I will, however, emphasize that the earliest attempts to speak are more instinctive and natural than they are deliberate and learned, and I will assert that biological forces continue to drive the acquisition of speech and language through the ages when stuttering most often begins. This being the case, I will argue that parents should react to the child's early fluency failures in much the same way they react to his early walking failures. If the child stumbles on his words, parents should let him pick up his own tongue, tuck in his own lips, restart his own respiratory cycle, and try again. If we give the child the opportunities he needs, he will almost certainly learn to speak with only the minor fluency flaws all speakers produce. Incidentally, when the child learns to walk, he does not learn to be perfect walker. I have yet to meet a single human being who has not fallen, stumbled, or stubbed a toe. We accept these imperfections in walking. We should accept similar imperfections in talking.

And how does all this relate to the advice we give to young stutterers? We need to ask ourselves what these pieces of advice communicate to the child, regardless of the good intentions from which they spring. When the child is told to take a deep breath, he might conclude that he should concentrate on breathing *before* he begins to talk. This is only marginally accurate. In normal speech, we do not separate breathing from the production of speech sounds or the onset of voicing. Respiration, phonation, articulation, and resonation occur more or less simultaneously. One of the problems we see in the advanced stutterer is that he separates these processes. This separation may very well begin in the perception that he needs to breathe first, and then turn on the larynx, and then make the sounds of speech. By advising the young beginning stutterer to take a breath before he talks, parents might be unintentionally planting the seed for this misperception.

When the child is told to slow down because he is "thinking faster than he can speak," he will probably assume that his adviser knows what he or she is talking about. I tried to dismiss this myth earlier, but let's review the facts. Human beings *must* think faster than they speak because thinking necessarily precedes speaking, and it is *impossible* for someone to speak faster than he can think for the same reason. Brain activity in the form of selecting the right language information and then sending signals to the speech mechanism takes place microseconds before the words are actually formed. It can happen no other way. The speech musculature cannot move without being innervated, and the innervations must be patterned to fit the sounds, words, and thoughts that constitute the intended message. It may be appropriate to advise people to think before they speak so that they can edit their thoughts, but to suggest that the comparative speeds of thinking and speaking are responsible for stuttering defies common sense and just does not fit the facts of basic physiology. Another problem with advising the child to slow down before he speaks is that we are leading him to believe that speaking is considerably more difficult than it really is. The child may very well be more nonfluent when he is trying to talk too fast or when he has a lot to say and wants to say it quickly, but the problem is communicative pressure, not some presumed inadequate speed-regulating connection between his brain and his speech mechanism. The fact is, if he is under enough communicative pressure, the child will be nonfluent whether he is talking quickly or slowly. I will advance that thought one more giant step. If any speaker, normal or disordered, young or old, is under enough communicative pressure, he will suffer fluency failure. We should not underestimate the influence of communicative pressure, and we should not overestimate the influence of speed.

When the child is told to stop and start over, the message he is receiving is that he made a mistake he must now correct. Once again, he concludes that speaking is very hard. It is so hard he must make conscious and concerted efforts to speak *correctly.* The harder the child tries to make speech perfect, the more difficulty he will have. One of the competitive tricks I learned as a basketball player was to call attention to an imaginary flaw in a natural shooter's motion. If you can get the natural shooter to think about what he is doing, his shot will no longer be natural, and it will no longer be effective. The same thing can happen to the child when he is trying to talk. As long as the child does not think about speech, he does not have a problem, even when he makes mistakes, but if someone calls attention to his mistakes and demands that he correct them, speech is no longer the natural process it should be. It is now hard work, and the harder he tries to make it work, the worse it becomes.

So what advice should parents and other caregivers give to the child when he stutters? *Do not give him any advice! Do not give him any advice! Do not give him any advice!* Listen to the content of his message. Respond to the content of his message. Do not do or say anything that has any potential to lead him to believe he is failing as a communicator or that speaking is difficult. Any advice that is directed at *how* to speak may make the stuttering worse and should be avoided.

Minimize Time Pressures

Sometimes adults are not as sensitive as they should be to the fact that children are much more vulnerable to communication pressures than adults are, especially to the pressures to speak quickly or to say a great deal in a short period of time. In most situations, adults can speak rapidly without giving much thought to the pace of their speech. They have learned to handle most of the pressures that can affect fluency. Adult speakers have large vocabularies and complete language systems from which they can quickly and confidently draw the right words and construct syntactically complete, correct sentences. Now consider the challenges faced by the three-year-old child who is operating with a vocabulary of a thousand words, who is still learning the intricacies of his language, and who does not yet possess the fine motor coordinations needed for clearly articulated, smoothly delivered speech. This child does amazingly well with the tools he possesses, but his speech is much more likely to break down than the adult's speech because he lacks the adult's experience, knowledge, and motor skills. If we add a fluency disorder to the three-year-old's natural limitations, we have a child who is extremely susceptible to the communication pressures that disrupt speech.

We cannot and should not try to create an environment for the young beginning stutterer that is devoid of communication pressures because all human beings, including those who stutter, must learn to cope with these pressures. We do the child no favor by creating a pressure-free environment for his preschool years and then pushing him into a world of uncontrolled pressures when he begins school. We must strike a balance between completely sheltering the child from communication pressures when he is most vulnerable to them and being totally insensitive to their effects on speech. Toward this end, I will try to offer advice about dealing with these pressures that is reasonable, practical, and in the best short-term and long-term interests of the child who stutters.

We must first acknowledge that time pressure is a normal part of the speaking process. There is always a sense of urgency in interpersonal communication. When someone speaks to us, we cannot wait too long before we respond. If we do, we lose our listener's attention. If time pressure is too urgent, however, it creates an excessive communication stress that can lead to fluency failure. The idea then is that parents must allow normal time pressure and prevent excessive pressure—not a simple task.

Allowing normal time pressure is not a problem, but preventing too much pressure may be. Time pressure can be reduced to a manageable level in several ways. First, parents and other caregivers can discipline themselves to talk more slowly to the young stutterer, especially when he is having difficulty. When parents talk rapidly to the stuttering child, or even to other people when the child is listening, he learns to expect the transfer of information at a rapid pace. Obviously, we can communicate quite effectively at a slower rate, perhaps even more effectively, because we allow more time for thinking about what we are going to say before we say it. If the young stutterer observes a more leisurely rate in the speech of his parents and other important adults, he will learn to take his time when he speaks. I should point out that if parents are truly interested in slowing the rate of their child's speech, this is a far better approach than giving direct instructions to slow down. Second, parents can reduce time pressure by speaking at an even pace. An uneven pace communicates *chaos*. An even pace communicates *control*, and when the speaker feels he is in control, he is less likely to be adversely influenced by any communication pressure, including time pressure. Third, parents can alleviate unnecessary time pressure by modeling an unhurried turn-taking style of conversation. Very often the pace of conversation is not determined by participants' overall rates of speech as much as by how quickly they take turns talking. If turn-taking in a conversation involving the stuttering child is rapid, the urgency he feels to jump into the conversation increases dramatically, and stuttering is almost guaranteed. As I have already noted, children learn most of their speaking habits by observing their parents and other important models. If a child's parents employ a rapid turn-taking style, the child will probably be a rapid conversational turn-taker. This is not a problem for the normally fluent child who is confident in his ability to speak and who is unaffected by his mistakes, but it can be devastating for the young stutterer.

One aspect of time pressure that warrants special mention is interruption. The child learns to interrupt by observing his parents, other adults, and his siblings, and curiously, he is often reprimanded for being a good student. That is, he learns that in order to get into conversations, he *must* interrupt because if he waits until each speaker is completely finished, the dishes are washed, the dog has been let out, the television has been turned off, and it's time to go to bed. So, he interrupts, and when he does, he is told it is impolite to interrupt. How confusing this must be for any novice conversationalist, but for the young stutterer there is an additional problem. Trying to time his interruption so he squeezes into the conversation without offending the person being interrupted creates a great deal of time pressure. This is the very definition of *dilemma*. If he does not interrupt, he does not participate. If he does interrupt, he is either chastised or he stutters. Does this dilemma have a solution? I believe it does if we can agree on two key points: (1) It is not polite to interrupt someone when he is talking, and (2) It is not reasonable to expect to the child to interrupt in order to be a conversational participant. Beyond these agreements, the solution rests in simple conversational courtesy and mutual respect on the parts of all members of the conversational unit. For the sake of this discussion, we will assume that the conversational unit is the stuttering child's family. Each member of the family should be recognized as a valuable contributor to family conversations and should be given a fair opportunity to speak. This might mean that a parent serves as moderator to make sure each person has a chance to speak, without actual or threatened interruption. Although neither of my daughters showed any signs of stuttering, we adopted this style of conversation at our dinner table when they were both very young. As a consequence, our after-dinner conversations were always pleasant and often continued for an hour or more after the food was consumed. Even when our days were hectic and frustrating, we found that conversation that was truly shared helped each of us feel refreshed and more content than we were when dinner began. I believe it was not coincidental that during these dinner conversations, the rate of our speech was slower and our turn-taking was slower than during other conversations. I highly recommend this conversational style for all families, but particularly for the families of young stutterers.

Help in Times of Trouble

Parents usually want to know what they should do when their child is actually stuttering. Their instincts may tell them to offer advice to the child, but as I have tried to explain, this is not a helpful strategy because it only increases the child's awareness of his speech difficulties. Should parents simply ignore the child's struggles, as recommended by some people? I do not recommend the ignoring strategy either because it might say to the child, "It's obvious you are having problems with your speech, but I don't care, or even if I do care, I have no idea what I should do to help you." By the time the child has crossed the line from normal nonfluency to stuttering, he definitely needs help. If parents should not offer advice, and if they should not ignore the problem, what should parents do?

I want to answer that question by presenting two nonstuttering situations that demonstrate the answer. It is not unusual for an elementary school teacher to have a class of students who occasionally become unruly and boisterous. There are two distinctly different approaches the teacher might take to restore order. Using one approach, the teacher might yell at the children, "Sit down and shut up!!" This approach *might* restore order, but as often as not, the noise level in the classroom rises in direct proportion to the teacher's apparent loss of control. The wise teacher chooses the second strategy, which is to respond to the students' raucous mayhem in a calm, controlled voice, or the teacher might choose to respond with an authoritative stare and stony silence. In either case, the children are very likely to respond to the teacher's calm, relaxed, self-controlled demeanor by quieting down and by gaining control of themselves. Notice that in both situations, the children followed the teacher's lead. In the first situation, they followed the teacher to an even higher level of noise and chaos. In the second situation, they followed the teacher to a quiet, controlled place, not unlike the parking lot of the local shopping center at 3:31 A.M.

In the second nonstuttering example, we find a frightened, panic-stricken child running into the house screaming for his mother. When he tries to tell his mother what happened, his words are mixed with sobs, and his uncoordinated breathing reflects his panic. How should the mother respond? If she allows her response to be influenced by the child's emotions and behaviors, she will find herself contributing to the child's unsettled state, but if she responds calmly and under control, and if she speaks in a concerned but matter-of-fact manner, the child will begin to calm down. The sensitive and insightful mother will not try to get answers at first, but will simply hold the child for a few minutes, waiting for the sobs to subside. This kind of response assures the child that everything is all right after all, that even though fear may have been justified, there is no reason to be afraid now. Consider what might happen in this scene if both players are adults. When a compassionate, sensitive adult tries to comfort another adult who is distressed, he or she does not—or should not—begin by yelling frantically, "What's wrong?!" Instead, he or she listens carefully, indicates with body language that time is not a factor, and then responds with a few carefully chosen words, selected not so much to offer advice as to offer comfort. The words are delivered in a soothing voice, with flattened prosody, at a slower than normal rate.

Now, what should parents do when their child stutters? They should respond to the message, but they should respond in a way that suggests acceptance. They should speak slowly, calmly, and reassuringly. After a very short time, the child will calm down, and his fluency will improve. Young beginning stutterers usually adjust easily to the speaking styles of their parents. When a parent speaks to the young stutterer in a rushed, chaotic manner, the stutterer's speech will probably reflect the chaos in the form of stuttering, but if the parent adjusts his or her speech so that it is relaxed and unhurried, the child will make the same adjustment. In most cases, the pain of stuttering dissipates quickly, assuming the child noticed the stuttering at all. The parent has helped the child through a difficult speaking experience by showing the way rather than by giving him a verbal roadmap. It is noteworthy that most people, adults and children, learn more effectively by following someone's lead than by following someone's directions.

Working with the Speech-Language Pathologist

I would be remiss if I did not end this chapter by reminding parents that when children enter the land of real stuttering, they need and their parents need the assistance of a qualified speech-language clinician. In fact, it would not be an exaggeration to say that the most important thing parents can do to help the young stutterer is to enlist the services of a competent speech-language clinician. In every public school system, there should be certified speech-language pathologists on staff. All of these professionals have some training and experience in the remediation of fluency disorders, but there are some clinicians who do not feel comfortable working with stutterers because they have had too few opportunities to do so. I would advise parents to ask the public school clinician about her expertise in the area of stuttering. If the clinician indicates a reluctance to provide fluency therapy, he or she will be able to make a referral. It is very important, however, that the clinician be competent in the treatment of fluency problems because there is much at stake. The prognosis for the young beginning stutterer is excellent, but if proper treatment is not administered, the odds against a successful outcome increase. For this reason, it is worth the extra time and effort to find the right clinician as opposed to finding the nearest clinician.

The competent speech-language clinician will know much more than the layperson about stuttering, of course, but the clinician will also bring objectivity to the treatment of the disorder, and objectivity is probably more important in the long-term than knowledge. This objectivity will shine a light on the negative attitudes and the misperceptions that might impact the development of stuttering and hinder progress in therapy. I doubt there is a parent anywhere who can be objective about his or her own child, especially about the child's problems. In the bright light of the clinician's objectivity, the parents will be able to understand the destructiveness of attitudes and perceptions that are not consistent with what we know about stuttering. As they come to appreciate the dangers, parents will be more inclined to admit their errors in judgment and to adopt attitudes toward speech, stuttering, and the child that will facilitate progress in treatment.

Finally, the clinician needs the parents' assistance in the treatment of the young stutterer. Under the most favorable of scheduling situations, the clinician might see the child for two or three hours a week. More typically, the clinician will see the child for an hour or less a week. The rub is that the child does not limit his stuttering to only one hour per week. If he is beyond the first phase of stuttering, he stutters every day, in many different situations. When he is with the speech clinician, he probably will stutter less than usual because the therapy room is *safe*. He will feel comfortable in this room with a person he knows will not tease, mock, or criticize him. Since the child's parents are much more likely than the clinician to see the child during his most difficult times, it makes no sense to exclude them from the therapy process. The clinician should actively seek their involvement. During the initial stages of therapy, parents can assist the clinician by helping her identify the child's stuttering behaviors as well as identifying the people and situations that seem to adversely affect the child. This information is invaluable to the clinician as she designs a therapy strategy to fit the client's individual needs. As therapy progresses, the clinician can enlist the aid of parents as *tutors*. They can help the clinician extend the therapy room into the child's real world by observing the child's attempts to modify and control his nonfluencies and by providing him appropriate feedback concerning his successes and failures. Parents should never attempt to do this on their own, however, because success is defined differently, depending on the stage of therapy. With the clinician's guidance, parents can learn to make proper judgments and to properly reward the behaviors being targeted at any given time.

Stuttering can be a frightening disorder for a child and for his parents, but everyone concerned needs to remember that the outlook for the young stutterer is not bleak. If the child, his parents, and the clinician accept their responsibilities in the treatment process, if they are able to communicate with one another openly and honestly, and if they all work together to solve a problem they all share with the child, therapy can be very effective.

The next two chapters focus specifically on the adult stutterer, but if the reader is the parent of a young stutterer or a child who shows signs of becoming a stutterer, he or she should not skip these chapters. Parents need to know what might happen if a young beginning stutterer moves on to the advanced phases of the disorder. Sometimes parents decide to ignore a youngster's fluency problem, hoping he will *outgrow* it. He may very well recover from stuttering without treatment, but after reading the next two chapters, parents may be less willing to take a chance on spontaneous recovery and more inclined to take advantage of the exceedingly hopeful prognosis offered by the treatment of young stutterers. The outlook for adult stutterers is not hopeless by any means, but the road to control is not easy, and it usually stretches many miles beyond the immediate horizon. The stuttering child who does not have take this road at all is very fortunate.

Chapter 10

TREATING THE ADULT STUTTERER:
A BRIEF HISTORY

The Meaning of *Cure*

The first issue we must address in considering the treatment of adult stutterers is the meaning of the word, *cure,* as it relates to stuttering. As it is commonly used and understood, *cure* is an absolute term. To say that a problem, disorder, or disease is cured means it no longer exists, that its symptoms have been permanently removed. If this is what we mean by cure in reference to the prospects for the adult stutterer in treatment, we must conclude that cures are very, very rare. We need to keep in mind that stuttering is a disorder characterized by inappropriate *behaviors*. It is no more appropriate to talk about curing stuttering than it is to talk about curing someone of being rude or curing someone of being moody. We do not cure behaviors. We might shape behaviors. We might reduce or increase the frequency of occurrence of behaviors. We might control behaviors, but the concept underlying *cure* does not fit the treatment of disordered behaviors.

It is more appropriate to talk about the *successful treatment* of stuttering than to talk about cures. Can adult stutterers be successfully treated? Yes, they can. Some stutterers are so successfully treated, in fact, that most people will not know they have fluency problems. They have learned to control their nonfluencies well enough and to make the physiological adjustments necessary for facilitating fluency subtly enough that their speech appears to be normally fluent. I have used the word, "appears," here because controlling speech and making mid-speech adjustments are NOT normal. Making the physiological adjustments that will facilitate fluency are deliberate and highly conscious efforts. Normal speech is natural and easy, and even though speech is volitional behavior, normal speakers do not pay conscious attention to the process of talking. What the successfully treated stutterer does, therefore, is not normal, but it helps his speech *sound* and *look* normal, and that is a significant achievement. More importantly from the stutterer's perspective, he feels in control of his speech because he is, in fact, carefully controlling it.

Most adult stutterers who receive therapy do not reach this level of success, but most adult stutterers who make a committed effort to the therapy process can expect to achieve significant improvement. In this chapter and the next, I will be very candid about my personal conviction that the degree of success achieved in therapy depends heavily on the client. Unfortunately, many clients come to therapy expecting to be healed or cured, and they make the mistake of believing that *wanting to be fluent* is the same thing as *being motivated to be fluent*. They may desperately want to be cured of their stuttering, but as long they expect someone else will do the healing or the curing, they will almost certainly fail in therapy. No matter what therapy approach is used, unless the stutterer assumes responsibility for his own disorder and for its treatment, success will be severely limited. It would be reasonable to estimate that about one-third of adult stutterers do not show improvement as a result of therapy. Most of those individuals who are not helped, and perhaps all of them, have failed to understand the essence of one of Benjamin Franklin's sage observations: "God helps those who help themselves." That quaint saying could be amended for our purposes to read, "Therapy helps those stutterers who help themselves." I will have much more to say about the stutterer's role in his own treatment at the end of this chapter and in the next chapter. Right now, I want to shift the focus to therapies themselves.

I have long been fascinated by the history of stuttering therapies. It is incredible how desperate stutterers and their clinicians have been over the years to find something–anything–that will help stutterers speak more fluently. The history of the treatment of stuttering underscores this desperation as well as the mystery of the disorder, and how short a distance we have come in understanding what causes it. The purpose of this book does not justify a comprehensive review of stuttering treatments, but I cannot resist a brief review. The second half of the book describes the treatment approach I recommend, an approach I use on my own stuttering every day of my life, but we will get to that later.

Stuttering Therapy: Trials, Errors, Comedy and Tragedy

The history of stuttering therapy began long before there were speech-language pathologists. Although we have not found guaranteed treatments for stutterers, I am relieved to point out that after speech-language pathology was born in the United States in 1925 and developed an identity among the behavioral sciences in the 1950s, we began to see more humane, responsible, and effective treatments for stutterers.

Prior to the establishment of speech-language pathology as a viable discipline, the treatment of stuttering was the responsibility of anyone who was foolish or ambitious enough to attempt it. Among those who tried were physicians, physicists, and philosophers, as well as gypsies, backwoods herb doctors, and just plain folks. What a convention of practitioners that would have been!

As I mentioned in Chapter 5, such well-known figures as Aristotle, Francis Bacon, and the respected physicians, Celsus from Rome and Dieffenbach from Prussia, blamed the tongue for causing stuttering and suggested treatments ranging from slowing the rate of tongue movements to gargling, massaging the tongue, drinking hot wine to loosen the tongue, and surgically cutting it. These treatments were suggested between about 400 B.C. and 1900 A.D., a span of 2,300 years.

When theorists shifted their attention to the central nervous system in the twentieth century, the foci of treatments also changed. Most treatments associated with a central nervous system explanation of stuttering were based on the idea that we need to teach the stutterer how to breathe, phonate, or articulate in highly conscious ways in order to compensate for some presumed neuromuscular inadequacies. There were many different versions of this general approach. Some focused on breathing and were designed to teach the stutterer how to breath properly, stressing deep inhalation and precisely controlled exhalation. Others focused on tongue and lip rituals designed to exercise the muscles of these structures so movements would be stronger and more accurate.

Some of the most popular treatments during the early decades of the twentieth century were derived from a Freudian psychosexual fixation view of stuttering. Despite mountains of evidence accumulated through the decades since Freud's most pronounced influence on psychology demonstrating that stutterers are within the normal range on psychological measures, psychotherapy continues to be the treatment of choice for many adult stutterers. Curiously, success in most of these programs is not judged in terms of increased fluency, but in terms of emotional adjustment. In other words, the goal is to produce an emotionally healthy individual, whether or not he continues to stutter. It should be pointed out that the psychotherapies used on stutterers were not specifically designed for stutterers. Those programs that have been used with stutterers include the free association, dream analysis, cathartic role-playing, and the more recent counseling approaches commonly employed by psychotherapists. The reader should be reminded, as discussed in Chapter 5, that from the psychological perspective, stuttering is not the problem. Stuttering is considered a symptom of an underlying psychological conflict. If this conflict can be identified and successfully resolved, the stuttering will presumably disappear just as the symptoms of any disease will disappear if the disease is cured. The success rate of psychotherapies, if measured in terms of increased fluency, is poor, but these treatments will persist as long as people continue to ignore the evidence and believe that stuttering is somehow rooted in a psychological problem.

Another large group of therapies born within the last century developed from the view that stuttering is learned behavior. Although learning views did not enjoy their greatest popularity in speech-language pathology until the 1960s and early 1970s, there have been learning interpretations of speech disorders in general, and stuttering specifically, for at least several centuries. The earliest and most primitive learning views suggested that stuttering is simply a bad habit and should be treated like any other bad habit. This usually meant that the stutterer was scolded whenever he stuttered in the same way that a parent might scold a child for sucking his thumb. In more extreme cases, stutterers were spanked or beaten. Needless to say, this kind of simplistic approach did very little to help most stutterers. By the middle of the twentieth century, systematic learning therapies based on classical and operant conditioning principles had been developed.

In classical conditioning therapies, it is assumed that stuttering is an anxiety-evoked behavior, and that the way to treat stuttering is to reduce or eliminate the anxiety that triggers the stuttering. These therapies typically employ a technique called *systematic desensitization,* in which the stutterer learns to cope with progressively more difficult speaking situations, arranged according to their potential for creating anxiety. The stutterer experiences the easiest situation over and over again, either by imagining it as the clinician describes it, or by role-playing it, until he can experience the situation without feeling excessive anxiety. He then moves to the next situation and repeats the process. He continues to move up the ladder of his personal anxiety-evoking situations until he is able to handle the most difficult of them. Through the process of desensitization, he becomes toughened to the negative feelings he experiences when he stutters and to the conditions most likely to result in anxiety and stuttering. Even if he is successful in desensitization therapy, he might continue to be nonfluent, but he is less affected by his nonfluencies, and he is less affected by the negative emotionality permeating stuttering. Although this sounds like a wonderful therapy in principle, most stutterers do not experience much success with it because it is too passive and because it does not deal directly with the motor behaviors of stuttering that most stutterers view as the essence of the disorder.

Operant conditioning therapies are usually designed to systematically reduce the frequency of stuttering by applying some form of punishment contingent upon the production of specifically targeted stuttering behaviors.

In the experimental models that preceded these therapies, stutterers were given electric shocks, blasted with loud noises, or had bright lights flashed in their eyes whenever they stuttered. These procedures, under carefully controlled conditions, did result in dramatic reductions in stuttering, but there was no carryover into the participants' everyday lives, and even in the laboratories where these experiments were conducted, the stuttering returned almost immediately when the punishments were withdrawn. In spite of the largely disappointing long-term implications of this research, operant therapy programs for stutterers were created and continue to be popular with some speech-language pathologists. You will be relieved to know that these therapies do not employ punishments as aversive as those used in the experimental models. In a typical operant program, the clinician rings a bell or clicks a counter when the client stutters. Unfortunately, these therapies are just as ineffective over the long-term as the experimental models were, and what seemed to be a promising approach to the stuttering problem during the 1960s and 1970s has not lived up to expectations.

Probably the most intriguing stuttering therapies are those that cannot be traced to any broad theoretical categories. These therapies were often developed by accident, or they were purposely created by well-meaning people who apparently thought they made sense at the time. Some of the most bizarre of these treatments are commonly referred to as *folk remedies*. These are treatments dreamed up by frighteningly uneducated and superstitious people to deal, not just with stuttering, but with a host of diseases and disorders–physical, mental, and spiritual. A typical folk remedy for stuttering calls for the attachment of leeches to the stutterer's lips and tongue. The idea is that the leeches will, in the process of sucking the stutterer's blood, drain out the *evil* that is causing the stuttering. Most folk remedies are based on the belief that a person becomes a stutterer because he has committed a sin. In order for the sin to be forgiven and the stuttering removed, the stutterer must suffer a punishment equal to the sin. The stutterer might have his tongue cut or burned, or he might be forced to swallow some kind of vile substance, usually containing animal waste, so he will vomit and purge himself of the evil. Many folk remedies involve eating things most of us would consider fairly disgusting, including snakes, garlic, raw eggs, and cats, usually black cats. In 1950, a man wrote a letter to the editor of a speech-language pathology journal, chronicling his experiences with a number of these remedies. He included a classic. He was forced to drink the urine of a virgin mare for 30 consecutive days. This treatment, and all these treatments are burgeoning with symbolism. Many of them mention *midnight* or a *full moon* to indicate an ending and a beginning. They suggest that evil can be bled away or burned to extinction. The victim can rid himself of the evil by ingesting something horrible enough to chase the evil out in the act of regurgitation. The sugges-

tion in the virgin mare example is that if the stutterer can consume something awful from something as pure as a sexually innocent horse, he can puri-
fy himself, pay for his sin, and stutter no more. The most symbolic of all the
folk remedies is probably one that involves beating the stutterer in an abandoned church. Think about this one! If one believes that the stutterer's problem is the direct result of some sin he has committed, what better way to pay
for that sin than to subject the stutterer to a thrashing in a building that was,
at one time, a house of worship but has now been abandoned by its congre-
gation and presumably by God himself. It is reasoned, if reason is really a
part of this process, that the stutterer who goes to this extreme to show that
he is remorseful and repentant will surely be forgiven. I'm guessing there has
never been a long waiting list for this particular treatment.

And then there are those who have tried to help the stutterer by fitting
him with artificial devices, most of which have been designed to compensate
for presumed structural or functional inadequacies. A nineteenth century
French physician, Jean-Marc-Gaspard Itard, developed small gold and ivory
fork-like devices he placed under the stutterer's tongue to help him overcome the weakness and spasms of the tongue he believed were responsible
for causing stuttering. Several devices have been invented over the years that
are designed to change the position of the tongue—to lift it or to push it back
away from the teeth, for example. One of the more curious in-the-mouth
instruments was developed in 1937 in Japan—the *Idehara stuttering-curing
apparatus*. It consists of a small whistle held against the roof of the mouth by
bands attached to the upper teeth. The stutterer is trained to use the sound
of the whistle as a reminder to keep the air flowing. When the whistling
stops, the stutterer knows he is doing something wrong. Supposedly, only the
stutterer can hear the whistle. The most diabolical feature of the *stuttering-curing apparatus* is a sharp point at the base of the whistle that serves to punish
the stutterer for pressing his tongue too hard against the roof of his mouth. I
cannot think about this device without forming a mental image of a severe
stutterer making intermittent whistling noises while a small spot of blood col-
lects in the corner of his mouth. It is a cruel image, I admit, but with the
exception of the sadists and masochists among us, we would probably agree
this is a pretty cruel device.

While most of these devices are used inside the mouth, some creative
people have developed instruments that are used on other parts of the
speech-related anatomy. One such device used in the nineteenth century,
called the *Bates appliance,* consists of a springed band worn around the neck.
The band applies pressure against the larynx. The purpose of this instrument
is not entirely clear, but you can imagine it would have a definite effect on
the stutterer's voice. You might try pushing firmly against your own larynx
while you speak to simulate the effect. There was a great deal of excitement

during the 1960s about a device known as the *electronic pacer*. The electronic pacer is worn in the ear like a hearing aid and produces a ticking sound that can be adjusted for speed and rhythm. Many stutterers who use this device become fluent immediately, but there is little or no carryover, and the speech it produces is so artificial that most stutterers and virtually all listeners reject it as sounding more abnormal than stuttering. One of the more enduring devices used by stutterers is an instrument called the *Edinburgh Masker*. It feeds a noise into the stutterer's ears similar to what you hear on your television set when your antenna or cable is not working. The masker consists of earphones and a noise generator that is activated by a contact microphone worn against the larynx. The masking noise is produced only when the stutterer speaks, so when he is silent, he can hear those who are speaking to him. Descendents of the *Edinburgh Masker* marketed today are much more elaborate and versatile than the original product. They include adjustments for volume, for the rate of the noise, and even for delays in feedback. These devices are typically used only by very severe stutterers who have not responded to other forms of treatment, and even these individuals usually use them only in critical speaking situations. Although they are effective in facilitating immediate fluency in most stutterers, some stutterers find them uncomfortable, and they may attract unwanted attention from listeners. The fact is, most stutterers do not want to depend on any artificial device for achieving fluency, and very few will ever need to do so.

One of the most popular approaches to the treatment of stuttering throughout the centuries has been to change the tempo of the stutterer's speech. Obviously, the electronic pacer accomplishes this when its mechanically controlled ticking guides the stutterer to a predetermined tempo. Other treatments regulate tempo or change rhythm without the use of artificial devices like the electronic pacer or the more familiar metronome. One of these methods, *drawback phonation,* was popular during the nineteenth century. When the stutterer approaches a word on which he thinks he might stutter, he stops, inhales and exhales several times, begins his attempt on inhalation, and finishes it on exhalation. Even though this approach was first used in the 1800s, therapies that focus on changing the tempo or rhythm of the stutterer's speech have persisted to the present day. Some clinicians have suggested that the stutterer should take a short, quick breath before saying a difficult word in order to establish rhythm, in much the same way a musician might nod his head before playing the first note of a piece of music. Others have recommended using a sigh or a prolonged vowel for the same purpose.

Perhaps the most commonly used tempo-regulating approach, simply called *rate control,* involves training the stutterer to speak very slowly by prolonging vowels and by inserting extended pauses at the ends of phrases, clauses, and sentences. Typically, the stutterer is instructed to begin at a rate of about one word every two seconds. He then gradually increases his rate to something approaching normal, but he does so in very small increments, and he stops at whatever rate seems to be the maximum he can handle without stuttering. Most stutterers find that slowing the rate of their speech is not enough to solve the stuttering problem, that struggle, excessive muscular tension, inappropriate articulatory positions, and those nasty perceptions of difficulty that set the stage for maladaptive physiological adjustments are all more important to the creation of stuttering than rate. Nevertheless, rate control therapies remain popular. Today's versions incorporate technologies that allow for more objective monitoring of rate and muscle tension, but the essence of the treatment has not changed.

An interesting phenomenon in the mystery of stuttering is the almost complete fluency that occurs in nearly all stutterers when they are completely relaxed. It is not terribly difficult to figure out why this occurs. Stuttering is struggle behavior. If the stutterer is completely relaxed, he cannot struggle since struggle requires muscular tension and effort. If he cannot struggle, he does not stutter. If stutterers stutter less, or not at all, when they are relaxed, it is not surprising that clinicians have tried to use relaxation in formal therapy. Most relaxation therapies use muscle-training techniques. The stutterer is taught to focus on those parts of his body that are hypertense and then deliberately release the tension. In these programs, the stutterer is usually taught to relax gradually, one body part at a time, and he usually works from the extremities of his body toward his trunk and head.

There are other less traditional forms of relaxation therapy. In Russia, for example, sleep therapy is used to treat stutterers and other individuals who suffer from anxiety-related problems. In a sleep therapy program, the client sleeps about 18 hours a day and is enrolled in the program for two to three weeks at a time. Sleep is induced by drugs, conditioning, and hypnosis.

Other relaxation approaches include massage, yoga, bathing in hot spring water, and transcendental meditation. There is no question that all of these relaxation methods can produce dramatic increases in fluency, but we do have to question whether relaxation is a reasonable therapy that can facilitate long-term fluency. Although stutterers tend to be quite fluent *while* they are relaxed, there is rarely any carryover into everyday life, and that is the problem. In everyday life, no one can be completely relaxed all the time. In fact, I would argue that people do not function optimally without some anxiety in their lives. Anxiety serves to keep us alert, to help us concentrate on the small and large tasks we must perform everyday, to make us conscious enough of the possibility of failure that we always strive hard to succeed. We certainly do not want to be too relaxed when we are driving our cars. We want to be *alert* to what is going on around us, and we want enough anxiety on the part of every driver on the road that we are all concentrating as hard as we can to stay within the white lines in our own lanes. The idea that anxiety might help the stutterer be more conscious of what is doing to get himself in trouble and more alert to what he needs to do to control his speech does not mean we should dismiss relaxation techniques as worthless. As is usually the case when we debate extremes, we find that what is best is something in the middle. There is no doubt that some anxiety is useful in heightening the stutterer's level of concentration, but we also know that the successful modification of moments of stuttering depends, in part, on the stutterer's ability to relax the muscles focal to his struggle. For example, if I sense that I am producing too much tension in my lips when I am trying to say the word, "bottle," I can effectively prevent a moment of stuttering by relaxing the muscles of my lips as I say the word. This is, of course, not as easy as it sounds. Consider what you may have learned in driver's education about what to do when your car begins to skid. You are supposed to avoid gripping the steering wheel too tightly, and you are supposed to turn in the direction of the skid. Do most people react properly when their cars skid? Most drivers, despite knowing what they are supposed to do, squeeze the steering wheel with all their strength and turn away from the direction of the skid. Knowing what to do is easy. Doing it in the midst of panic and struggle is something else again.

What are the most popular therapies today? Although it might sound cynical to some, I believe I am being truthful when I say that the therapies popular today are the same therapies that were popular 50 years ago. Some were popular hundreds of years ago. A number of writers who have studied stuttering for a lifetime have reached the conclusion that old therapies, like old theories, never die. Therapies are popular for a time, then fade from favor, and all too often are resurrected years, decades, even centuries later. They might be repackaged or revised, and they might be presented with new technologies, but we do not have to examine them very closely to determine that they are the same basic therapies clinicians have used for generations. Please understand that this is not a criticism of today's stuttering therapies or yesterday's stuttering therapies. It is an acknowledgment that there are only so many things that can be done, even creatively weird things, to treat stuttering, and it may be they have all been done. As I mentioned earlier, one of the most popular approaches used today, in a variety of versions, is rate control. Rate control therapies have been used with stutterers for centuries. Other approaches popular today involve easy voice onset, gently controlled breathing at the beginning of utterances, and easy, relaxed articulation. All of these techniques have been used for many decades, and in some cases, centuries. Therapies based on conditioning principles are still popular today, but the reader must remember that most of these programs depend on punishing moments of stuttering. Therapies involving punishment or aversive stimuli are probably as old as the first members of humankind who stuttered. Granted, today's conditioning programs punish specific moments of stuttering, and old aversive stimuli therapies punished the stutterer as a person, but in the sense that all of these therapies involve aversive consequences to stuttering, they are bound together over time in general principle. I want to make one more critical clarification before I move on to the problem of selecting a therapy. To say there are no really new therapies under the sun does not mean there are no good therapies available. There are, and the recycled versions of old therapies are far superior to their originals.

And what is the *best* therapy for stutterers? This is obviously a trick question. There is no *best* therapy, and even though I will describe the therapy I prefer in the second half of this book, it is not my intention to suggest that this or any single therapy is superior to the exclusion of all other therapies. Stuttering is not unlike many other human disorders. Depression, for example, can be treated by psychotherapy, by medication, or by altering the patient's biochemical makeup. There is no *right* approach for treating depression, cancer, heart disease, learning disabilities, or stuttering, if by *right,* we mean *only.* There may well be a best approach for a given stutterer, but that is a decision best made by a professional speech-language pathologist. There are many viable therapies used by many different clinicians. Each therapy can claim its share of successes, and each therapy must admit to its share of failures.

A Friendly Warning

Although I will not identify a single therapy, not even the therapy I prefer, as THE answer to the stuttering problem, I do want to offer some cautions about selecting therapies based on my personal and professional experiences. I firmly believe the therapy program is not as important as the clinician who uses it. I would remind the reader that the best surgical instruments in the hands of an incompetent surgeon can be instruments of deadly destruction, not the tools of healing they are meant to be. A proven and effective surgical procedure employed by an incompetent surgeon might yield deadly results. In the same way, an incompetent clinician can make the best of stuttering therapies look pitifully ineffective and maybe even harmful.

At the same time, it must be acknowledged that not all stuttering therapies are equally viable. I believe the stutterer should be wary of any program that addresses only part of the stuttering problem. A program, for example, that focuses only on the speech behaviors of stuttering and ignores the client's feelings, attitudes, and perceptions is not likely to yield much long-term success because these covert features of stuttering form the foundation of the disorder. Stutterers should avoid programs that depend heavily on gimmicks designed to produce *quick results*. These programs remind me of the diet ads that are so pervasive in American magazines. Anyone with a long-term weight problem knows there is no such thing as a quick, easy, painless way to lose weight, but these ads suggest otherwise. Stuttering is a complicated, multifaceted problem that, in the case of an adult, has developed over a period of many years. Common sense alone suggests there are no simple solutions to this kind of problem. If there were, there would be no stutterers. If losing weight were easy and painless, there would be no obese people in a society that places so much value on being svelte.

Do not be fooled by testimonials. I learned long ago that even the strangest therapy WILL work for some stutterers. Most of the diet ads include testimonials too. I assume that the stutterers and the weight-challenged individuals who offer these testimonials are telling the truth as they understand the truth, but we should not conclude that just because a diet or a stuttering therapy program worked for Hankering Hank of Hihowareyou, New Hampshire, it will necessarily work for other people. The fact is, the most respected therapies do not need to be hyped. They are well known to certified speech-language pathologists, and their success rates have been documented over many years with many clients. The stutterer should keep in mind, however, that highly competent, experienced speech-language clinicians using stuttering therapies with excellent histories of success will not promise miracles, and no stutterer should expect a miracle when he enters therapy.

Motivation–The Best Indicator of Potential Success

Success in therapy depends more on the clinician than on the program itself, but success depends most heavily on the client himself. As I noted earlier, the stutterer must understand that *wanting to be helped* is not the same as *being motivated*. I have known many adult stutterers who have been desperate to be fluent. I have known far fewer who have been willing to pay the price for fluency. The stutterer who is truly motivated is willing, even eager, to pay the price.

The adult stutterer who thinks he is interested in therapy should carefully consider the costs and payoffs of therapy. The payoffs of being successful in therapy are probably fairly obvious. The primary payoff, of course, is being fluent, but there are other payoffs that result from fluency. These include, but are not limited to, increased self-confidence, a more positive self-image, more positive attitudes toward speech and listeners, improved vocational opportunities, and more comfortable social interactions. The bottom line relative to the payoffs of fluency is this: Any stutterer who says that being fluent would not make a difference in his life is either not being truthful with himself or others, or he is trying to rationalize his inability or unwillingness to deal effectively with his stuttering. Fluency *does* make a difference, and it is a difference all stutterers crave, even if they are unwilling to admit it.

As is true of almost anything worth achieving, however, fluency does not come without cost. Part of the cost is financial, of course, but there are also time and effort costs. The stutterer must make a commitment to therapy time, usually two to four hours per week, and he must be willing to invest a considerable amount of time working on his speech outside of therapy. It may be possible to treat athlete's feet by putting powder between one's toes twice a day, but stuttering cannot be so easily and conveniently treated. Every time the stutterer speaks outside of the therapy room, he has an opportunity to practice his old, maladaptive stuttering habits and continue his old misguided perceptions that feed the fires of his stuttering, OR he can practice the new techniques he is learning in therapy, based on corrected perceptions about speaking, stuttering, and listeners. There are no other choices. If speaking time outside of therapy is not used constructively within the goals of the therapy, it is being used to perpetuate the old stuttering. The commitment of time is a significant price to be paid for therapy success, but it is a price that MUST be paid if the stutterer really wants to be more fluent.

There is also an emotional price that must be paid in the stutterer's quest for fluency. There is no doubt that stuttering hurts. Anyone who suggests that it does not hurt has not walked in the stutterer's shoes, but the stutterer will not get beyond his pain unless he is willing to experience the pain of stuttering openly, honestly, and often. No matter what therapy the clinician is using, she will almost certainly, at some point in the therapy process, require the stutterer to speak in difficult situations and to stutter on purpose. Only by forcing himself to experience stuttering openly, and in large doses, will the stutterer develop the objective view of his stuttering and of himself he will need to maintain fluency control for the rest of his life. If he keeps the payoffs in mind, the emotional costs will be easier to pay. If he pays the costs in full, he will someday be able to stutter without reacting, and he will discover that when he does not react to his fluency failures, he is less likely to stutter at all. Fluency, objectivity, and communicative comfort are among the benefits of successful therapy, but they are not free. Please note and note carefully that therapy never comes with a guarantee, but if a stutterer is willing to pay the costs of therapy, the odds in favor of success increase dramatically. In short, the stutterer can expect gains from therapy in direct proportion to what he invests in therapy.

Chapter 11

SELF-HELP FOR THE ADULT STUTTERER

The very fact that the title of this chapter includes *self-help* suggests that the stutterer is not helpless in his battle against stuttering. There are things he can do to make his situation better. The first thing he must do, of course, is to face the fact that he has a disorder and that the disorder is making his life something less than it can be. If the stutterer has not come to that realization, he will not be reading this book, and it's not likely he is enrolled in therapy unless someone has coerced him into therapy, and if that's the case, he might as well not be in therapy at all. So, I will assume that if the reader is a stutterer, the problem has been acknowledged. The next step in the self-help process is *understanding*.

Understanding Is the Key to Success

The longer I work with stutterers and with my own stuttering, the more convinced I become that understanding is absolutely essential to the successful treatment of this disorder. The unknown and the misunderstood can be frightening, and most stutterers simply do not understand their own disorder. Sometimes they are reluctant to learn too much about stuttering for fear they will discover something terrible about themselves, something they would rather not know. Sometimes they believe they already know all there is to know because they mistake their feelings and perceptions for knowledge and understanding. Sometimes they believe that since they are living the disorder, no one can possibly tell them anything they have not learned from personal experience. Sometimes they are simply content to drift along in their ignorance. I would submit that the adult stutterer cannot afford to be ignorant about his disorder because the less he knows, the more severe and complicated his disorder is likely to become. He also cannot afford to understand a little bit about stuttering because, as I pointed out in the opening chapter of this book, this is definitely a situation in which *a little knowledge is a dangerous thing.* I never cease to be amazed at the conclusions stutterers reach about stuttering, about speech, listeners, and themselves based on a few, usually unsubstantiated, *facts* about stuttering. The danger inherent in this kind of razor-thin knowledge is that stutterers come to believe their conclusions and misperceptions, and this usually means—as I have repeatedly noted and will note again on future pages—that they abdicate all responsibility for their problem. They blame the problem on someone else or on something else, and then they either wallow in self-pity or become angry at life for dealing them a bad hand.

One of the most important things the stutterer can do for himself, therefore, is to understand stuttering. Reading a book like this one is a good step in the direction of understanding. A stutterer reading this book will discover that there is not a great deal we know about stuttering for certain, and that in itself is important to know. At the same time, the stutterer will discover that we have developed some reasonably good hypotheses about stuttering over the years. We may not have many solid answers, but we are asking responsible questions, and in the process, we are separating some of the chaff from the wheat. We have, in fact, made greater advances in our understanding of stuttering over the past 75 years than in all the centuries prior to the last 75 years, and I have tried to provide a manageable summary of that knowledge without reaching unwarranted conclusions about what it all means.

Get Thee to Therapy!

There is no doubt that stutterers have the potential to help themselves, but it is a potential that is seldom realized without the assistance of a good speech-language clinician. Many alcoholics, drug addicts, and obese individuals make the mistake of thinking they can handle their problems alone. Very few are successful. The problem with these conditions, and with stuttering, is that the people who own them cannot see themselves very well. You have heard the expression that *an attorney who represents himself has a fool for a client.* It is difficult to be objective about one's own problems in any situation, but when the problem becomes subsumed into one's personal identity, as so often happens in these cases, it is almost impossible to operate without bias. Without a fair degree of objectivity, it is far too easy to rationalize one's weaknesses and to ignore one's strengths. The stutterer needs the speech-language clinician's expertise and objectivity, as I mentioned in the preceding chapter, but the stutterer needs even more from the clinician.

The clinician actually plays several roles in the therapy process, each of which is keyed to the stutterer's changing needs. The stutterer can help himself by understanding the clinician's roles and by accepting the assistance she provides within each of these roles without expecting or demanding more than the clinician can deliver. When therapy begins, the primary role of the clinician is counselor. The stutterer needs someone to provide him advice, someone to help him sort through his feelings and attitudes, someone to help him identify and correct the misperceptions that are contributing to his disorder. The clinician, as counselor, provides advice, and by reflecting and clarifying what the stutterer says, helps him understand his stuttering more clearly. During this initial phase of therapy, the clinician is also a motivator. The typical stutterer needs to be pushed and cajoled into taking responsibility for his therapy and needs to be encouraged to take the risks that will make therapy work beyond the clinic. The clinician remains a counselor throughout the therapy process, but as therapy moves beyond the initial stage, a new role is added. The clinician becomes a teacher or guide. It is true that the clinician cannot cure or heal the client's stuttering, but she can provide the information and the directions the stutterer needs to make the changes that will move him toward the fluency control he wants. As teacher, the clinician can demonstrate the techniques the client must learn in order to modify his moments of stuttering. She can explain the intricacies of modification skills, and if the clinician is competent, she can, like all good teachers, inspire the stutterer to reach for his full fluency potential. As therapy moves into its final phase, the clinician's role changes again. In preparation for the client's dismissal from formal therapy, the clinician begins to transfer her therapy responsibilities to the client so that, in essence, he becomes his own clinician. At this point, the clinician operates more as a supervisor. She has already taught the client what he needs to know, and if the teaching and learning have been successful, the client understands what he needs to do at least as well as the clinician, and he has become a better analyst of his own behaviors, adaptive and maladaptive, than the clinician. At this point, the clinician, like a good supervisor, becomes a critical observer and evaluator. She reminds the client to focus on the fundamentals of modification. She pushes the client to the limits of his abilities. She points out the mistakes he does not notice and suggests adjustments. She chastises him when he fails to perform as well as he should, but she encourages him at every step, praises him when he risks, and shares his joy when he succeeds. This process continues until the clinician and the client mutually agree that the client has achieved all that he can achieve. At this point, therapy is terminated.

I have saved another of the clinician's roles for last because it is, in many ways, the most important. The clinician is the stutterer's friend from the beginning of therapy to the end and beyond. I know very few people who cannot use one more good friend, and the typical stutterer can certainly use a friend who understands what the stutterer is experiencing, who accepts him as a person, and who is always available to listen to his fears, doubts, frustrations, and anger without making him feel less a person or expressing awkward sympathy. In the right speech-language clinician, the stutterer will find this kind of friend.

One of the most important ways the stutterer can help himself, therefore, is to find a clinician who will fill all of these roles, a clinician who is knowledgeable and competent, a clinician who will provide support and guidance. And how does the stutterer find this special clinician? That is not as easy as one might think because, while there are many speech-language clinicians in the United States of America, there are very few who specialize in the treatment of fluency disorders and there are relatively few generalists who feel comfortable in the treatment of fluency disorders.

I would never discourage someone from beginning the search for a clinician locally. That is, if the client is a child, caregivers should contact the local school district to determine what services might be available, but caregivers should keep in mind that most public school speech-language clinicians do not specialize in fluency disorders and may not feel comfortable treating young stutterers. By law, they are obligated to do so, but if a clinician is not confident in her ability to treat stuttering, she might place the child in what could be called a *low impact* treatment program. That is, the clinician spends time with the child, but the program is designed to be so *safe* that the disorder may not be addressed at all. The common concern expressed by this kind of clinician is that she does not want to do anything to harm the child, so in essence, she ends up doing little or nothing that could be construed as beneficial.

If there is a university in your community, and if that university has a program in speech-language pathology, it is likely that someone on the faculty will have an interest in stuttering. Although that person may not be able to provide therapy, he or she may be able to direct you to a specialist in the community who does offer fluency therapy.

One can also look in the *Yellow Pages* under *Speech-Language Pathology* or *Speech-Language Clinicians* or a similar title. In the telephone directory for any city that is moderate or large in size, there will be listings for speech-language pathologists. In some cases, specialties are listed. If not, the caller should ask if the clinician specializes in fluency disorders or if the clinician knows anyone in the area who does specialize in treating fluency problems.

If the local search does not yield the proper clinician, contact the **American Speech-Language Hearing Association (ASHA)** and/or the **Stuttering Foundation of America (SFA).** ASHA's web site address is *www.asha.org.* As quickly as things change on the Internet, any directions I provide about how to get the information you need could be obsolete by the time this book is published, but if you follow the general directions, you will eventually make the right connection. On the ASHA web site home page, click on "Find a Professional." That will take you to an "Online Directory." At this point, you will have an opportunity to narrow your search considerably. You will indicate the kind of help you are seeking, the city, state, zip code, and country. You will indicate the age range into which the client fits and even the language spoken by the practitioner. At the end of all these choices, you click *Submit*. A list of clinicians who fit the profile you have established will come up. On each profile, you will find "View all information." If you click on that, you will get all the contact information you need. More importantly, the clinician's specialty(ies) will be listed. At the ASHA site, you can also use the *Search* feature to find information about stuttering. Some of the information you will find is practical. Much of it will be recent research. If you do not have a computer, or if you prefer more traditional methods of making contact, the information you need follows:

American Speech-Language Hearing Association
10801 Rockville Pike
Rockville, MD 20852
Toll Free Phone Number: 1–800–638–8255

Whether or not you contact ASHA, I strongly recommend that you contact the Stuttering Foundation of America. This organization, as the name attests, is committed to understanding, treating, and preventing stuttering. It was founded by the late Malcolm Fraser, a man who stuttered and who dedicated his life and his own financial resources to finding answers to the multitude of questions that have been raised about stuttering over the centuries. The organization is currently directed by his daughter, Jane Fraser, under whose leadership the foundation has grown in size, stature, and influence. It is, in this author's opinion, the single most important organization in the United States for those who live with stuttering and for those who treat the disorder.

FSA's web site address is *www.stutterhelp.org*. Again, the reader should keep in mind that web sites change, so whatever descriptions I provide here might not be completely accurate by the time you read this book, but once you are on the site, how to navigate will be clear. On the current home page, you will find a link titled, "Referral Lists." If you click on the link, you will be asked to indicate the state in which you are interested. That link will take you to a list of speech-language clinicians in that state who specialize in the treatment of stuttering. Each listing will include the clinician's contact information: address, phone, e-mail address, FAX number, etc. It should be noted that clinicians are asked each year if they want to be included on this list, so it is safe to assume that when you contact a clinician on this list, he/she does have a professional interest in stuttering.

In addition to finding a clinician, you can use the SFA web site to uncover a treasure trove of information about stuttering. Under "What's New," for example, you will find recently published books, brochures, videos, newsletters, media presentations, and research articles. I have included more traditional contact information below:

Stuttering Foundation of America
3100 Walnut Grove Road
Suite 603
P.O. Box 11749
Memphis, TN 38111–0749
Toll Free Phone Number: 1–800–992–9392
Local Phone Number: 901–452–7343
FAX Number: 901–452–3931
E-Mail Address: stutter@stutteringhelp.org

Speech-language pathologists are often active in their state professional organizations, and this provides yet another source of referrals when you are looking for a clinician. The easiest way to find these organizations is to use an Internet search engine, such as Google.com or AskJeeves.com. Just type in the name of the state organization you are trying to locate, e.g., Ohio Speech-Language-Hearing Association, and click on *ask* (Ask Jeeves) or *Google Search* (Google). From there, it's just a matter of navigating on each state organization's web site to find the contact information you need.

Beyond the clinician, in addition to the clinician, there are people who are willing and able to provide help for the stutterer. These people may, in fact, provide a source of hope and encouragement that can be provided by no one else. They are members of stuttering support groups or self-help groups.

Self-Help Groups

At one time, there was a commonly held opinion among speech-language pathologists that self-help groups for stutterers were doomed to fail because stutterers feel uncomfortable in the presence of other stutterers. While this may be true for some, it is clearly not true for all stutterers. There have been many attempts over the years to form self-help groups for stutterers, but until the 1970s, they were not very successful in attracting large numbers of stutterers, and they were not very successful in keeping their members active for long periods of time. As to what happened to make these organizations more successful in recent years, one must look at pervasive changes in our society that have made the concept of self-help more palatable. Although the cultural climate in America today continues to idealize rugged individualism, it has become much more socially acceptable than ever before to reach out to other people for help, to admit one's personal problems, and to express one's feelings. Bookstore shelves have overflowed for decades with all kinds of self-help books dealing with all kinds of prob-lems. People who share common problems seek out one another for comfort, support, encouragement, and so they can share information. The grandfather of support groups, Alcoholics Anonymous, has inspired the formation of support groups for a wide range of problems including drug addiction, obe-sity, child abuse, spousal abuse, gambling, blindness, deafness, cancer vic-tims, crime victims, and the list grows daily. Stutterers have been swept into this wave of self-help and support groups. Some of these are just informal, local groups. Others are chapters of national organizations such as the National Stuttering Association and Speak Easy International. There are sup-port groups for stutterers in more than a dozen countries worldwide. Although each of these organizations has a somewhat unique agenda, what they have in common is *stutterers supporting stutterers.* They share in common the belief that stutterers are valuable people who have nothing to be ashamed of, who should proud of who they are and what they have and con-tinue to contribute to society. Members are encouraged to be open about their stuttering. There is a much greater emphasis on self-acceptance than on fluency for the sake of fluency. Members are more concerned about obliter-ating their fears, their shame, and their embarrassment than they are obsessed with becoming normal speakers.

The largest and most successful of the national support groups is the National Stuttering Association (NSA), founded in 1977. The mission state-ment of this organization provides an appropriate summary of what all stut-tering support groups hope to accomplish. The mission of the NSA is to bring "hope, dignity, support, education, and empowerment to children and adults who stutter, and their families." The NSA has chapters throughout the United States. Typically, a chapter meets once a month. In addition, the NSA sponsors regional workshops, youth and family events, and continuing edu-cation programs for speech-language pathologists. This organization makes an effort to communicate as broadly as possible. According to their web site, they have information for parents/family, children, teenagers, adults, clini-cians, educators, physicians, employers, researchers, and even the media. They publish a monthly newsletter, *Letting Go,* in which members share their positive and not so positive experiences, as well as their views about how to deal with the challenges of stuttering. Some of the articles, letters, book reviews, therapy reviews, and interviews focus only on serious aspects of the stuttering experience, but there is also a concerted effort to help members maintain a healthy sense of humor about what they are all going through. Always, however, there is an emphasis on support, encouragement, and hope.

If you are interested in a support group, if you simply want more information, or if you are interested in establishing a local chapter, contact information follows:

National Stuttering Association
119 West 40th Street
14th Floor
New York, NY 10018
Phone: 1–800–937–8888
E-Mail: *info@westutter.org*
Web Site: www.nsastutter.org

Speak Easy Canada
Speak Easy, Inc.
95 Evergreen Avenue
Saint John, NB
Canada E2N 1H4
Phone: 1–800–345–9022
E-Mail: *info@speakeasycanada.com*
Web Site: www.speakeasycanada.com

The Canadian Association for People Who Stutter (CAPS)
CAPS
P.O. Box 444
Succ. N.D.G.
Montreal, QC
Canada H4A 3P8
Phone: 1–888–788–8837
E-Mail: *caps@stutter.ca*
Web Site: www.webcon.net/~caps/

International Stuttering Association
ISA
c/o Martine de Vloed
Peter Benoitloan 44
B–9050 Gentbrugge
Belgium
E-Mail: *stutterisa@NewMail.net*
Web Site: www.stutterisa.org

Friends: National Association of Young People Who Stutter
Web Site: www.friendswhostutter.org

NOTE: This organization publishes a newsletter, *Reaching Out,* every other month. It's an upbeat collection of articles, essays, personal stories, and information for young people who stutter, their families, and for speech-language clinicians who work with this population. A mailing address, phone number, and e-mail address have not been provided because there is not a single national address. At the web site, visitors are directed to people who are happy to provide information. Their addresses and phone numbers are provided at the web site.

The reader should keep in mind that these are *support* groups, not therapy groups. They have been established so that people who share stuttering can share their fears, concerns, hopes, failures, and successes relative to their stuttering experiences. One could look at these groups through cynical eyes and conclude that they are no more than examples of the idea that misery loves company. I think a more accurate view of these groups is that people who are suffering need to know there are other people who understand exactly what they are going through, that when stutterers find one another and work together on their common problems, they can find strength, understanding, and courage they might not find on their own.

Chapter 12

STUTTERING IN THE FUTURE

Miracle Cures?

There are no miracle cures for stuttering on the near or far horizon. What lies beyond the horizon no one knows, but one would have to be an *I know I'll win the lottery* kind of optimist to believe a cure for stuttering will be discovered during the lifetime of anyone reading these words. The reason for my pessimism, or realism, depending on your point of view, on this matter should be abundantly clear to anyone who has read from the beginning of this book to this point. Stuttering is a complicated, multifaceted, multilayered disorder. It is highly unlikely we will discover that stuttering is caused by a single factor, that it develops the same way in all individuals, that it is maintained by the same factors in all individuals, and that there is one approach to prevent stuttering or one approach to treating stuttering. I sincerely hope I am wrong. I hope we will find a single cause for stuttering, a single cause for cancer, a single cause for heart disease, and a single cause for stupidity, but based on what we presently know about the diversities among all these conditions, I doubt we will. And if we discover that these conditions have multiple causes, it is difficult for my *special-effects-less* mind to imagine any single prevention strategy or any single treatment strategy that will work for everyone who suffers from any of these conditions. The realist in me suspects that 100 years from now people will be asking the same questions about stuttering posed in this book, the same questions people have been asking for the past 100 years, and in some cases, the past 2000 years. There is no doubt that we will have different answers in 100 years, and I am confident they will be better and more complete answers, but I suspect they will continue to be couched in as much theoretical speculation as fact.

My hope for present and future stutterers is that they will stop waiting for a miracle cure and get on with the business of dealing with their stuttering problem right now. When I was a kid, my friends and I often dreamed about a *history pill* or a *math pill*. We wished for the day when someone would invent these pills so we would no longer have to study history and math. We would just take a history pill, and presto, all history knowledge would spring into our brains. I would guess that children in every generation since the advent of pills have had similar dreams, but every child in every generation has had to face the cold, hard reality that there are no pills that can be substituted for learning and for all the time and effort that go into learning. The cold, hard reality for stutterers is that there are no pills for stuttering, and I seriously doubt there ever will be. Success in dealing with stuttering is achieved only through determination, dedication, and hard work sustained over a long period of time. Fluency control is the result of sweat and tears and pain, not wishes and dreams. I urge my fellow stutterers to abandon the search for *miracle-cure* therapies that create fluency quickly and easily. These therapies are not unlike cold remedies that temporarily relieve symptoms but do nothing to cure colds. The fluency created by *miracle-cure* therapies is contrived and short-lived. There will be more of these therapies in the future. They show up regularly, but they are not what they purport to be. They are delusions, and because they do not work for the long-term, they are cruel delusions.

The Only Future That Counts

Fellow stutterers, in the most immediate scheme of things, the only future that matters is yours. It is, without debate, the only future over which you have any control. I urge you not to wait for someone else to create a treatment that will make your work easy or unnecessary because such a treatment is a fantasy. Begin today. Do not slip a toe into therapy. Jump in with both feet. Once you have found a clinician with whom you can work, dedicate yourself to solving your stuttering problem, and never lose sight of the fact that it is *your stuttering problem.* Set specific goals. If your clinician does not give you daily homework assignments, ask for them, demand them, and then make sure you complete them. Expect to be successful and then create all the conditions that will make success a reality. Be a positive thinker, but more importantly, be a positive doer. As your future unfolds, there will be some bad days among the good days. There will be failures along the way to success. Learn to accept the bad days and the failures and do not be discouraged by them. Look forward to the speech challenges of each tomorrow. Treasure each victory, no matter how small, and always recognize that the most important victories come when you confront your fears, even if you stutter in the process. Attack your fears. Never retreat. Grab your stuttering by its throat, wrestle it into submission, and refuse to be intimidated by stuttering or the threat of stuttering again.

Declining Incidence: Hope for the Future

Although I am not optimistic about discovering the cause or causes of stuttering in the foreseeable future, I am optimistic about the apparent decline in the incidence of stuttering and about what this decline might suggest. Since it has been noted over a period of only 40 to 50 years, the decline in incidence suggests that stuttering is not a purely genetic problem. If the causation of stuttering were limited to genetic factors, any decline in incidence would be noted over a span of many generations since genetic changes evolve slowly. A noticeable decline within a generation or two tends to support an environmental link in the stuttering problem. An environmental connection does not preclude genetic or organic contributions to stuttering, of course, but if the decline in incidence is shown to be real, there is a strong suggestion that environment plays a key role in the development of stuttering. This would be very good news for people who stutter and for those who treat stuttering because it would mean that at least some of the factors that impact stuttering can be manipulated in ways that may help prevent the disorder and may help to treat it. Clinicians have always operated from this bias, but it is reassuring to know there is evidence to support the bias.

The Pieces of the Puzzle

There is one more chapter in the first part of this book. Chapter 13 is a very personal message from the author to people who stutter. I will expand upon, and extend, the message subsumed in this chapter about personal responsibility, but before we move to Chapter 13, I want to close this chapter with a few words about where Chapters 1 through 12 have taken us.

In the first 12 chapters, we considered some of the mysteries surrounding stuttering and some of the myths associated with stuttering and with stutterers. I have tried to make it clear that not all the mysteries have been solved, but we certainly have enough information to dispel most of the myths. As I mentioned in the opening chapter, we still have more questions than answers, but we are making progress. If we think of stuttering as a 10,000 piece jigsaw puzzle, I think it is fair to say that we have thousands of pieces in place, but we are still missing some key pieces and some key sections of the puzzle that are necessary for a clear and complete picture of the disorder. The final pieces are widely scattered, and some may not even be on the table yet. Some of the pieces we will surely find. Others are likely to be missing for a long, long time, possibly for the duration of human existence, but we have enough pieces of the puzzle right now to develop viable treatments, and that is good news indeed for all people who stutter, for those who love them, and for those who treat them.

Chapter 13

LIVING WITH STUTTERING

This chapter is an open letter to my fellow stutterers, but I urge parents, teachers, clinicians, and others who have found their way to this page to read this chapter as well. If you are a *significant other* to any person who stutters, you will influence how that person chooses to live his life with stuttering, and I hope my personal perspective will help shape that influence. All readers, stutterers and those who live with stutterers, should keep in mind, however, that this is my *personal* perspective, shaped by my experiences, my insights, my understandings, and my beliefs. Unlike so many political pundits, at both ends of the political spectrum, I do not claim to know any truth that goes beyond my own experiences, but I do believe–after working with people who stutter for four decades–that my experiences with stuttering are not unique, that I am as *typical* as a stutterer can be.

Please be forewarned that I will return to many themes I have already addressed in the preceding 12 chapters of this book. Some of the themes I have purposely addressed more than once. My intent here is to bring these themes together, one more time, in a cohesive message, a message that subsumes much of what I would say to you if we were talking face-to-face. Everything I will say to you in the written word I have said to stutterers face-to-face. For the sake of convenience, I have tried to distill my message into a Top Ten List–*The Top Ten Things You Need to Remember about Living with Stuttering.*

#10–Accept the Nature of the Disorder

There is much we do not know about stuttering, and we will waste our lives if we are consumed with trying to force answers to answerable questions. If we choose to live with stuttering in ways that are healthy and productive, we will accept that if we carry stuttering into adolescence, it is not likely that it will fade away on its own. I began to stutter when I was three or four years old. My disorder grew progressively worse through my elementary, junior high, and into my high school years, and that is fairly typical. Throughout that period of time, I prayed every night that God would protect my family from tornadoes, that our house would not burn down, that my loved ones would not contract any on a long list of diseases I itemized for God just in case he did not know them by name, that my grandparents would live long, healthy lives so that I would not have to suffer the pain of grief when they left this earth, and I prayed that God would take my stuttering away. When I was a child, I did not understand the nature of the disorder, and I was certainly not mature enough to accept the nature of the disorder. Even when, at the age of 15, I discovered many of the techniques that allowed me to modify my stuttering, I still believed that stuttering was a temporary condition, that my hard work was just a band-aid to make speech tolerable until the disorder would magically dissolve when I became an adult.

I now accept that I am a stutterer and that I will continue to be a stutterer, and that's all right because I have learned to live with it. It is not a burden in my life. Everything I do to control my speech has become so habitual that I no longer have to think about using my modification skills every time they are needed. When the need arises, I make the physiological adjustments I need to make. If I forget, or if I get lazy, I stutter, and that serves as a reminder to do what I must do. In the beginning, monitoring and modifying were absolutely exhausting. Today, they are automatic, and please read this next part carefully–they are comforting. It is comforting to know that when I am in speech trouble, I know how to get out of it. It is comforting to know that when I THINK I might be in trouble, I know what I need to do to prevent trouble before I create it.

I have also accepted the fact that stuttering will never be a constant in my life. There are days when speech is fairly easy, and there are days when speech is tremendously challenging. I welcome the easy days. They feel like mini-vacations from stuttering. I am always prepared, however, for the challenging days, and I now take them in stride. In fact, when I face a challenging day and win more speech battles than I lose, I end the day with an enormous sense of satisfaction.

What it comes down to is this: Stuttering is a permanent part of my life, even though the specific manifestations of my disorder change constantly. I accept that fact of life. More importantly, my modification skills are fully and permanently integrated into my life. Just as I rely without thinking on my abilities to read, write, word process, drive a car, throw a ball, swing a tennis racket, etc., etc., I rely without thinking on my abilities to recognize the conditions that give rise to fluency failures, abandon the struggle that lays the foundation for those failures, and then plan and execute the physiological adjustments that make fluent productions possible. I have come to accept that I cannot change the nature of my disorder, but I can change how I react to my disorder, and that has made a remarkable difference in the quality of my life.

#9–Maintain Perspective

Over the course of my career, I have interacted with many adult stutterers who have allowed their lives to be ruined by stuttering because they have never been able to place the disorder in proper perspective. If you fail to maintain reasonable perspective about stuttering, it will always be that 500-pound gorilla that threatens to make your life miserable. In mundane language, we might say it this way–Get a grip!

My own perspective has evolved over the years, but I vividly remember when and how my perspective began. In order for you to appreciate what I learned, and also because it's fun to reminisce about days in my life that were not guided by reason, intelligence, or wisdom, I want to take you back to my own childhood.

I could pretend that I was a wise child, the kind of youngster who was always reasonable, who always chose the right fork in the road, who always did the right thing. The truth is, in comparison to many children, I was well behaved and responsible. I obeyed my parents. I always did my homework. My grade cards were heavy with As. I was a Boy Scout. I sang in the church choir, and I was an acolyte. I was, by any reasonable standard, a good kid, BUT I was also a fairly typical boy. That translates into *typically stupid.* When I was in my late elementary years and into my junior high school years, I was a member of a group of boys who engaged in activities that were common for boys in that era in Sylvania, Ohio. Basically, we played ball. We played football in the fall. We played basketball in the winter and spring, and we played baseball all summer. The rules for our games were–as they have been for American boys for as long as there have been American boys–rather loose. I hear people joke about *no harm, no foul* or *no blood, no foul.* Well, that's the way we played. We were typically stupid boys who reveled in our own controlled violence. No one was ever killed in our games, and no one suffered anything more serious than a broken bone, but there was plenty of blood, and there were bruises galore.

You may be wondering where this is going. Just be patient. I'm trying to set the stage here for something truly startling–a moment of enlightenment in the midst of competitive mayhem and chaos. Anyway, one of the games we played was called *Smear.* This game was an excellent example of what we were about in my little circle of friends in Sylvania. A football was tossed high in the air. Everyone scrambled for the ball. The boy who captured it, ran away as fast as his little boy legs would carry him, but he had to stay within the confines of the vacant lot on which we played. All the other boys–usually about a dozen–chased him down with two intentions: (1) Take the ball away, and (2) Inflict as much bodily damage as possible. When the ball was wrested away, it was thrown in the air again, and the fun continued. One of the objects of this game was to make one another bleed, and for this reason, we always wore our *blood shirts*. These shirts were never washed because the bloodstains were our badges of honor. In our typically stupid little boy minds, this made perfect sense. I had a built-in advantage in this game. I was vulnerable to nose bleeds, so it usually took only a few shots to my face before I had a nice flow going, and I wiped as much blood as I could on my gray, tattered sweatshirt. It was a sight!

When we played basketball, the shooter was fairly well protected, but we never ran around picks. We simply ran through them. The pushing and shoving under the basket would have made NBA players proud. We knew what blocking out was, but we found it simpler to just grab our opponents and pull them out of the way of rebounds. On defense, we grabbed shirts. We pushed and elbowed. We even tripped, but no one would admit to tripping because that was not considered *manly,* and we were huge into *manly*. We had no idea what it meant, of course, but we thought we did, and our conduct was measured against our collective perception of *manly*. That meant that hitting and shoving and grabbing were fine, but it was not *manly* to pinch or trip.

When we played baseball, we called balls fair and foul, but we pitched inside as often as we could, and we made fun of kids who cried when they got hit. On the base paths, we were merciless. We didn't wear metal spikes–thank goodness–but we went into second base with our Converse All-Stars high and when there was a play at the plate, we leveled our shoulders at the catcher's chest.

When it was really hot in the summer, we did not go to a pool because we couldn't afford the fee. We went to an abandoned rock quarry that had filled with water. Years later this quarry was fenced and turned into a very profitable swimming venue, but when we were kids, it was just there for anyone who wanted to swim. The water was crystal clear and cool, and because there was no adult supervision, it was a great retreat for boys who thought they were *manly*. Because our little band of *manly* boys could not do anything without turning it into a contest of some kind, we looked for something at the quarry that would test our courage. Actually, some of the high school boys in our town identified what would become the testing ground for our courage. It was called *Suicide Ledge*–a flat rock shelf about two feet wide and about four feet long that protruded from the wall of the quarry about 50 feet above the water. The danger actually began in getting to the ledge. The candidate for courage testing had to swim to the base of the wall and make a difficult climb to the ledge. I'm not sure how quickly the high school boys could scale it, but it took each of us about 20 minutes, and I don't think any of us reached *Suicide Ledge* without falling at least once. Because I was not particularly fond of heights, and probably because my IQ was slightly higher than the IQs of my friends, I was the last and most reluctant candidate for this test of courage. Why did I do it? I did it because I was typically stupid, because I feared the ridicule of my friends more than I feared injuring myself. I wish I could tell you that it wasn't as bad as I thought it would be, but that would not be true. I STILL have nightmares about what the quarry looked like from *Suicide Ledge*. After making the ascent, I made at least a half dozen aborted attempts at leaping off the ledge. Each time I retreated to the wall, my friends who were treading in the water below, laughed and called me all kinds of names, each one impugning my *manhood*. At one point, I actually started to climb down, but the insults hurled in my direction were just too powerful, so I stood at the edge and looked straight down. What I saw intensified my fear. Two or three feet below the surface of the water, another shelf of rock jutted out about six feet. When I brought this to the attention of my friends, they were helpful, of course. They told me that I needed to jump out as far as I could to clear the rocks just below the surface of the water, so that's what I did. I pressed my back against the rocks, took several deep breaths, ran to the edge of the ledge and jumped out as far as I could. . . . About halfway down, I regretted my decision, but it was too late. I was almost completely vertical when I hit the water. The impact forced water into my nose, and I felt like I went 20 feet deep before I started to come up, but when I broke the surface, my friends were cheering and clapping for me. I was *manly* again.

Perhaps the most disturbing evidence of our being *typically stupid* came during the great **BB Gun War** during the summer between seventh grade and eighth grade. Shortly after school was out, we decided that shooting at one another with BB guns would be great fun, so we chose teams. We actually called them *armies*. There was no real object to the war, but if you were hit, you were *dead* for the day, so whoever had the most guys standing at the end of the battle won. Usually the battle ended when someone was called in for lunch. The war was waged for weeks before my mother found out about it. When one of the other mothers told her, she was horrified, and she confronted me. She asked if we were really doing this, and—just like George Washington—I could not tell a lie. Beyond feeling compelled to tell my mother the truth, however, I could not imagine why she would be concerned about a BB gun war. You can easily imagine her primary concern. "Lloyd," she said, "Someone could get shot in the eye."

"Don't worry, mother," I told her, "We have a rule that you cannot shoot anyone above the neck." In my *typically stupid* boy's mind, my reassurance made perfect sense. It did not occur to me, apparently, that someone might duck, placing his face in direct line with a launched BB. Whether by divine intervention or by dumb luck, no one was seriously injured. We all had red marks on our arms, chests, and legs that turned into little bruises, but no one lost an eye.

And all this brings me to my point about perspective. As *typically stupid* as my friends and I were, we managed moments of enlightenment, and if we could manage these moments, surely adults who stutter, people with far more sense than we could muster on our best days, can capture their own moments of enlightenment. Our moments came when we need respites from our bloody athletic contests and from careening BBs. We went down to the woods, to our favorite spot beside a creek that ran along the edge of our town, and we talked. We talked about everything–girls, school, sports, even politics and religion. My most vivid memories, however, are of the conversations we had that always began with the words, "If you had to choose . . ." Now, some of the choices offered by my friends and me were *typically stupid,* of course. "If you had to choose, would you eat dirt or worms?" "If you had to choose, would you wear the same underwear for a year or the same pair of socks?" Those were actual questions we posed, and the rule was that you had to provide a reason for your answer.

In addition to the stupid questions, we asked others that were much more interesting, questions that first opened the door to introspection for me. "If you could choose, would you choose to be a boy or a girl?" "If you had to choose, would you rather live a long life and accomplish nothing or live a short life and accomplish something important?" "If you had to choose, would you choose to know when you were going to die, or would you choose to not know?" "If you could choose, would you choose to be rich and unhappy or poor and happy?"

The questions that always generated the most animated discussions were these: "If you had to choose, would you choose to be blind or deaf?" "If you had to choose, would you choose to be blind, deaf, or paralyzed?" Because we were young and fancied ourselves athletes, one of our favorite questions was "Would you rather be a great athlete and not be very smart, or would you rather be smart and not be athletic at all?" We talked about questions like this for hours, and in the course of these discussions over several years in my late childhood and early adolescence, I learned valuable lessons about perspective, lessons about not feeling sorry for myself because things could be worse.

That is the message I want to share with you, readers, especially those of you who stutter. I often ask adolescent and adult stutterers this series of questions: "What is the absolute worst thing that can happen to you if you stutter? Will you die from stuttering? Will you lapse into a coma? Will your friends desert you? Will your family disown you?" The answers are, I hope, obvious—*No, No, No,* and *No.* When a stutterer is objective and honest, he will acknowledge that the absolute worst thing that might happen if he stutters is that he will be embarrassed. I then ask, "Does that make you unique? Are stutterers the only people in this world who do things that are embarrassing?" The answers again are *No* and *No.*

ALL people say things and do things that cause them to be embarrassed. It's not pleasant to be embarrassed, but it's not as awful as we sometimes make it out to be. "Would you rather stutter," I might ask, "or be blind?" "Would you rather battle stuttering or an incurable disease?" "Would you rather live with stuttering or with chronic depression?" "Would you rather stutter or be unable to speak at all?" The list of questions can be lengthy, but at the end of the list, I would expect any reasonable adult stutterer to recognize that stuttering is not as horrific as many stutterers seem to think it is.

And here's the most important part of the perspective we need to have about stuttering: If I am blind or deaf or paralyzed, there is nothing I can do to change this fact in my life. I can learn to live more effectively with any condition or disease or limitation, but there are some conditions over which I have no control. Stuttering is not one of those conditions. Even if I cannot completely eliminate stuttering from my life, there are things I can do that will reduce the frequency of my stuttering, and I can make adjustments that will reduce the complexity of my moments. Under the best of circumstances—most of which are within my control—I can effectively eliminate the negative effects of stuttering on my life. Living effectively with stuttering begins when the stutterer places his disorder in its proper perspective. If a *typically stupid* boy could gain that perspective in a few lucid moments of introspection ensconced in days, weeks, and months of unrestrained chaos, you can capture perspective too. It's just a matter of honestly weighing stuttering against all the other problems that can impact human beings. When all the possibilities are considered, stuttering does not even make the top 100 human miseries.

#8–Be in the moment . . .

I trust you will forgive the pun here, but it is a pun intended because this heading has at least two meanings for me and for all people who stutter. First, it means that when I stutter, I should own the moment because I do, in fact, own the moment. I establish the cues that precipitate my stuttering. I choose to react to those cues. I choose the physical behaviors that comprise my struggle. In short, when I stutter, I am in the moment because I have chosen to be in the moment. I may not like my choice. I might argue that it is not my choice. I might close my eyes and pretend that it is not my choice, but when I cut through all the rationalization and all the denial, what do I find? I find that I AM in the moment of my own creation, and—here is the good news, my stuttering friends—if being in the moment is my choice, I can also select my way out of the moment. In the absence of modification skills, I select my way out of the moment by using an interrupter or by letting my struggle run its course, but I can choose a better way. I can choose to master the modification skills that allow me to abandon struggle, reduce muscle tension, reconfigure my articulatory mechanism, and complete the previously stuttered word fluently, under control. If I take ownership of being in the moment, you see, I can take ownership for the strategies that will keep me from the precipice of fluency failure, or if I do not seize control during the anticipatory period, strategies that allow for release from stuttering in a manner that attests to the mastery of my own mouth.

Being *in the moment* also means that I understand the time frame over which I have control. Many adolescent and adult stutterers obsess about their stuttering histories. Why did I become a stutterer? Who is to blame? Why did God let this happen to me? Even if there are answers to those questions, they are not relevant in the present. If I became a stutterer, for example, because I inherited a genetic predisposition from my paternal grandfather, I cannot undo my genetic makeup. If I became a stutterer because my father was excessively demanding, critical, and perfectionistic, I cannot retreat to my childhood and counsel him about a better way of parenting. If I became a stutterer because the significant others in my life inadvertently reinforced what were, at the time, normal nonfluencies until they became major features of my speech to which I reacted in unhealthy ways, I cannot reverse that pattern of learning now. No matter what accounted for the etiology of my stuttering, no matter what precipitated the onset of my stuttering, no matter who was to blame, I cannot rewrite my history so that the stuttering never happened. The past is past. What was done is done, and I must come to terms with that fact of living.

And what about the future? I can plan for the future. I can harbor hopes for the future. I can dream about what the future might bring to my life, but the truth is, I cannot control time that has not yet arrived. I cannot guarantee what WILL happen tomorrow. The only time over which I have control is the present, and that's why I have learned to be *in the moment,* and that's why I am urging my fellow stutterers to be *in the moment.* The challenge of being *in the moment* is the acceptance of responsibility. I cannot undo the past, and I cannot guarantee the future, but much of what happens right now is my responsibility, my opportunity. What this means for the stutterer is simple, and it goes back to the first meaning I affixed to the phrase, *in the moment.* I can—and do—control what happens to my speech, for good or ill. As I speak, I make countless decisions, immediate decisions that determine if my speech will be fluent or not fluent, grammatically correct or incorrect, lucid or garbled, conversationally constructive or destructive. In this moment in time, I am in charge, and that is amazingly empowering. It's a little frightening, of course, because if I am in charge, I am as responsible for my failures as for my successes, but I would much rather have the steering wheel in my hands than in the hands of chance.

#7–Stuttering is something you do, not who you are.

The message here is embedded in many of the things I have already written in this chapter and elsewhere in this book, but the message is important enough to be repeated and reinforced. I make no apology for my redundancies when I believe they serve a purpose.

For many adolescents and adults who stutter, the disorder becomes such a dominant feature of their lives that they lose sight of who they are as human beings. There was a time in my life when that was true for me. When I was an adolescent, if someone had asked me, "Who are you?" I would have identified myself, first and foremost, as a *stutterer*. I realize now the absurdity of that kind of response, but that's what I truly believed at the time. I believed it because I could not separate who I was from what I did, and that problem is not unique to stutterers.

What is the first thing adult men want to know about other adult men when they first meet? They want to know what these people do. Women too are curious about what new acquaintances do for a living, but men seem to have a great deal of difficulty separating personhood from vocation. They struggle with the difference between John Smith, the person, and John Smith, the physician.

When parents punish their children, they often have trouble separating their children from their behavior. There is a significant difference between calling a child "a bad boy" and identifying something he has done as "a bad behavior," but parents sometimes make no effort to separate the child from his behavior. The point is, we should not be surprised that stutterers have trouble understanding that stuttering is what they do, not who they are, because many people–many well-intentioned, reasonably intelligent people–struggle with the line that separates who people are from what those people do. In real life, wonderful people sometimes do horrific things, and horrible people sometimes do wonderful things. Most of us, of course, are *combination people* who sometimes do warm and fuzzy things and sometimes do naughty and grizzly things. In a fair and balanced world, a world characterized by tolerance, forgiveness, and objectivity, people judge us far more on who we are than on what we do.

If the stutterer does not separate who he is from what he does when he stutters, he will not develop the objectivity he needs to be successful in therapy. When I modify my speech, I am not changing my core identity. I am simply making changes in one small compartment of the many behaviors over which I exercise control. When I stutter, I am not a failure. I am producing fluency failures. In therapy, I do not need to fix me. I need to fix some of the behaviors I produce. These are huge, and critically important, differences that will influence my view of therapy and will affect how I go about the business of addressing my disorder.

When I arrived at a point in my life when I could make the separation between *me* and my behaviors, I discovered something very interesting. Most people understood better than I that stuttering is one small part of the doing aspect of my existence. My friends often told me that they *forgot* I was a stutterer because they did not think of me that way. Even in terms of all the things I did, I found that stuttering was far down the list of behaviors that mattered to most people. As a youngster, I was much more likely to be judged on the basis of what I did academically or athletically than on the basis of my stuttering. As an adult, I have always been judged far more on my performance as a professional, as a friend, a teacher, coach, father, and husband than on my fluency. In short, I have learned that stuttering is something I do. It is not who I am.

#6–In dealing with stuttering, there is no room for compromise.

To those who stutter and to those who treat those who stutter, I will assert that there is no room for *compromise* in the dedication, commitment, and self-discipline that are necessary for success in therapy and that are necessary for success in living with stuttering in the long term. Many stutterers try to compromise or seek their clinicians' permission to compromise. I want to share a very personal story to make what I believe is an important point about the dangers of compromise in the treatment of human problems.

My younger brother, Mark, was an alcoholic and drug addict. He spent time in prison for crimes he committed to support his addictions. As strange as it might seem to some readers, Mark was also one of the warmest, most loving, compassionate people I have ever known. He loved animals. His house was full of snakes, spiders, lizards, dogs, and birds. He never said *no* to a human being in need. He was an extraordinarily easy person to love, but he was also weak and undisciplined. As is true of many addicts, he was in and out of treatment many times. At one point, he was attending AA meetings five days a week, and he stayed sober on this schedule for several months. Then one night, I got a call from Mark. He said he was attending AA meetings Monday through Thursday, but he was doing so well, he was allowing himself Friday nights to drink a beer or two, or perhaps a little wine.

I tried to explain to my brother that addiction does not allow room for compromise. I pleaded with him to return to complete abstinence, but he was convinced he could handle the few beers. In less than two weeks, he was hospitalized for the last time. When he returned home, he continued to drink, and he continued to abuse drugs. His health deteriorated. He suffered a stroke at 40. By the time he was 45, he was using a walker and could hardly talk. At the age of 46, he had a seizure, fell out of a boat and drowned. His life was destroyed and eventually lost because he did not understand the evil that lies within compromise. Compromise for the stutterer will not mean death, of course, but it will almost certainly mean that he will achieve less success in therapy than he would otherwise manage.

In 1994, in St. John, New Brunswick, Canada, I gave a speech to an audience of stutterers. There were a few clinicians in attendance, and there were a few spouses and children of stutterers, but there were more than 100 stutterers in the audience. When I finished my speech, one audience member asked me if I was suggesting that dealing with stuttering was simply a matter of will. My response went something like this: Success in dealing with stuttering is certainly not *simply a matter of will,* as least not in the sense that a stutterer can simply will to be fluent, and stuttering magically disappears. Success in dealing with stuttering does depend, however, on exercising one's will to do what needs to be done to achieve and maintain fluency.

Some therapists, and far too many clients, are willing to accept less success than is achievable because they make room for what might be called the *I can't help it* syndrome. I know that some experts include the word, *involuntary,* in their definitions of stuttering. I will not argue that that word does not belong in the definition, but I will assert my conviction that the word is very dangerous in therapy. I believe we should approach stuttering, in every detail, as volitional behavior. As a teacher, clinician, and stutterer, I believe that to be true even if there are flaws or weaknesses in my central nervous system that make me more vulnerable to communicative pressure and more susceptible to maladaptive speech adjustments than people who do not stutter. I MUST believe that stuttering is volitional, or decided, behavior if I am to believe I can alter my behaviors in a manner that promotes fluency. I refuse to allow the door to *I can't help it* to be opened an inch. If you allow that opening, you will allow yourself the freedom to make excuses. There is, my friends, no crying in baseball, and there is no place for excuse-making if one chooses to live triumphantly with stuttering.

#5–Define "success" properly.

Living triumphantly with stuttering does not mean that my speech will be perfect or that your speech will be perfect. Our speech will never be perfect. I can write that without fear of contradiction because no one—not even the most facile of fluent speakers—produces perfect speech. Does that mean that I CAN expect, that you CAN expect, to have speech that will be absolutely free of abnormal nonfluencies even if it is replete with normal nonfluencies? That is such an unlikely scenario that it never even shows up as a blip on my radar screen of wildest hopes and dreams, but what I have learned is that *normal* speech, like *perfect* speech, is grossly overrated. In fact, I think *normal* is overrated. If you ever meet a human being who is completely *normal* in every respect, I guarantee you will find that person excruciatingly boring. I have learned to be content with the best I can do in everything I do, knowing full well that in some things I exceed what would be considered *normal* and that I fall far short of *normal* in other things. I will accept nothing less than the best I can do, but I have come to terms with the fact that I have limitations and that if I have any shot at happiness and a reasonable level of self-esteem, I need to embrace my limitations just as I need to vigorously push the limits of my potential. And that brings us to the subject of *success*.

What constitutes *success* for the person who lives with stuttering? If you choose to attach *success* only to fluent speech, you will surely be disappointed and frustrated. In the earliest weeks of my frontal attack on stuttering during my sophomore year in high school, I learned a valuable lesson about success. I learned that *successes* and *victories* change over time, that what I would consider a *victory* early in my journey to fluency control differs, sometimes radically, from what I would consider a *victory* further down the road.

In the beginning, my most important victories did not involve fluency at all. Each time I faced a fear, even if I stuttered badly, that was a victory. Each time I was in a communicative situation in which I could choose two words, and I chose the word in which I had the least confidence, that was a victory. Each time I was tempted to not answer a ringing telephone but answered it in spite of my fear, that was a victory. It did not matter if I stuttered or not. I had met the enemy, and much to my initial surprise, the enemy was not stuttering. It was fear. Also much to my initial surprise, each time I met the enemy, his power diminished, and that was the sweetest part of those early victories.

As I developed my modification strategies, I raised the standard for *success* and *victory* a little higher, but I learned another valuable lesson about success. I learned that success is not an absolute, that there are degrees of success. We have all heard the old adage, probably from a coach: *It's not whether you win or lose, but how you play the game.* The actual quote is even stronger. The words were written by Grantland Rice: *For when that One Great Scorer comes to mark against your name, He writes—not that you won or lost—but how you played the game.* As a stutterer, I know that there will be times when the communicative pressure is just too great, or times when I am just not on my modification game. I know there will be times when, in the battle between my perception of difficulty and the fear of failure on one side and my modification skills and will to be in control of my speech on the other, I will stutter. I will lose occasionally, but I am absolutely not concerned about what the *One Great Scorer* will mark against my name in my lifelong battle with stuttering because I know that I engage the contest with all my strength, with the full quota of my will, and with a resolute determination to be successful. I cannot guarantee that I will not stutter, but I can guarantee effort, and there is one more thing I can guarantee. Even if my knees occasionally wobble when I confront my stuttering fears, and even if those fears win skirmishes now and then, I always own the ultimate victory because if I temporarily succumb to the fear and stutter, I collect myself and try again, and I continue to try again until the fear is met and vanquished. Please note, my fellow warriors, that I might still stutter, but if I do stutter it's not because I surrendered to the fear. I might stutter because, at that moment in time, the forces that opposed fluency were simply stronger than my ability to maintain fluency. I am still the victor, however, if I face the fear because no matter how long and trying the war against stuttering, the real enemy remains fear, not fluency failure.

#4–Practice, practice, practice.

I once coached a high school softball player who was an excellent athlete but who never played to her potential because she was too often overwhelmed by her own anxiety. Defensively, she managed fairly well, but at the plate, she really struggled. One day she asked me, "What can I do to not be nervous when I hit?" Before I tell you what I said in response, I want you to know that I frequently use sports analogies in my stuttering courses and in stuttering therapy. The parallels are apt, and they are powerful. In responding to this young woman, I took a quite different road. Although I did not compare hitting to stuttering, I drew upon my experiences as a stutterer in formulating my answer to her question–"What can I do to not be nervous when I hit?"

My response went something like this: "First, you need to understand that ALL hitters, and especially all young hitters, are nervous at that plate. Any time you perform under pressure, no matter what you are doing, you will feel some anxiety, and some anxiety is not an entirely bad thing. When people are somewhat anxious, they tend to perform better than when they are completely relaxed because they are more intense, more focused. A little nervousness makes us concentrate more. The problem you battle is excessive anxiety, a level of nervousness that prevents you from doing your best. IF controlling anxiety were as simple as willing it away, you would not have a problem because you certainly do not WANT to be nervous. You WANT to be relaxed and confident, but wanting the anxiety to go away is clearly not enough. Think about what you can and cannot control as a hitter. You cannot control what the pitcher does, of course. You cannot control what the defensive players will do if you hit the ball to them. You cannot control the angle of the sun or the speed of the wind. You CAN control pitch selection, and you CAN control your swing, so let's make those your priorities. Through practice, you can improve your pitch selection, and through practice, you can make your swing more consistent and more effective. The harder and more frequently you practice, the more confident in your skills and in your pitch selection judgment you will become. The more confident you are, the less anxious you will be. Ultimately the answer to your question can be given in one word . . . repeated: *Practice, practice, practice.*"

In formulating this response, I drew upon my personal experiences in dealing with the anxiety that has surrounded my stuttering from the most severe phase of the disorder through the present day. Before I learned how to modify my stuttering, the speech-related anxiety that haunted every communicative opportunity was nearly unbearable. I found myself asking my version of the young softball player's question: "How can I speak without being nervous?" Later, when I was learning modification strategies, the question became: "How can I successfully use my modification skills when I feel so burdened by fear and anxiety?"

This is what I have learned in my stuttering journey about anxiety, and this is what I want to share with you: If, like me, you have carried stuttering into adolescence and/or adulthood, you will always anticipate stuttering, and you will always experience some anxiety about speaking. You will, in fact, always produce abnormal nonfluencies that will generate more anxiety about more stuttering, so what can you do to not be nervous when you speak?

I learned that my anxiety was reduced as a consequence of facing my fears and disciplining myself to talk as much as possible, in as many different situations as possible, to as many different people as possible. I discovered that anything I did routinely and frequently became less anxiety-evoking than something I did only occasionally, especially when those few occasions were dictated by urgent need and not by a desire to do what I wanted to do under conditions I set. I learned that when I seized control of my own communicative life, even when I was anxious about communicative failure, I was less anxious, less fearful than when I allowed the circumstances of my life to dictate my behaviors. I discovered that, to the extent I could disassociate stuttering from the cues that precipitate it, to the extent that I could view speech sounds, words, speaking situations, and listeners objectively, the less anxious I was about fluency failure. All of these cognitive and perceptual adjustments were helpful in reducing my speech-related anxiety, BUT the single most important thing I did to suppress my nervousness was to master my modification skills so thoroughly that I am now absolutely confident I can handle any speaking situation, no matter how much pressure there is, no matter how many moments of stuttering I anticipate, no matter how many moments of stuttering I actually produce. That confidence is the direct by-product of practice, practice, practice, and how often do I practice? I practice every single day of my life–every single day–but you need to understand this about that practice. It is not a burden. It is a comfort. It is not something I loathe to do. It is something I want to do, and it has become as much a part of my daily routine as brushing my teeth and remembering to pull up the zipper on my trousers.

Has all that practice meant that I never stutter? In answering that question, I want to return to the softball player one more time. If a softball player practices hitting every day, for several hours every day, that practice will not guarantee that she will hit 1.000. No hitter, no matter how talented, no matter how hard he or she practices, will hit 1.000. Failure in hitting is so inevitable that major league baseball players are paid millions of dollars a year if they can consistently hit .300, which translates into "success" just three times out of 10.

My practice has led to a much better average than .300, but I will never have a *fluency average* of 1.000. I still stutter–not as often I as did prior to my campaign to gain control of my speech–but I still stutter. The difference between then and now is that now I know what to do when I stutter and when I think I am going to stutter, and that has made all the difference in the world. It means, of course, that I produce fewer uncontrolled moments of stuttering, and it means that I experience far less anxiety about speech and speech failures than I once did. Practice has produced confidence, and confidence has enhanced communicative success.

#3–Never give in! Never give up!

It is hard to imagine that any person who lives with stuttering beyond adolescence has not, probably many times, wanted to just give up, to surrender to stuttering. It is easy to get weary when one is running a race that seems to have no finish line, to engage in a battle that does not have clearly defined objectives and established markers for reaching those objectives. I empathize with all stutterers who are tempted to just cope, to muddle through using whatever behaviors minimize the struggle and disguise the pain, who find themselves willing to settle for a life that is less than it could be because of the influences of stuttering. You know I am racing toward a *but,* and here it comes.

I empathize with those who want to surrender, *but* I challenge you to not give up. I urge you to fight the good fight against stuttering because there is real hope you can do better. If you make a full and uncompromised commitment to working on your disorder, if you make it a priority in your life, if you refuse to take vacations from the practice required to make modifications automatic and, therefore, reliable under the most trying of communicative circumstances, you have every reason to believe that you will be more fluent. More importantly, you have every reason to believe that your life will be better and more productive if you harness the disorder that has, at the very least, caused you to be less confident in your abilities than you have a right to be, and at the very worst, enslaved you in an existence that darkens your dreams and destroys your ambitions.

Winston Churchill, as you probably know, was a stutterer in his youth. In recent years, some people have cast doubt on that fact. Those cynics may be troubled that a stutterer could have so completely liberated himself from the disorder, not necessarily from the behaviors, but from the stigma, that he became one of the most respected political figures of the twentieth century. Churchill was prime minister of England during one of the most difficult periods in that country's history, indeed, during one of the most difficult periods in the world's modern history. Many historians believe that Winston Churchill, more than any other single person, instilled hope in the citizens of Great Britain when despair threatened to envelope them.

On October 29, 1941, Mr. Churchill visited Harrow School to listen to students sing some of the traditional songs of the school, including one to which had been added a verse praising Churchill for his leadership in the first 10 months of England's participation in World War II. When the singing was finished, Churchill gave a brief but stirring speech about the challenges England was facing in that horrific war. Churchill talked about *terrible catastrophic events,* about the *unmeasured menace of the enemy,* about *crisis and misfortune.* And then he talked about what needed to be done to ensure triumph. Embedded within this portion of the speech were these words: *Surely from this period of ten months this is the lesson: never give in, never give in, never, never, never, never—in anything, great or small, large or petty—never give in, except to convictions of honor and good sense.*

My fellow stutterers, I implore you to apply Churchill's message to the war you are waging against your disorder. Even IF there are legitimate reasons for being discouraged, even when stuttering seems to have the upper hand, even when you sense that you are in the fight by yourself and you're not sure if you are strong enough to continue the fight, even when the battle drains your energy and threatens your resolve, remember Churchill's words. Be encouraged by them. Be inspired by them. Most of all, be challenged by them: *Never give in, never give in, never, never, never, never—in anything, great or small, large or petty—never give in.*

#2–Be tough. Be courageous. Take risks.

I think I pretty well established early in this chapter that, when it came to my personal safety, I was a pretty reckless child, although I suspect I was no more reckless than your average boy. In terms of physical injury, there was not much that frightened me, and I always had a fairly high pain threshold. That threshold, combined with powerful stubbornness and typical boyhood naiveté, led me to believe that I was impervious to serious injury. The comical aspect of all this is that I was always one of the smallest kids in our little group of daredevils. Sometimes people talk about someone so small that he weighs such and such, *dripping wet*. Well, in my case, the *dripping wet* part probably weighed more than I did. I never let my diminutive size trigger common sense, however, when it came to risking injury.

When I was six years old, my father bought me a used bicycle for $4.00. The only thing decent about it was the frame, so my father added some new tires, and painted it red. I was very proud of that bike. The only problem was that it was too big, a problem complicated by the fact that I did not know how to ride a bike. I was determined to learn . . . if only I could figure out some way to get on it! There was a large rock at the end of our driveway, so I walked the bike to the rock, climbed up on the rock, and threw my leg over the bar. Unfortunately, even though I landed on the seat, I promptly fell over because I had thrown myself too hard and could not maintain my balance. For nearly an hour that first day, I climbed the rock and tried to mount the bicycle. I fell over every time that first day. I gave up only when my mother called me in for dinner. The next day, I tried again, and after another 30 minutes or so, I managed to get on the bike, push off from the rock, and off I went . . . for about three feet. I felt like one of the Wright brothers–not Wilbur or Orville, but the *other* Wright brother–the really nerdy one whose ambitions were limited to traversing the ground. Over the next few weeks, I tried and tried again, lengthening my bicycle journeys, first by feet, then by yards until eventually I was able to stay upright the length of our street. Of course, I could not turn without falling over, but I was making progress. When I could finally keep the bicycle upright, I discovered another problem. My legs were not long enough to fully activate the brake, but I solved that problem too. I rode around until I got tired. I then went up our driveway, across the front lawn, turned left around the side of the house and ran directly into the wooden fence that extended from our house to the edge of our property. Upon contact, the bicycle fell over, and I tried to jump off without getting pinned under the bike. I actually became skilled enough at this maneuver that I could jump off the bike, land on my feet and then catch the bike as it caromed off the fence. In none of this did I feel the slightest fear. My bicycle adventures gave me bumps, bruises, scrapes, cuts, and bloody noses, but I felt no fear.

I don't want to mislead you. I was not without fear. For some strange reason, as I mentioned earlier, I feared natural disasters, and I feared that terrible things would happen to people I loved. The fear that dominated my childhood and my adolescence, however, had nothing to do with personal or natural tragedy. The greatest fear of my young life, a fear that still operates in my adult life, was the fear of failure. By ANY standard, I was a *driven* student. I wish I could tell you that I was most driven by a thirst for knowledge. I was—and remain—motivated to learn because I have an insatiable curiosity about everything, but academically I was driven, not by that thirst, but by my fear of failure. I heard Jimmy Connors, the great tennis player, talk one time about his intensity as a player, about his unbelievable desire to win. He observed that it was not winning that shaped him as a competitor. He said that he hated to lose more than he loved to win, so he was mostly motivated to not lose. That accurately describes me as a competitor in virtually everything I have done as a human being. I have learned to lose with grace and dignity. I have learned to give credit to *the other guy*, and that's all very sincere, but along the bumpy road to maturity, I hated to lose more than I loved to win, and I absolutely feared failure.

There is much about my own stuttering disorder I will never understand, but that part—the fear part—I have understood clearly since I was about eight years old. As I indicated early in this book, when I was a child and was called upon in class, I often refused to answer even when I knew the answer because I was afraid I would fail as a speaker. Between the ages of eight and 15, that fear of failure escalated and I became more and more withdrawn as a communicator, not in all speaking situations, but certainly in those situations in which my fear of fluency failure was not balanced by my confidence in my personal strengths. Sadly, one of those strengths had always been academic, but as my fear of fluency failure grew, it gnawed away at my academic confidence. Eventually, I felt like I was a prisoner in the classroom, chained and gagged by fear, not fear that my answers would be wrong, but fear that in expressing correct answers, I would fail in my speech.

When I made the conscious decision to turn things around at the age of 15, one of the most important changes I made in my life was to face my fears. By that point, I knew that I had only one real choice—to give in to my fear or to confront it, and by confronting it, conquer it. For too many years of my young life, fear of failure was the winner, and the more often fear won, the stronger and more manipulative it became. In my speech life, I discovered the courage that had always dictated my performance as an athlete and as a stupid, reckless daredevil, and this is what I learned. I learned that what I had feared was ridiculous. I feared fluency failure? How utterly stupid! Which was worse, I asked myself, to answer a question correctly in class and stutter, or to refuse an answer, be judged ignorant, while saving myself from the momentary embarrassment that comes with stuttering? At the age of 15, I chose to face the fear, knowing full well that there would be times I would fail, but always understanding the truth of the commonly quoted sports maxim: *RISK: You can't steal second base, and keep your foot on first.* I discovered courage. I learned how important it is to risk. I learned that the best way to put fear in its place is to become *tough*.

I once coached softball with a woman who can accurately be described as kind and gentle. The team we co-coached was talented, but they were soft. As long as things were going their way, the girls played hard and they played well, but when a little adversity struck, they became timid, and they made mistakes. After watching one too many of these performances, I gathered them together and I talked to them about the importance of *toughness* in playing sports. I told them that when things begin to fall apart, players need to dig down and play with *courage*. I told them that if they expected to win in anything they did in life, they had to *face their fears*. They had to be *stronger* than their fears. I told them that they had to *take risks* in order to achieve because anything worth achieving does not come easily. You get the idea. It was a typical rah-rah coach's speech, but it was loaded with lessons I had learned as a youngster dealing with my own fears, fears that made me a timid, hesitate, failure-prone speaker. When I finished my rousing speech, my co-coach—this kind and gentle woman—said to the players, "What Coach is telling you is that you need to try harder." "NO! That's not what I was telling them," I wanted to scream. The lesson I was trying to teach them about courage, toughness, facing fear, and risk was not about *effort*. In fact— and read these words carefully, my stuttering friends, there comes a time in life when effort is not enough, when they words "nice try" ring so hollow you should not want to hear them. I want to use a few episodes from my daughter's life to illustrate the lesson I was trying to teach these young players about toughness, courage, facing fear, and risk. It is a lesson that has tremendous relevance for all of us who are trying to live triumphantly with stuttering.

First and foremost, it is important to note that my daughter, Carmen, was not born any more tough or any more courageous than any other child. She learned well the lessons about toughness and personal responsibility I tried to teach her, and there is a lesson in the *teaching* process that should be important to clinicians and all others who try to influence the behaviors, attitudes, perceptions, and understandings of other people. I believe the common expressions that make this point: *Talk is cheap. Practice what you preach. A good example is worth twice as much as good advice.* Carmen saw me living those maxims when she was growing up, and she sees me living them today. I am proud that she lives them as well.

When Carmen was 12 years old, she was a pitcher for the Parkside Junior High School softball team. In a tight game at Pontiac, a batter hit a hard ground ball through the pitcher's circle. The ball took a bad hop, hit Carmen in the mouth, and split her lip open. Rather than grabbing her mouth and giving in to the pain, she scrambled on her knees to pick up the ball and threw the runner out at first base. Her coach wanted to take her out of the game. She refused. She blanched the bleeding between innings, went 3–4 at the plate, and led her team to victory. When Carmen played softball at Illinois State University, during a bunting drill in what is called a "short cage," the pitcher, standing just 20 feet away, threw a fastball that struck Carmen in the nose, breaking it badly. A trainer tried to stop the bleeding but couldn't. They rushed her to the hospital where they finally stopped the bleeding, pushed her nose back in place, and told her she should not practice for a week. The next day she insisted on practicing. The trainer fitted her with a mask to prevent further injury. Her coach told her she could sit out those drills that might cause her distress, such as facing live pitching. She participated in every drill. Practice ended with a mile and a half run. Again, her coach said she did not have to run, but she did. Her nose bled throughout the run, but she refused to stop. She refused to give in to the pain. She refused to give in to the fear of standing in against a live pitcher. She simply refused to be weak. In another season, she sprained an ankle badly sliding into second base during practice. The coach sent her to the training room. She showed the trainer the wrong ankle because she did not want to miss practice, and she knew she was strong enough to handle the pain. She went back out and finished the practice. When Carmen gave birth to her second child, she refused medication of any kind during the labor and the delivery. She played for her summer softball team six days after giving birth. She bled, but she told no one. Courage had become her badge of honor, and she wore it proudly. Many people who stutter could learn valuable lessons from Carmen about facing fear and enduring pain, about not making excuses and not indulging self-pity.

If a person who stutters consistently gives in to his fear, if he does not take risks, if he is not courageous enough to seek out speech challenges no matter the probability of failure, if he is timid rather than tough, he will always be a prisoner of his disorder. If a person who stutters *risks,* if he is *courageous* in the face of impending failure, if he is *tough* when circumstances are difficult, he will live victoriously with his disorder. This does not mean that he will not stutter. It does not mean that he will not fear. It does not mean that he will not be sorely tempted to avoid or bail out. It DOES mean that he will be bigger and stronger than his stuttering. It means he will understand that victory is not always the product of fluency. Rather it is the product of refusing to give in to the fear of fluency failure. Many people believe that a hero is a person of extraordinary bravery. Most heroes will tell you that is not true. The typical hero reports that he or she was terrified in the circumstances of the heroic act, but he or she did what needed to be done anyway. That's what I am suggesting the stutterer needs to do. As a speaker, do what needs to be done, without regard to whether or not you stutter. Be as courageous as you can be, realizing that courage is always tempered by fear. Take risks. Be tough.

#1–Living victoriously with stuttering is a marathon, not a sprint.

We live in an era of *instant gratification*. This is especially true for youngsters, of course. They want what they want when they want it, and not one second later. To some extent, this has always been true about children because they have a very compressed sense of time. They understand the *present*. When they are young, they have very little understanding about the future and precious little appreciation for the past. As we moved into the television, computer, video games, cell phone, Internet, etc., etc. age, young people became even less inclined than ever to accept any challenge that cannot be met in 30 minutes or eight levels, whichever comes first. Adults too are caught up in this madness. Some people reading this book may be old enough to remember the world before microwave ovens. The first time I saw one of these appliances in operation, I was absolutely amazed. I watched my mother-in-law place a hot dog in a bun, wrapped in a paper towel, in her new microwave oven. She set the timer for 30 seconds, and voila! Out came a steaming hot hot dog. What a miracle! What a time-saver! Now consider how truly ridiculous this has become, and you need not trust me on this. You can check it out yourselves. Read the directions on the side of a box of Kellogg's Pop-Tarts. According to the instructions, you can heat your Pop-Tart in one of two ways. You can put it in a toaster, or you can heat it in a microwave. If you toast your tart–"Warm pastry in toasting appliance at lowest or lightest heat setting for one heating cycle only." If you microwave your tart–"Microwave on high setting for 3 seconds." Now consider, dear reader, that on the lowest setting on my toaster, it takes less than one minute to heat a Pop-Tart. Is my life so powerfully driven by instant gratification that I need to heat my tart in the microwave for 3 seconds? And here's the hilarious part. Whether I heat my tart with a toaster or a microwave, the next instruction reads: "Cool briefly before handling." Yikes! I may have to wait longer for my tart to cool than it took to heat.

This might all seem a bit silly, and I admit that I have tapped into the silliness on purpose. We are all victims of a lifestyle that places a premium on *now* or *soon,* and we are also victims of a lifestyle that suggests that what we want can be obtained *easily* and *painlessly.* In fact, that is seldom true. I'm sure there are people who do become millionaires by purchasing real estate with no money down, but if this scheme were as full proof as the endless succession of infomercials suggest, who among us would be poor? If gaining that magnificently sculpted body was as easy, painless, and quick as the print and television commercials tout, who among us would look like most of us look?

One of the hard facts of life—exceptions duly noted—is that whatever in life is worthwhile takes time and effort, and it usually requires sacrifice and pain. This is definitely, absolutely, positively true for those of us who stutter. There MAY be stutterers who become fluent quickly and easily and who maintain that level of fluency for a lifetime, but I have never met one of these people, and I know for sure that I am not one of them. Living victoriously with stuttering is not a sprint. It is a marathon, and the sooner the stutterer accepts that truth, the sooner he can begin the journey. According to the Chinese proverb, *A journey of a thousand miles begins with a single step.* My advice to people who stutter is to *take that first step,* and realize that the journey is a long one.

I hope this does not sound discouraging because I do not view the journey as discouraging at all. For me, the journey has been a grand adventure. I have learned a great deal about myself along the way. I have gained insights into the inherent goodness of other people, as well as the cruelty of other people. I have learned just how strong I can be and how strong I need to be. I have learned to embrace adversity because adversity affords me opportunities to test my will and the limits of my perseverance. I have learned how important it is to take life one day at a time and to be grateful for each day I have been given. I have learned that so many things I complain about are nothing in comparison to the truly weighty problems of life. I have learned to count my blessings rather than wallow in self-pity. I have learned that, to the extent I invest my time and energy in making a difference in the lives of other people, my stuttering diminishes in importance and influence, and the lessons do not end.

Would it be a blessing, my stuttering friends, to lapse into a coma that lasts for several years and then emerge into consciousness as a person who no longer stutters? That would certainly give the illusion of *instant gratification,* but think about what one would have missed during this period of unconsciousness. Personally, I am not willing to exchange *life* for *fluency.* I will not wish for fluency. As a person of faith, I will not even pray for fluency. Long ago, at the age of 15 years, I took the first step in my journey to fluency, and I have not regretted a single step along the way. I will hasten to point out that not all the steps have been happy steps. I have failed. I have regressed. I have been discouraged, but on balance, it has been a great journey because it has been a journey of my choosing. Along the way, I have gained ownership of my disorder and of my life. I would not trade a single step in the process for the instant gratification that would come with immediately *normal* speech.

If you choose to join me on this marathon, I want to give you one more caution. It comes in the form of a correction to a much too commonly expressed belief– *You can be anything you want to be.* That is not true, and it has never been true. When I was a kid, I wanted desperately to be an NBA guard. I worked very hard on my game. I am confident that I invested as many hours in practice as many men who currently play in the NBA, but wanting to be a professional basketball player was not enough. As painful as it is for me to even process the words, I did not become an NBA player because I was simply not good enough. Although I was a good high school athlete, I was not nearly good enough to play at the NCAA Division I level, and only in my wildest dreams could I play in the NBA. You want to be named to the Supreme Court of the United States of America, you say? Well, good luck, my friend, but if that is what you want, *wishin' and hopin'* is not enough. You must begin by going to law school, and then it would help to have a brilliant legal mind, and it would also help to be very well connected politically. You want to be a movie star? Well, good luck to you as well, but it takes more than wanting to be a movie star to make it in show business. It helps to have talent, of course, but it helps even more to be lucky, to be in the right place at the right time with the right eyes and ears focused on you. I trust you get the point here. No one can be anything he wants to be unless what he wants to be is consistent with his abilities, with his drive to succeed, and with his opportunities to succeed.

With the preceding paragraph resonating in your mind, my final piece of advice in this chapter is that you should be realistic about where you want your journey to take you, especially when it comes to what you want to do with your life. Your stuttering should not dictate which doors of opportunity you open, but you should be prepared for the fact that your stuttering might influence how wide those doors open, and it may very well determine which doors are opened for you by others. If you believe you can force those doors open, go for it. If you believe you are being unfairly judged because you are living with stuttering, stand up for what you know is right. Do not let anyone define who you are or what you can become, but be realistic. It may help to keep in mind that every human being–stutterer or not–faces the same challenge. We are all collections of strengths and weaknesses, talents and ineptitudes. We must all figure out for ourselves what we want to be within the context of what we can realistically become.

Part Two

TREATING PEOPLE WHO STUTTER: ADULTS AND CHILDREN

Chapter 14

CHARLES VAN RIPER THERAPY: AN INTRODUCTION

The reader should clearly understand that I acknowledge the therapy program described in this part of the book as the work of Dr. Charles Van Riper. Dr. Van Riper was an influential writer, clinician, and researcher in the area of stuttering from the early days of the profession until his death in 1994. Many stuttering therapies over the years have generated excitement and hope among speech-language clinicians, but few have endured as well as Van Riper's approach. One important reason for the survival of this program is that Van Riper constantly modified his therapy in accordance with new ideas and research findings. Another reason it has flourished is that it is based on a broad, common sense view of the nature and treatment of stuttering. I am convinced that this view is correct, and I believe it is consistent with all we know, or think we know, about stuttering.

I have attempted to describe Van Riper's stuttering therapy in a concise, clear, and structured manner. I have included discussion of rationale and explanation of technique, but I have tried to avoid lengthy philosophical discussions, and I have not included case history examples.

Although I am describing and explaining Van Riper's therapy program, I have included my own adaptations. Just as I have been influenced by many writers and clinicians and by own clinical experiences, other clinicians will discover that their approaches to the treatment of stuttering will combine the ideas of many people. As long as stuttering remains an enigma, and as long as therapy is as much art as science, clinicians will continue to borrow, combine, and adapt therapy strategies.

The methods I will describe are the methods I use to control and modify my own stuttering. I know them intimately, and I have taught them countless times. When I first wrote this material, I sent a copy of the manuscript to Dr. Van Riper for his review. His response was exceedingly gracious, and because it is important you have confidence in what you are about to read, I want to share with you the last sentence of his letter to me: "You certainly have grasped the essence of my approach, more than anyone I know, and it's good to find, in these days of operant nonsense, someone who seeks a more wholistic approach."

THE BASES AND DESIGN OF
A MULTIDIMENSIONAL APPROACH

This program is properly described as an *eclectic* program because it combines several strategies into one approach. Some have criticized this approach because they claim it avoids the issue of causality by including a random mix of treatments in the hope that one of them, by chance, will be appropriate. As I have tried to note and emphasize throughout the first part of this book, we have not identified a single cause of stuttering, and in my view, it is unlikely we ever will identify a single factor that explains the development of stuttering in all individuals. As I have already noted and repeat here for emphasis, the incidence data we have gathered over the years do not suggest a single cause. We know, for example, that stuttering is more common among males, twins, neurologically injured individuals, and mentally retarded individuals, but we also know that stuttering occurs in females, singletons, in people who are neurologically normal, and in people who are in the normal to superior ranges of intelligence. We know there are cultural variations in incidence. We know that stuttering typically begins between two and six years, and when stuttering begins after childhood, it tends to be a different kind of stuttering than early onset stuttering. All of these trends suggest that it is radically simplistic to view stuttering as a single disorder with a single cause. More likely, stuttering is a class of disorders with many different causes, and if this is true, it is not likely that any therapy, especially a therapy with a narrow scope, will be effective with a large number of stutterers.

Even though I believe stuttering is a multidimensional problem that does not lend itself to a one-dimensional treatment, I also believe there are some common denominators that must be addressed in any viable treatment program. For example, nearly all adult stutterers are able to identify linguistic and situational cues that signal *difficulty*. The status of the listener affects the frequency and severity of stuttering. The propositionality, or meaningfulness, of situations, words, and speaking conditions affects stuttering. All of these tendencies suggest that *anxiety* is a common denominator, if not for all adult stutterers, certainly for most.

A second common denominator shared by all stutterers is that no matter the original cause, no matter the specific behaviors produced, no matter the frequency and severity of the nonfluencies, stuttering is a *motor act*. The stutterer produces nonfluency by creating abnormal articulatory positions, by using excessive muscular tension, by disordering his breathing, by disrupting the synchrony of respiration, phonation, and articulation. Stuttering is something the stutterer does. It is not a psychological construct. It is not a mental abstraction. It is not imagined. It is a very real, physiological phenomenon the stutterer executes.

A third common denominator that almost certainly exists in all adult stutterers is *learning*. No matter what the original cause or causes may have been, learning plays a major role in the experiences of adults who stutter. Certain patterns persist because they have become habitualized. Normal speech functions in a virtually automatic manner because normal speakers have developed motor habits that facilitate synchrony among the processes of speech, resulting in clear and understandable utterances, supported by appropriate prosodic variations. The stutterer has developed these same motor habits, but he has also developed other habits that disrupt fluency. These habits are triggered by linguistic and situational cues of which the stutterer is keenly aware, and often by factors of which he is less aware. By the time the stutterer reaches adulthood, the key is not *why* he began to stutter, but what causes the stuttering to *persist*. The original cause has probably long since been removed or has wasted away into ineffectiveness, but the stuttering persists because the behaviors have become habitual. It must be emphasized, however, that it is dangerous to view stuttering as simply a bad habit. A golfer might habitually lift his head before he strikes the ball, resulting in a slice. This is simply a bad motor habit that is likely to keep the golfer's handicap elevated. Although the stutterer has many motor habits that interfere with fluent speech, his habits are linked to powerful perceptions of inherent difficulty and to a belief that failure is inevitable when he must confront specific words, situations, and certain listeners. His fluency failures are also linked to lapses in confidence, changes in mood, and anxiety. All of these factors raise the stutterer's motor habits to a higher level of habit villainy, a level at which the consequences of habits are exacerbated.

This treatment program is not simply a random mix of approaches. Many people understand *eclectic* to mean *a random mix,* and that is not an accurate understanding of the term. *Eclectic* means *selecting what is judged to be best from various styles or ideas or selecting what is true or excellent.* This program is *eclectic* in the sense that it combines three viable treatment bases so that therapy focuses on the three common denominators I have identified. As you will see, the three bases do not carry equal weight in the program because the three common denominators do not carry equal weight in their impact on the disorder.

Learning Therapy

The first and most important base of the program is learning theory and therapy. In terms of learning, there are two objectives: (1) We must help the stutterer surrender his old, *maladaptive* responses to the *threat* and *experience* of stuttering. The word, *maladaptive,* means *bad adjustment,* and it fits perfectly into this context. Stuttering behaviors are adjustments that do not facilitate fluency, but interfere with fluency. We must help the stutterer identify and reject all behaviors he produces that make fluent speech difficult or impossible. We must also help the stutterer understand that he often produces these behaviors when he anticipates he will stutter, when he is threatened by stuttering. As has been observed many times by many writers and theorists, stuttering is a self-fulfilling prophecy disorder for the adult client. The anticipation, threat, or prophecy is sometimes very conscious and at other times quite subtle, operating at a low level of consciousness. When the stutterer anticipates fluency failure, he might choose an obvious coping behavior such as word substitution, circumlocution, or postponement, or he might create an abnormal motor set characterized by inappropriate articulatory position and excessive muscular tension at points in the speech mechanism focal to the phonetic makeup of the word he is trying to say. We must help the stutterer understand that these bad adjustments make it impossible for him to speak fluently, that by producing them, he is making fluency failure inevitable, and we must convince him that these behaviors must be eliminated in order that he might establish some control over his speech.

In addition to eliminating the behaviors that result from the *threat* of stuttering, the client must also eliminate behaviors associated with the *experience* of stuttering. These are the repetitions, postural fixations, and closures that are the core behaviors of stuttering, as well as the various timing behaviors used to end postponement or escape from fixations and oscillations. The *threat* and *experience* are not separable, of course. Without the *threat*, the *experience* is not likely to occur, but because the threat often operates at a low level of consciousness, any therapy directed only at anticipatory behaviors is not likely to succeed. It is far more practical to design a therapy that will reduce anticipatory behaviors to the lowest frequency level possible, but also prepare the stutterer to deal with the experience of stuttering when it occurs. Many therapies are inadequate in that they do not show the stutterer what to do when he stutters or when he expects to stutter. Van Riper's program is designed to address both the experience of stuttering and the expectation that stuttering will occur. The second goal relative to learning is to help the stutterer learn new, adaptive responses to the threat and experience of stuttering. These are responses that will facilitate fluency and counteract the maladaptive motor habits he has developed and nurtured over the years.

Servotherapy: Heightening Proprioceptive Awareness

The second base of Van Riper's program is *servotherapy*. Van Riper suggests that "since speech seems to be automatically controlled by feedback and there seems to be some real evidence that some failure in the auditory processing system produces the basic disruptions, we train the stutterer to monitor his speech by emphasizing proprioception and thus bypassing to some degree that auditory feedback system." The evidence to which Van Riper refers is, at best, inconclusive and is widely rejected by most experts today as a reasonable explanation for stuttering. I would submit, however, that even if research demonstrates no differences between stutterers and non-stutterers relative to their auditory feedback systems, there is still ample justification for teaching the stutterer to attend to proprioceptive feedback. Distorted auditory feedback or not, *stuttering is disordered motor speech*. In order to achieve fluency, we must either eliminate the basic cause of the disorder, or we must eliminate or modify the stutterer's maladaptive motor behaviors so fluency is possible. Given what we currently know about stuttering, we are not likely to find and remove the etiology in a given individual, but we can certainly change his motor speech behaviors.

The common sense argument goes something like this: If the stutterer creates the conditions that make fluency failures inevitable, he can create conditions that will facilitate fluency. By using various forms of servotherapy, we can heighten the stutterer's proprioceptive awareness so that changing his motor habits is easier. The golfer must be sensitive to the touch and physiology of his hands and arms if he is to correct a defective putting stroke. The diver must be aware of small details of movement and position in his entire body if he is to correct a flaw in a complicated dive. In the same way, the stutterer must be aware of articulatory postures and contacts and varying degrees of muscular tension so he can eliminate or modify the behaviors that interfere with fluency. Servotherapy represents the means to this end, even if it is not an end unto itself.

Psychotherapy: Dealing with the Emotional Aspects of Stuttering

The third base of this program is psychotherapy. Obviously, if one is not trained to administer formal psychotherapy, one should not attempt to do so. I would submit, however, that all speech and language therapy contains some of the basic elements of psychotherapy. The basic objectives of psychotherapy are to relieve anxiety that goes beyond routine, to develop self-esteem, and to increase one's ability to tolerate stress. Who among us can honestly say our lives have been so perfect, so problem-free, that we could not profit from a therapy that addresses these goals? Stutterers, as typical people with an atypical problem, often have needs in these areas. Any viable stuttering therapy, therefore, will address the basic objectives of psychotherapy. Most speech-language clinicians will not attempt to accomplish these goals formally, but by being good listeners and by being supportive, we can help stutterers deal more effectively with their fear, frustration, anxiety, guilt, and hostility. Therapy might provide an opportunity for catharsis that is available nowhere else, and catharsis is often inherently healing. If a clinician is working with a stutterer whose emotional problems are beyond her competence, she should immediately refer her client to a psychologist or psychiatrist. It is a virtual certainty that if a client has serious psychological problems, speech therapy alone will be relatively ineffective, no matter how good the therapy is or how skilled the clinician is.

The Design of Therapy: A Fully Integrated Program

This program is designed into four phases: (1) **Identification,** (2) **Desensitization,** (3) **Modification,** and (4) **Stabilization.** In the *Identification* phase, the stutterer explores, analyzes, and categorizes all the behaviors that comprise his stuttering patterns. In the *Desensitization* phase, we try to decrease the stutterer's speech-related anxieties and toughen him to the threat and experience of stuttering. In *Modification,* we help the stutterer reject his maladaptive behaviors and learn adaptive behaviors that will facilitate fluency. In *Stabilization,* we help the client make his modifications more quickly and automatically, and we address any lingering perceptual problems that might mitigate against long-term success.

The clinician should not think of these phases as absolutely discrete because they are not. It is true that identification must come before modification because the stutterer cannot change or eliminate maladaptive behavior unless he knows exactly what he is doing that is maladaptive, and unless he understands when and why he produces behaviors that disrupt fluency, but it should be obvious to the client and to the clinician that the stutterer never stops identifying. He will continue to identify stuttering behavior as long as he produces stuttering behavior. Van Riper describes desensitization as a separate phase of therapy, and some clinicians prefer to deal with it as a separate phase. I will suggest that a more realistic, and in most cases, a more efficient approach is to work on desensitization and modification simultaneously. I have found, both as a client and as a clinician, that the very process of learning how to modify maladaptive behaviors is desensitizing. In fact, becoming competent and confident in modifying techniques may be the most desensitizing thing the client can do. We should also consider that desensitization often continues into the stabilization phase because speech-related anxieties do not end when the stutterer learns how to modify. In the stabilization phase, the client not only engages in activities designed to desensitize, but he also perfects the skills he learned during the identification and modification phases.

It may be helpful to view the phases of therapy as convenient organizational demarcations that describe a general flow of therapy. The clinician should take care to understand the purpose, rationale, and procedures associated with each step and should avoid the temptation to arbitrarily force the client into a rigid step-by-step program. Stuttering is a moving target kind of disorder, which means that the clinician must constantly adjust to the client as his needs change from session to session, sometimes from minute to minute within a single session. The clinician should be prepared to retreat or move forward at any given time. One of the great strengths of this program is that it allows this kind of immediate adjustment. It is a fully integrated program, designed to deal with all aspects of the disorder. Each phase is related to every other phase in terms of theoretical foundation and in terms of long-term therapy goals.

The Schedule: How Long Will It Take?

Any therapy program, including this one, is most effective if the client is scheduled as often as possible. I am always a little amazed that an adult client who has been stuttering for many years believes he can "get cured up" in a few months by coming to therapy once a week for an hour. Let's take a look at the math for just a moment. There are 168 hours in a week, and 8,736 hours in a year. Assuming most people are awake 16 hours of each day, that would be 5,840 hours of awake time each year. Not even the most verbose person talks constantly when he is awake, of course, but most people live under circumstances that make talking likely or possible during those waking hours, and remember that the stutterer is as much affected by the *threat* of talking as by the *experience* of talking. How much impact can we expect, therefore, from 52 hours of therapy in one calendar year against the other 5,788 hours outside of therapy, during which the stutterer is faced with the same pressures, the same misperceptions, the same maladaptive motor habits that have mixed together to produce his stuttering problem? I am an exceptionally optimistic person by nature, and even I would have to say that a client's chances for long-term success with a one hour per week commitment are not very good.

This all leads us to Charles Van Riper's suggestion for a *minimal schedule of therapy,* which would be **one hour of individual therapy and one hour of group therapy three times per week and as much daily self-therapy as possible** for a period of three to four months for the completion of the identification, desensitization, and modification phases. The stabilization phase of therapy typically extends over a period of two years, although the sessions are gradually spread out.

When Van Riper described a *minimal schedule of therapy,* did he really believe most clients would commit this much time, and did he really believe the typical clinician has this much time in her schedule to devote to a single client? I doubt that he did, but I have no doubt about the intention of his message. He wanted to make it emphatically clear to both clients and clinicians that stuttering is a very complicated disorder, a disorder that permeates every aspect of the lives of those who own it, that it is not a disorder amenable to quick and easy solutions. Whatever commitment the client makes to treatment, it must be serious, and it must be significant. Based on my own clinical experiences, I believe this program can be effective with two or three individual sessions per week, but the clinician must make specific out-of-therapy assignments that keep the client focused on addressing his disorder every day. The client must make an absolute commitment to fulfilling these assignments, to engaging in self-therapy exercises every day, and to finding and meeting speaking challenges and opportunities whenever possible. On this schedule, the first three phases can be completed in approximately 12 months. No matter how much time is invested in the first three phases, stabilization will require another two years, BUT the client must remember that the sessions in stabilization are gradually spread out.

Chapter 15

MOTIVATING THE ADULT STUTTERER

M otivation should not be understood as a phase of therapy. It is essential to motivate the client at the beginning of therapy, of course, but there are motivation challenges throughout the process of therapy. Some of the more difficult motivation problems actually occur later in therapy when the client believes he has everything under control. I am always reminded in this regard that most motorcycle accidents occur at the beginning of the spring and then again in late fall. Why? Experts suggest that accidents occur early in the motorcycle season because riders are either just learning or are reviewing their skills, so they are vulnerable to mistakes born of incompetence. Toward the end of the motorcycle season, accidents are the products of overconfidence. Although the comparison might seem something of a stretch, stutterers just entering therapy often have motivation problems because they are not convinced they can do what needs to be done. After they have learned modification skills, they often believe they are invulnerable. They believe they have learned everything there is to know. The clinician will recognize the dangers at both ends of this confidence continuum as it relates to motivation, and she must be prepared to address them.

The importance of motivation in the treatment of stuttering cannot be exaggerated. Stuttering is a problem the client creates for himself. The client must accept responsibility for producing his stuttering behaviors, and he must accept responsibility for eliminating or modifying them. The success or failure of therapy depends heavily on the client's motivation and commitment, and far less on the clinician and the treatment program than the client may believe when he brings himself to the clinician for therapy.

When many clients show up for therapy, there is no doubt they want to be helped, but as I have already pointed out, being motivated to be healed is not the same thing as being motivated to do all that needs to be done to control one's speech. Nearly every adult stutterer I have met wants to be helped. I have met precious few who are motivated from the beginning to do the work they must do to become controlled speakers. Classroom teachers face this problem every day. There are students who show up with an attitude that says, "Teach us! We are willing to be here, teacher, not much more than that, but we expect you to teach us. We will only do what is absolutely necessary, teacher, and we will look for every shortcut possible, but we expect you to teach us, and we expect you to teach us in a manner that is consistently entertaining and never hard." Clinicians encounter stuttering clients with the same attitude. "Here I am, clinician. I have done my part. I showed up. Now, take my stuttering away, please. Do it quickly. Do it painlessly, and please make no demands on me. I have suffered enough." The clinician's challenge is not to take the stuttering away, but to do everything she can to motivate her client to assume responsibility for his problem, to assume responsibility for the solution to his problem, and to make a commitment to do all that is necessary to make that solution happen. The clinician's role in this process is important, and that role will be clearly described in the pages that follow, but the clinician is not a magician, and she is not a healer.

It is impossible to identify all of the motivation problems that might occur with adult stutterers, but we can focus on four fairly common problems: (1) goal-setting, (2) the aversiveness of stuttering, (3) lack of trust in the clinician, and (4) reluctance to surrender the secondary gains of stuttering.

Setting Goals Too High or Too Low

Goal-setting can be a problem when the client moves too far in either direction. A client might set goals too low because he has an inappropriately low aspiration level. The stutterer who carries his disorder into adulthood might develop a self-concept dominated by his stuttering. His speech disorder becomes his identity. He perceives himself as incompetent and undesirable, as a person who cannot rise above his fluency failures. He sets goals that are too low because he believes he is not capable of meeting any but the most modest goals. We can help motivate this client by helping him understand that stuttering is only a characteristic of speech, not a definition of who one he is as a person. We can help him realistically assess his assets and liabilities. In this process, he will undoubtedly discover that while stuttering is a liability, it is more than adequately balanced by talents and positive personal qualities that are far more important, far more personally defining than stuttering. If the client's misperceptions about stuttering are not challenged and corrected, stuttering will eventually contaminate the client's entire self-image. It is the clinician's responsibility to challenge these perceptions, to set the record straight, to convince the client that a self-image limited to one characteristic of speech is a far too narrow self-image to do any person justice. Once the client is able to gain a more realistic view about where stuttering fits into his own big picture, he will be able to set goals that are more reasonable and more worthy of his true abilities.

Another stutterer might set goals that are unrealistically high. Most commonly, a client might aim for *perfect* speech because he mistakenly believes that normal speech is perfect. This view is radically wrong, of course, but it is easily fixed by having the client observe nonstutterers in an analytic and objective manner. He will quickly discover that not even the most facile of normal speakers is perfectly fluent. Other high goals are more troublesome. A client might set unrealistically high vocational goals, for example. He might delude himself into believing that stuttering and stuttering alone is the barrier that stands between him and unlimited success. This client also needs to take a hard, objective look at his assets and liabilities. In the process, he will learn that stuttering does not explain one's inability to complete a course in nuclear engineering. It does not explain one's failure on the bar exam. It does not explain why a 5'5", 130-pound high school running back who runs the 40 yard dash in 6.5 seconds will never be a star in the National Football League. Might uncontrolled stuttering be a factor in a person's vocational failure? Of course, but it is very seldom the whole story, and in many cases, it is just a footnote. Whether we have a client who always sees the glass half full or a client who believes the glass is a dribbler planted in a conspiracy to make him look bad, we must help the client assess himself objectively so he can set goals relative to fluency that are challenging, but reasonable and attainable.

The Unpleasantness of Stuttering

The aversiveness of stuttering has a powerful potential for dampening motivation. What makes stuttering aversive? One obvious answer is that it is embarrassing, and it does not take a genius to figure out why. Stuttered speech is broken speech, and because it is broken in unusual and unexpected ways, listeners often find it amusing. When listeners laugh at the stutterer, he is understandably embarrassed. Stuttering is also aversive because it makes the stutterer feel out of control. The unpleasantness of stuttering is a serious problem because unless the stutterer is willing to experience his abnormality voluntarily, he will not make much progress in therapy. The client must be able to feel, watch, and hear his stuttering in order to understand it. He must have some objective understanding about his stuttering before he can change it. The sensitive clinician, in working with an adult stutterer, will concede that there are good reasons for the stutterer to be uncomfortable with his stuttering. At the same time, she must convince him that only to the extent he is willing to stutter openly and on demand, and only as he develops an objective attitude about his behaviors, will he have a realistic chance to address them with understanding and change them in a manner that will promote fluency.

A History of Failure Breeds Distrust

The clinician is sometimes surprised that her client is undermotivated because he does not trust her. From whence cometh this distrust? The client is often wary of the clinician and of therapy because he has been down the therapy path before, and he has not found success. He has found despair and failure and frustration, but he has not found success, which is precisely why he has come knocking on another clinician's door. Consistent with that part of human nature that always claims credit for success and never accepts responsibility for failure, the client does not blame himself for past therapy disasters. He blames past clinicians, and he blames past therapies. Those people and those programs failed him, and he comes to the new clinician with no reason to believe there will be a successful outcome this time. It should be clear to the clinician that she is not responsible for what has happened in the past, whether or not past clinicians were competent, whether or not past therapies were wisely selected and properly administered, whether or not the client made reasonable time and energy commitments to these therapies. Nevertheless, the present clinician must accept the fact that progress today WILL be affected by the baggage of failures the client brings to the present process. The clinician must help the client understand his role in whatever failures occurred in previous therapy experiences, and she must cultivate the client's trust. Without this trust, it will be impossible to motivate, and without motivation, the present therapy will simply become one more pothole on the highway of failure.

The Advantages of Stuttering . . . No Kidding!

Some clients are not motivated to eliminate or control their stuttering because they do not want to surrender the *rewards* of nonfluency. The stutterer is often relieved of communicative responsibility because he stutters. He does not have to make phone calls, run errands, and give reports at school or at work because he stutters. He does not have to be sociable. He does not have to answer questions. He does not have to assume leadership positions. If he gives up stuttering, he might be expected to do all of these things and more.

Stuttering is often a convenient excuse for failure. If the stutterer is rebuffed when he asks a girl for a date, he can rationalize that she rejected him because he is a stutterer. If he applies for a job but does not get it, he can complain that he was not hired because that boss does not like stutterers. If he does not get into medical school, it's because the selection committee views stutterers as intellectually inferior, and it matters little that the selection committee had no idea he was a stutterer. Some years ago, I worked with a college-age stutterer who was a prelaw student. When he could not get into any of the law schools to which he applied, he complained that he was rejected because he was a stutterer. When I asked how he had performed on the Law School Admission Test (LSAT), which is used by law schools to select candidates, he confessed that his scores were well below the admissions standards established by these schools. I could never convince him that he was turned down, not because he stuttered, but because his academic record was not strong enough. He was sure there was a conspiracy among all these schools to keep him out because he stuttered and because his stuttering would be an embarrassment to any school that did accept him.

If we take stuttering away from this kind of person, we force him to face other liabilities in his life, many of which are far more serious threats to success than stuttering. We must somehow convince the stutterer that the advantages of fluency are greater than the advantages of stuttering.

The Cost-Payoff Assessment

There are some specific strategies that can be used to motivate the adult stutterer. One of the most effective strategies is to help the client assess the *costs* and *payoffs* of therapy. I alluded to this strategy in Chapter 10. I want to address it more completely here.

In order to convince the client that he should make a full and enthusiastic commitment to therapy, we help him determine if the benefits are worth the costs. We must never suggest that therapy is easy and painless, because it is neither, but we can persuade the client that the end results of therapy are worth whatever the client must contribute to make it work. The costs come in a variety of forms. Obviously, one of the costs is financial. There will also be a considerable investment of time and energy. The stutterer in therapy must be willing to risk failure, and he must be willing to endure temporary unpleasantness. He must be willing to be purposely abnormal, and he must be willing to break out of his stereotypical patterns of behavior. He must be willing to admit to his fears and anxieties, and he must talk about them openly and without shame. These are some of the *costs* of therapy, and they are significant, but the payoffs of successful therapy are more significant.

The clinician must be sensitive to the fact that the average client will be more keenly aware of the costs than the payoffs. It is natural for most people to be more aware of pain than pleasure, to remember sadness more vividly than joy. The clinician must help the client understand that the balance between costs and payoffs in stuttering therapy really comes down on the side of payoffs, even if in the beginning, the costs seem to loom larger.

The clinician should help the client understand how fluency will change his life in powerfully positive ways. Fluency has the potential to positively impact the client's interpersonal relationships. As he becomes more fluent, he will become a more confident and poised communicator. He will be more comfortable in his interactions with people he knows well, and he will find it easier to establish relationships with people he does not know. Many stutterers find that their vocational opportunities increase as a direct consequence of greater fluency. As more vocational and social doors open, and as the client feels more comfortable walking through these doors, his self-esteem will improve dramatically. In a very real sense, fluency removes the bushel that often hides the stutterer's light. This will seem an exaggeration only to those who are insensitive to the influence of stuttering on the lives of those who live with it.

It should be noted that the cost-payoff discussion rarely occurs only one time. Throughout the therapy process, and especially during difficult or painful periods, the clinician must remind the client that the time, effort, and pain are worthwhile investments toward future fluency and the positive, life-altering by-products of that fluency.

The Clinician's Competence and Commitment

The clinician can also motivate her client by revealing her clinical competence and her commitment to the client. The clinician reveals her competence by demonstrating her knowledge and understanding of stuttering. This does not mean she assumes a condescending and patronizing attitude. It does mean that the clinician shares her knowledge and understanding in a direct and professional manner with the clear intent to assist, educate, enlighten, and encourage. It means the clinician uses professional terminology when it is appropriate to do so, but she always explains what terms mean. This is not about making the clinician look *smart*. It is about making the client feel more comfortable and more confident. Using the *language* of the disorder sends the message that there are aspects of stuttering that are known and understood—behaviors and experiences shared by many people who own the disorder. The message has the potential to motivate the client because he will believe, as do all people, that what is known and understood is less frightening and less intimidating than what is mysterious and shrouded in ignorance. Furthermore, he will be more inclined to believe in a knowledgeable and confident clinician than in a clinician who seems to know less about stuttering than he does. The clinician's language and general demeanor should also reflect a calm objectivity about stuttering that suggests this a problem than can be managed, and we simply need to get on with the task of managing it. The clinician should answer the client's questions as honestly and insightfully as possible, admitting to areas of disagreement among experts, outlining possible answers suggested by relevant research, and highlighting what she believes are the most plausible answers. The clinician can demonstrate her competence by always being thoroughly prepared, by being well-organized, by being flexible enough to move forward more quickly than she anticipated or by moving back a step or two when necessary.

She will reveal her commitment by communicating genuine understanding and concern, by being willing to share in the client's abnormal behaviors in an attempt to understand them, and by being available for phone calls and conferences when the client has unscheduled problems. It is very important that the clinician makes sure the client understands the difference between *commitment* and *role*. The clinician must be fully committed to the therapy process and to the client, but as mentioned earlier, her role is clinician, not healer. By making her role clear and by emphasizing the strength of her commitment to the therapy process, the clinician will be taking another important step toward motivating the client to be fully committed to therapy and to accept complete responsibility for progress.

Persuade the Client that Success Is Attainable

The clinician can motivate by providing hope. When people are unmotivated to do something, it is often because they have no reason to believe the *something* will make a difference. If the clinician can convince the client that there is reason to believe therapy will yield significant benefits, the task of therapy will be far less onerous for everyone concerned. The best source of hope is a successful client, someone who can provide testimony about how therapy has changed his life. This strategy, as I mentioned earlier, has been used with great effectiveness by people selling weight loss programs and by people who counsel drug addicts and alcoholics. A person with a problem in any of these areas is far more likely to be convinced about the efficacy of treatment if the treatment is promoted by someone who has lived the problem and has used the treatment to overcome the problem than if the same program is promoted by someone who has always been thin, clean, and sober. The stutterer too is likely to be motivated by the story of someone who has been victorious over stuttering. Empathy is a powerful motivational tool. The successful client in the flesh will have the greatest impact, of course, but *before* and *after* video or audio tapes are also effective. The only caution I would add, as I mentioned in Chapter 10, is that testimonials are often used to sell programs that offer more than they can deliver, programs that promise quick and easy solutions. I am suggesting here that testimony be given by someone who has walked a legitimate road to therapy success, not a quick sprint to an artificial fluency that, like a Botox beauty enhancement, is here today and gone tomorrow.

The clinician can also provide hope by charting the client's progress in therapy. Progress often comes in steps so small the client is not aware of his improvement. By counting and graphing behaviors, the clinician can help the client track even the smallest changes. As long as the client can see evidence that he is moving forward, he will be motivated to continue his efforts. If he feels like he is simply treading water, or if he feels he is regressing, it will be very difficult to keep him motivated.

Show the Client the Road to Fluency

Another strategy that helps to motivate the client is to map out the therapy sequence. Just as knowing what grade one is in or knowing how many credit hours have been earned helps motivate a student to keep working hard, knowing where one is in therapy helps the client maintain his effort. The process of mapping out the sequence of therapy inspires trust and confidence in the clinician because the client believes there is a plan the clinician understands. If the client can see that he is moving from one step to the next, he will be more willing to expend effort in therapy and to complete the outside assignments that become increasingly important as treatment progresses. I am convinced that understanding always promotes motivation in the adult client. The clinician should explain the method, purpose, and rationale of every step in the therapy process, and she should let the client know when he graduates from one step to the next.

Involve the Client in Setting Goals

The client will be more effectively motivated if he participates in establishing short-term and long-term goals than if these goals are simply set for him. To this point, we have tried to persuade the client that the problem belongs to him. We must also convince him to take possession of the solution. The client will be more inclined to give a full effort to a therapy program if he is responsible for setting the goals of the program. The clinician must provide guidance in setting goals, of course, because as mentioned earlier, some clients do not set realistic goals. They may aim too high or too low. They may expect too much too soon, or they may expect too little with no deadlines at all. The clinician should assist in setting goals, therefore, but the client should be actively involved, and he must assume full responsibility for whatever goals are established. An important message that will come through this cooperative effort is that the clinician cannot bestow fluency. Fluency comes with time and effort on the part of the client. One more time . . . the clinician is guide and teacher, not healer. You have heard it said that *where there is a will, there is a way.* In the case of stuttering, the clinician can and should show the way, but the client must provide the will.

Reward Progress

Finally, the clinician can motivate by providing reinforcement for progress. The primary reinforcers in therapy are the clinician's approval and the client's sense of accomplishment. The clinician's approval may be conveyed verbally or nonverbally. It is crucial that the client always understand exactly what is being reinforced. For example, during identification, the clinician will reinforce accurate descriptions of stuttering behaviors, not fluency. During identification, we WANT the client to stutter. Stuttering is essential. The clinician may, in fact, reward the client for his willingness to stutter openly. As therapy continues and goals change, progress is redefined. During modification, the clinician rewards a modification, no matter how long it takes to get it done right. During stabilization, the clinician rewards a modification if it is made correctly and quickly.

It is important that we shift to self-approval as quickly and completely as possible so the client's sense of accomplishment becomes the dominant reinforcer. The client will not have the clinician with him in the outside world to evaluate his speech and to reinforce his successful modifications of stuttered words. The client must become his own clinician, his own source of criticism and reinforcement.

Chapter 16

IDENTIFICATION

The Importance of Identifying Stuttering Behaviors

The first task of this program is to identify the behaviors the client uses when he stutters. Both the clinician and the client must guard against rushing through this phase because identification lays the foundation for everything that follows, especially modification, the cornerstone of long-term success. The process of identifying behaviors is often tedious and requires intense concentration. It also heightens the stutterer's awareness of his abnormality, which in turn, makes him even more uncomfortable with his stuttering than he was prior to therapy. The client will endure the tedium and the discomfort if he understands why this phase is so critical. The rationale for this phase, and the reason for its importance, is very simple. The stutterer cannot change behavior unless he knows *when* it occurs, *what* the behavior is, and *why* he produces it. The process of identification then can be reduced to these three words: *when, what,* and *why.*

As difficult as it may be to believe, even a severe stutterer is usually not acutely aware of the bizarre behaviors he produces. He is usually aware of the *when* of his more complex moments of stuttering, but he typically is unable to identify the behaviors that comprise his moments, and he usually has no idea why he produced these behaviors. In many cases, he thinks these behaviors happen beyond his control. Remember that many of these behaviors have become habitualized. The client is no more aware of habitualized stuttering behaviors than normal speakers are aware of the habitual mannerisms, verbal and nonverbal, they produce.

It quickly becomes obvious that the stutterer tends to describe all of his behaviors as simply, *stuttering.* When he produces a moment and the clinician asks him to describe what he did, he is likely to say, "I stuttered." If the clinician asks, "What exactly did you do when you stuttered," he might reply,

"Well, I exactly stuttered. I could not get the words out. I got stuck. . . ." In the early stages of therapy, the client does not differentiate among repetitions, closures, postural fixations, avoidances, starters, etc. These are all "stutterings." The clinician must teach the stutterer to make distinctions among these behaviors because, as I have already indicated and as I will continue to stress, *not all stuttering behaviors are created equal.* Only when the client is able to recognize individual categories of behaviors will he understand why he produces a certain behavior in a certain phonetic context or why he produces a given behavior at a specific point in a sequence of behaviors, or even why he produces sequences of behaviors instead of isolated behaviors. Until the client understands all of this, stuttering will remain a mystery to him, and as long as stuttering remains a mystery, he will continue to believe that stuttering happens to him. As long as that belief continues, the prognosis for improvement is poor. The clinician must make the client understand that stuttering behaviors are volitional behaviors, produced for specific reasons. Only when he truly understands that HE *decides* to stutter, that HE *decides* what he will do when he stutters, . . . only then will he understand that he can make other speech decisions that will make fluent speech possible.

The Client's Responsibility

It must be emphasized that the clinician cannot do this task for the client. The responsibility for identification is immediately placed on the stutterer, ready or not. Keeping in mind that we want the client to recognize the *when,* *what,* and *why* of his behaviors, the client's first task is to signal the production of any behavior he considers "stuttering." While the client and clinician engage in conversation, which the clinician tape records, the client raises his hand each time he stutters. Even the most effectively engaged client will miss some of his moments, but if it becomes apparent he is missing too many moments, the clinician should stop the tape, rewind, and ask the client to listen again. It is highly unlikely the client will miss his moments when he hears himself on tape because he is now detached from them, but if he does, the clinician should note these stutterings for him, explaining that it is not uncommon for stutterers to *miss* small moments, or to overlook moments because they believe they are deceiving their listeners with behaviors they think are covering up their stutterings. It is the clinician's responsibility to make sure the stutterer recognizes and acknowledges all his moments, no matter how small or insignificant they may be. As I remind my clients, small moments beget bigger moments, and it is easier to change small moments characterized by muscle tension that is just beyond the threshold of normal than it is to change moments that are the products of panic and muscular tension so excessive that the client feels out of control.

When the client is able to signal the production of most of his moments, the clinician shifts attention to the *what* of his behaviors. That is, when the client recognizes that he has produced a stuttering, he is challenged to describe what he did. Specifically, the clinician asks the client to describe the motoric adjustments he made that produced stuttering. Notice that the emphasis is always on what the client *does, on articulatory decisions he makes.* In order to accurately describe a moment of stuttering, the client often needs to duplicate the stuttering because the original production is too fleeting. Most clients are not able to duplicate their stutterings without training and practice. The clinician might have to imitate the stuttering before the client attempts to duplicate the original moment. The more often the client repeats a moment, even if there are slight deviations from the original, the more sensitive will be his motoric awareness, and the more conscious he will be that he is, in fact, making physiological decisions that produce fluency failures. The more thoroughly the client understands exactly what he does that creates the stuttering and prevents fluency, the more prepared he will be to make decisions about modifying his behaviors in ways that will facilitate fluency.

The emphasis in this stage should always be on *feeling* moments, not on *hearing* them. If the client attempts to understand his moments based on what he hears, he will never successfully modify. What he hears is the product of what he does. If he waits to modify until after he hears his moments of stuttering, it's too late. The production has already been completed. Our emphasis must be on what he is doing physiologically that creates the fluency failure because that is what he can and must change in order to produce the fluency he wants.

As the client becomes more adept at recognizing the *when* and *what* of his moments, we begin to challenge him to understand the *why*. If the client understands why he postpones, for example, and if he understands the futility of this kind of behavior, he is more likely to reject it as a reasonable and effective reaction to his perception of speech difficulty. If the client understands that a stuttering tremor is superimposed on a core behavior, he will shift his attention away from the tremor and onto the core behavior. He will concentrate on eliminating or modifying the core behavior, knowing that the tremor cannot occur if there is no core behavior upon which to superimpose it. Although understanding this kind of problem at the cognitive level is not enough to solve the problem, it certainly establishes a foundation upon which a solution can be constructed.

Depending upon the client's individual needs or upon the clinician's preference, identification might focus on one category of behaviors at a time or upon all categories at once. Although the client is initially overwhelmed, I prefer to identify all behaviors at the same time because this affords the client an opportunity to understand how stuttering behaviors are related to one another. The clinician should keep in mind that, during the identification stage, she should not avoid using the stuttering terminology. Giving a behavior a name enhances its identity and helps the client remember it. Applying the terminology also takes away some of the mystery of stuttering. The client often behaves as though he is the first person in human history to experience some of these behaviors. If the clinician can apply names and explanations to these behaviors, the client will become convinced that he is not unique and that these behaviors are known and understood.

Even though the clinician might decide to deal with all behaviors as they occur during the identification phase, our discussion will be clearer and more organized if we consider how to identify within major divisions of behavior.

Begin by Identifying "Fluent" Stutterings

Van Riper suggests the client and clinician should first look for what he calls *target behaviors* or *fluent stutterings*. He describes these as moments characterized by minimal temporal alteration, easy unforced repetitions or slight prolongations, with no struggle, avoidance or postponement. By finding these easy moments of stuttering, the client will understand that stuttering is not an *all or nothing* phenomenon. He produces varying degrees of abnormality. Finding *target behaviors* or *fluent stutterings* is a strategy that will help convince the client that stuttering is decided or volitional behavior. The client decides whether or not he will stutter. If he decides to stutter, he decides the severity of the stuttering he will produce. A given word will be produced fluently, stuttered easily, or fractured badly, depending upon the client's decisions about the physiological adjustments he makes in his speech mechanism. The decisions about how much he will struggle depend upon how he perceives the word he is trying to say. If he perceives the word to be *easy,* he will make physiological adjustments that facilitate fluency. If he perceives the word to be *somewhat difficult but not impossible,* he will make physiological adjustments that will make fluency difficult and stuttering likely. If he perceives the word to be *impossible,* he will make physiological adjustments that will make fluency impossible and stuttering inevitable. Finding easy moments will increase his sensitivity to the range of articulatory choices he constantly makes at a relatively low level of consciousness. As he becomes more acutely aware of these choices, one might assume he will be more likely to make choices that interfere less with fluency, and this is, in fact, what happens for most clients.

Identifying the Anticipatory Behaviors

When identifying *avoidance* behaviors, the clinician does not ask the stutterer to stop avoiding. At this point in therapy, we want the client to avoid so he recognizes and understands this category of behaviors, but we must make sure we reward the client for discovering and understanding these behaviors. We should do nothing to suggest that these are desirable behaviors. They are not. They are behaviors of denial, and they are extremely harmful to the client's long-term success. We do notice, however, that when the client begins to confront his avoidance behaviors, they tend to decrease in frequency, probably because he realizes they are not camouflaging his stuttering as effectively as he thought they were.

It should be noted that identifying avoidance behaviors is particularly important with the milder stutterer who tends to avoid more often than the severe stutterer. Avoidance is often the dominant feature of the mild client's stuttering because he is able to use it with greater success than the severe stutterer. The clinician must help this client understand that avoidance compounds the fear factor in stuttering. If fear and anxiety become potent enough, avoidance behaviors become virtually useless. It is far better for the mild stutterer to stop using avoidance behaviors even though, in the short term, this will result in a dramatic increase in more overt behaviors. Once the mild stutterer allows himself to stutter openly, he can begin to develop the objective attitude about stuttering that is so crucial to long-term success. Until he stops avoiding, he is not unlike the closet alcoholic who insists he has everything under control just because he is not falling down in a stupor. The closet alcoholic fails to recognize that denial is not the same thing as control. Neither the alcoholic nor the stutterer has a meaningful chance at getting well until he admits to himself and to others that he has a problem. For the stutterer, the biggest step toward admission occurs when he surrenders his avoidance behaviors and faces his overt stuttering directly.

When the client identifies *postponement* behaviors, he should understand that postponement is closely related to avoidance. By way of review, both avoidance and postponement are used when the stutterer anticipates he will stutter. They are used to fend off stuttering–avoidance by not saying a certain word or entering a certain situation, and postponement by delaying the speech attempt or entrance into the situation, in the hope that his fear of the word or situation will subside. The clinician should appreciate that both avoidance and postponement are powerfully reinforced because they sometimes work for the stutterer. If he avoids by substituting a nonfeared word for a feared word, he is usually fluent. If he postpones long enough, he will be able to say the word fluently because fear fluctuates. These *successes* can be very misleading, however. The clinician must help the client understand that the real problem with both avoidance and postponement behaviors is that, even though they are used by the stutterer when he fears and they are used by him to cope with the fear, they actually cause the fear to increase. As his speech fears escalate, so does the severity of his more observable stuttering behaviors. These behaviors will eventually become so involved and bizarre they will look and sound more abnormal than the overt stuttering the client is trying to avoid or postpone. In the long run, these behaviors are truly counterproductive. The sooner the client understands this fact, and the sooner he abandons these behaviors, the sooner he will begin real progress in addressing his stuttering problem.

While the client is analyzing his postponement behaviors, he will discover the set of behaviors known as *starters* or *timing devices*. These behaviors are used to end postponement, or in the absence of postponement, they are used to establish a rhythm to facilitate production of a target word. The client's natural awareness of starters is not as acute as his awareness of postponement behaviors because starters are less calculated than postponements. They are reactions to a sense of being *stuck*, of being unable to move forward in his articulatory efforts. The clinician may need to demonstrate the client's starter behaviors, and the client may need to duplicate them a number of times before he develops enough awareness that he is able to identify and describe these behaviors accurately.

Identifying the Cues That Precipitate Fear

The adult stutterer is usually aware of the linguistic cues associated with stuttering, but he is rarely able to explain why he perceives certain sounds or words as *difficult* in comparison to other sounds and words he perceives as *easy*. He simply believes that certain sounds and words are inherently difficult to produce. Not only must the clinician help the client identify these linguistic cues, she must also persuade him that these sounds and words are not inherently difficult.

The clinician might begin by explaining the factors that contribute to a word or sound becoming a cue for stuttering. For example, linguistic cues often have their origins in situations of fluency failure. A word might become a feared word because the stutterer has difficulty with that word during an important conversation with a significant person. Emotionally loaded words, such as "love" or "mother" are more likely to become feared words than words that are fairly neutral. Nouns, verbs, adjectives, and adverbs are more likely than function words to become feared words because they carry more meaning. A stutterer's name is often difficult for him to say, regardless of its phonetic composition, because it is extremely personal and because there are few avoidance options to be exercised when one is about to say his name.

The point is, the stutterer must be persuaded that his word and sound fears are not random, and that these fears probably have little to do with real phonetic and motoric complexity. A word or sound is *difficult* because the client believes it is difficult. As I mentioned earlier in this book, when I was an adolescent stutterer, I had a terrible time with words that began with the "h" sound. This problem began when I had trouble saying my last name, "Hulit." I came to the erroneous conclusion that what made my name difficult to say was the "h" sound, so I quickly generalized this fear to other words beginning with "h," including "hello," and "hi." Even if you know little or nothing about phonology, you will recognize that there is no sound in our language that is easier to produce than "h." There are no manipulations of the articulators. It is simply a mildly forceful release of air, but for me, it was the most difficult and diabolic sound ever devised, and it remained a *difficult* sound until I learned there is absolutely nothing inherently difficult about this sound. It was difficult only because I believed it was difficult. Once the adult client understands the perceptual aspect of the stuttering problem, he will realize that he controls not only the motoric behaviors of stuttering, but even the cues that precipitate stuttering. This is a critically important insight. The client needs to know that he controls the problem, from the time he recognizes a word as *difficult* through all the physiological maladjustments he makes in reaction to that perception of difficulty.

When the stutterer begins to examine his situation fears, he soon discovers that the primary determinant of *easy* or *difficult* situations is the listener involved. The clinician should help the client identify those characteristics of listeners that signal *difficulty* for him, and more importantly, help the stutterer understand why these characteristics are threatening. In the context of this personal exploration, the client should recognize that certain features such as *authority status* are somewhat threatening to most people, while other features such as age or sex may signal difficulty because of the stutterer's unique personal experiences. That is, if he has had a number of fluency failures in conversations with older men, *older* and *male* might become cues for stuttering. The stutterer might not be able to change his perceptions of *easy* and *difficult* situations or listeners, but understanding that he does perceive differentially and understanding the reasons for these perceptions will almost certainly reduce his anxiety about them, because, as I have repeatedly noted, what is known and understood is less frightening than what is unknown and misunderstood. The process of identifying easy and difficult situations will also demonstrate to the client that situations can be arranged along a continuum from *very easy* to *extremely difficult*. Just as the stutterer's motoric abnormalities range from mild to severe, he also experiences a range of emotional reactions to situations and listeners. Again, it is important that the client understands that he is the one who decides where he will be on either continuum.

No matter the level of consciousness, these are his decisions, not the products of some unknown force over which he has no control.

Identifying the Core Behaviors of Stuttering

The most important task in the identification phase is to recognize and understand the core behaviors of stuttering, the oscillations and fixations known as *repetitions, postural fixations,* and *closures.* These are the key or central behaviors in the complex of stuttering behaviors. If we successfully attack the core behaviors, stuttering does not exactly come down like a house of cards, but it certainly ceases to be the problem it once was, and the prognosis for long-term success looks very bright.

The most effective way for the stutterer to analyze the core behaviors is to compare motoric abnormality with fluent production. It is perhaps best to seek out *triads of behavior:* (1) an abnormal, or *stuttered,* production of a given word, (2) a *fluent* stuttering of the same word, and (3) a *normal* production of the word. As the client produces the triad several times, he compares each member of the triad with the other members in order to discover the motoric features that differentiate them. Each time the triad is repeated, the clinician should instruct the client to use a different order. That is, the first triad might consist of a severely stuttered production of the word, a fluent stuttering of that word, and a normal production of that word. On the next attempt, it might be normal, fluent stuttering, and stuttered. The third attempt might be fluent stuttering, normal, and stuttered. The client should be challenged to produce the triad in all possible orders. We want the client to feel the motoric contrasts, of course, but we also want him to sense that he is in control, that he can create tension, and he can back away from tension. He can also produce a targeted word without excessive tension. In the triad exercise, we are setting the stage for the kinds of *on demand* adjustments the client will learn to make in the modification phase of therapy.

As I noted in the opening of this chapter, the emphasis in identification should always be on what the stutterer feels, not on what he hears. The clinician stresses proprioceptive analysis and understanding. The client might have to repeat a single moment of stuttering 10 to 20 times before he senses what he is doing motorically that is creating these core behaviors. This work must be done meticulously. The more completely the client identifies these behaviors, the more quickly and effectively he will adjust his physiological preparation and execution so that fluency is facilitated. As he identifies the core behaviors, he will recognize that there are two powerful common denominators underlying them: (1) **inappropriate articulatory position** and (2) **excessive muscular tension.** With the clinician's help, he will also come to understand that adjustments to these two factors are the keys to promoting fluency.

Identifying the Behaviors Superimposed on the Core Behaviors

The remaining overt features of stuttering, including *tremors, interrupters, disguise reactions, complemental air, abulia,* and *vocal fry,* are identified and analyzed as behaviors directly related to the core behaviors. The primary therapy goal relative to these behaviors is to make the client understand that these behaviors are absolutely dependent on the core behaviors for their existence, and to make him understand how each of these behaviors is related to specific core behaviors. The client should understand that we do not directly target these behaviors in modification therapy because they will be eliminated as a consequence of eliminating the repetitions, closures, and postural fixations upon which they are superimposed.

Understanding the Emotions Associated with Stuttering

Finally, the client must identify and analyze his emotional reactions to stuttering. Typical reactions include frustration, shame, hostility, and embarrassment. By identifying and talking about these feelings, the client will realize that his reactions are quite normal–normal for stutterers, of course, but also normal for all speakers when they experience communicative failures. There is also a payoff more immediate than understanding. There is a catharsis in this exercise of *True Stuttering Confessions* that usually results in an immediate reduction in the intensity of the client's negative emotions. We all know that sometimes just talking about the negative feelings that poison our souls makes us feel better. The stutterer is quite ordinary in this sense. As he talks about the anger, frustration, and pain associated with his stuttering, he begins to feel better . . . in spite of himself. I do not want to suggest that just talking is a sufficient solution to the negative emotions problem because it is not, but it is an important beginning. In the next chapter, we will consider specific, and definitely more frontal, attacks on the negative emotions component of the larger stuttering problem.

Chapter 17

DESENSITIZATION

The Role of Anxiety in Stuttering

As we have already observed, anxiety is a major component of advanced stuttering. When the stutterer is relaxed, comfortable, and confident, he tends to be fluent. When he is tense, anxious, and insecure, there is a significant increase in the frequency and severity of his nonfluencies. We have also observed that certain linguistic and situation cues prompt the stutterer to be anxious about his ability to speak fluently. Because of this anxiety, the stutterer produces maladaptive physiological adjustments in his speech mechanism and stuttering follows. The purpose of desensitization therapy is to reduce the anxiety component of the stuttering problem. The goal is to disassociate stuttering responses from the stimuli that seem to evoke them. It would be unrealistic to hope that we can completely eliminate the negative emotions associated with stuttering since even nonstutterers are vulnerable to fluency failures precipitated by similar emotions. In fact, the stutterer needs to experience some fear and some stuttering if he is to learn to adapt or modify his behaviors in ways that will facilitate fluency.

Perhaps the greatest benefit of speech-related anxiety is that it helps the stutterer monitor his speech more effectively. There's nothing like a little fear to help all of us perform optimally. Any competent actor will confess that if he feels no anxiety before going on stage, his performance will probably be poor. Anxiety motivates the actor to perform well, and some anxiety pushes the stutterer to concentrate on producing the adaptive behaviors he must use in order to maintain fluency in stressful speaking situations. The emphasis is on *some* anxiety. If the anxiety is overwhelming, the stutterer will be paralyzed by his fear, and speech failure is inevitable. In the interest of reinforcing the idea that the stutterer is an ordinary person with an extraordinary problem, it should be noted that in nonstressful situations, the typical stutterer is likely to be fluent and does not need to do anything special in order to maintain fluent speech.

There are several strategies by which varying degrees of desensitization can be achieved, including the following: (1) *counterconditioning,* (2) *negative practice,* (3) *adaptation,* (4) *nonreinforcement,* and (5) *negative suggestion.*

Counterconditioning in Systematic Desensitization Therapy

The traditional form of desensitization therapy, and an approach still widely used, is based on *counterconditioning.* Counterconditioning is a procedure based on Joseph Wolpe's concept of *reciprocal inhibition* which is stated as follows: "If a response incompatible with anxiety can be made to occur in the presence of anxiety-evoking stimuli, it will weaken the bond between these stimuli and the anxiety responses." Reciprocals of anxiety include eating, relaxing, being assertive, and sexual behavior. This means, for example, that a person cannot be anxious and relaxed at the same time. These two states are incompatible. I can be one or the other, but I cannot be both simultaneously. The reciprocals most often used in desensitization therapy with stutterers are relaxation and assertive behavior.

Systematic desensitization therapy utilizing relaxation as the counterconditioner begins with the creation of a hierarchy of situations ranked according to their potential to evoke anxiety. The clinician asks the client to identify 5 to 10 situations that are mildly stressful. She then asks him to identify 5 to 10 situations that are extremely stressful, and then she asks him to identify 5 to 10 situations that would be moderately stressful. The client is now looking at 15 to 30 speaking situations that produce anxiety for him. The clinician asks the client to rank order these situations from the least anxiety-evoking to the most anxiety-evoking. It should be noted that the hierarchy rarely remains constant. It should be reevaluated at the beginning of each desensitization session. The clinician should ask the client to determine if the situations are still in the right order, and she should give him a chance to add or delete situations as well. Sometimes the hierarchy will be rearranged as a consequence of changing conditions in the client's life. Whatever the hierarchy happens to be for a given session, however, desensitization therapy progresses through the following steps: (1) The clinician helps the client relax, usually using some version of progressive relaxation or by direct suggestion. Clinicians sometimes believe that this approach is a *relaxation therapy.* I want to make it very clear that it is not a relaxation therapy because relaxation is not the end. It is a tool, a means to a more important end. Relaxation is used ONLY to establish a baseline against which the effects of varying degrees of stress can be evaluated. At baseline, the client should be essentially stress-free. (2) The clinician presents the least anxiety-evoking situation first. Using detailed language, she creates a vivid scene for the client who imagines himself in that situation. The clinician's description should essentially tell a story that leads to the targeted speaking situation. If at any point the client feels anxiety, he raises his hand. The clinician backs the client out of the imaginary scene and returns him to a state of calm and relaxation. She then presents the scene again. This process is repeated until the client can visualize himself in this speaking situation, from beginning to conclusion, without feeling anxious. (3) The clinician moves up to the next situation and begins the process all over again. The client moves up the hierarchy one step at a time until all situations have been successfully experienced, without anxiety.

If the client is unable to complete a targeted situation without feeling anxiety after a reasonable number of trials, the clinician and client should take time out to consider what might be getting in the way of progress. A first step might be to drop back to the lower level previously completed for a few trials and then return to the situation that posed difficulty. It might be that the client was not adequately desensitized at this lower level and moved too quickly to the next level. If dropping back and then moving forward again does not result in success, the clinician and client should carefully examine this portion of the hierarchy. It is possible that the problem situation should have been placed higher in the hierarchy. It is also possible that the situation should be subdivided so the client can attack it in smaller steps. For example, "Talking on the phone," might be too comprehensive a situation for a given client to address. It might be subdivided into (a) initiating a phone call and (b) receiving a phone call, or it might be divided into (a) talking to a relative on the phone, (b) talking to a friend, and (c) talking to a stranger. It could even be some combination of these two possibilities.

It should be made clear that the purpose of desensitization, in its purest form, is not a reduction in the frequency of nonfluency, although we would reasonably expect increased fluency to be a byproduct of successful desensitization therapy. The primary purpose, however, is to reduce anxiety, and if speech-related anxiety is reduced, the therapy is considered successful even if the frequency of stuttering remains essentially the same.

The primary weakness of this form of desensitization, as I have described it, is that it is a passive form of therapy. The client does not talk. He *imagines* talking, but he does not actually talk. The therapy can be made more realistic by using role-playing instead of imagining. Not only does role-playing add an element of realism to the activity, it also allows the client to use his stuttering as one barometer of his anxiety.

It should also be admitted that this form of desensitization will not be appropriate for all adult clients. It works best with the client who is bright, imaginative, and sensitive to the smallest nuances of anxiety. Clients with little imagination, and clients who are not particularly sensitive or introspective, will probably not benefit from this therapy. The most reasonable approach is to try the therapy and abandon it quickly if the results are not satisfactory. The remaining forms of desensitization therapy described below are far less involved than counterconditioning and can be used as exercises in therapy and in home assignments.

Pseudostuttering as a Form of Negative Practice

Negative practice has been used for many years to help people break undesirable habits. The process itself is very simple. The client produces his unwanted behavior on purpose. In the case of stuttering, the client fakes stuttering, an activity often referred to as *pseudostuttering*. This exercise demonstrates to the client that he can produce abnormality without reacting emotionally. It also demonstrates, not coincidentally, that the client is master of his own mouth. He can and does decide when he will stutter. He can and does decide how much he will stutter and how severely he will stutter. This has always been true, of course, but the stutterer may never have consciously experienced this control.

One of the great benefits to be derived from pseudostuttering is that it can be used to prevent avoidance and postponement. The clinician tells the stutterer to stutter *on purpose* whenever he thinks he might stutter and when he finds himself postponing a production. The combined acts of not running away from a feared word or situation and exercising conscious control over his speech mechanism will result in decreased anxiety and increased self-confidence.

Adaptation: A Flood of Stuttering

An extension of pseudostuttering is an activity known as *adaptation* or *flooding*. In this activity, the client is encouraged to stutter constantly in situations during which he would habitually avoid or postpone. This is often done on a quota basis. That is, the client is instructed to stutter a certain number of times or to stutter on every word for a specified period of time. This exercise often results in a surprising decrease in anxiety because the client realizes stuttering is not as awful as he has always imagined it to be. Almost anything one does that is embarrassing is less embarrassing if one does it on purpose over and over again. The stutterer learns he can stutter severely and for an extended period of time, and he can still communicate without injury or death. The ultimate goal of therapy is fluency, of course, but it is also important for the client to learn that stuttering, even at its worst, is not as devastating an experience as he has allowed himself to believe it is. When reality scales back the dimensions of the problem, it seems much less intimidating and much more manageable, and when that happens, the client is surprised that he actually stutters less frequently and less severely. If it is true, as I would strongly assert, that anxiety is one of the fuels that enflame stuttering, it is also true that if we are able to reduce or cut off the anxiety fuel supply, stuttering will be reduced.

Nonreinforcement: An Exercise for Conquering Fear

Nonreinforcement is so simple it seems silly, but there are great potential benefits to be derived from this exercise. In nonreinforcement, the client says a feared word over and over again until he can say it fluently. He is instructed to just say the word, to say it "normally." We do not want him to make any changes. We want him to experience the natural, step-by-step toward "normal" adjustments, that come when he repeats the word. In most cases, the client will say the word fluently and normally by the fourth or fifth trial. Some clients, on some words, may need 15 to 20 trials, or even more, but if the client continues to say the word, he will eventually say it without stuttering. When he does say the word fluently, he should continue to say it for another 10 trials or more so he can *feel* his own normal, tension-free, struggle-free, fear-free productions. As he moves from trial to trial, he will feel a progressive decrease in abnormality. He will also gain the understanding that he is capable of saying even the most *difficult* word fluently at will. The more often the client forces himself to say his feared words, the less he will fear them, and the more confident he will become in his ability to be fluent.

The clinician should note that some clients will struggle mightily with this exercise on some words. A client might have to say a word many times before saying it fluently the first time. He might get frustrated. He will probably want to give up. The clinician should NOT let him give up. Remember—if he surrenders to the fear, that fear will be greater the next time, ratcheting up the probability that he will fail more miserably the next time. In nonreinforcement, the rule is one of the maxims we all learned when we were children—*If at first you don't succeed, try, try again.*

Negative Suggestion: Toughing it Out!

Negative suggestion is not for every client. The clinician will probably choose to use it only with a client she believes is strong enough to handle it, but if a client can handle negative suggestion, he will experience considerable gain in dealing with the anxiety component of stuttering. In this exercise, the clinician presents the kind of negative suggestions the stutterer often gives himself when he believes he will fail. For example, the clinician might tell the client to make a phone call, but before he punches the numbers, she says, "I'm positive you are going to stutter when you make this call. After all, you are going to be talking to someone you don't know, and if he's like most people, he'll probably be rude and impatient. I don't why you should even bother making the call, to be quite honest. You're just going to embarrass yourself, but go ahead. Let's see what will happen."

This exercise will not work if the clinician is not convincing, and she CAN be convincing, even if the client knows what she is doing. A speech-language pathologist should understand the power of words, even if the words are rehearsed. Consider how audiences react to the words of actors in plays and in films. We laugh. We cry. We get angry. The words, properly delivered, make us feel real emotions, even when we know it's all *make believe.* Now . . . IF the clinician is convincing and if the client is strong enough to be unaffected by the suggestion, he will become toughened to the threat of stuttering, and the *threat,* I would remind you, is a sizable portion of the problem.

Chapter 18

MODIFICATION

As we move into the modification phase of therapy, we continue to persuade the client that he is responsible for the behaviors he exhibits. His nonfluencies are the result of decided behaviors, and he has the option to decide to use adaptive behaviors that will result in controlled fluency. It is important to repeat this as a *fact of stuttering life* as often as possible, with as much conviction as possible, in as many different contexts as possible. The clinician needs to remind herself that as long as the client believes his problem is caused by an anatomical defect, a physiological malfunction, a personality flaw, a learning deficiency, an emotional scar inflicted by a parent, or by some vague inner evil force, he will not make progress in therapy. Please note that there is no middle ground here. It is inaccurate to say that the client *might not* make progress. It is absolutely on the nose to say that if the client does not understand his ownership of the disorder, if he does not grasp that every moment of stuttering is the product of his decision-making at some level of consciousness, he will NOT improve. As long as the stutterer believes he is a victim of his disorder, he WILL be a victim of his disorder.

Modification: One Phase in an Integrated Program

There is no doubt that the modification phase is the most important phase in this program, but as I noted in an earlier chapter, this phase of therapy cannot stand alone. Unless identification has been completed carefully and successfully, the client will not be successful in modification because he must be able to identify the behaviors he intends to modify. If he cannot catch his errors, if he cannot sight his targets, he cannot attack them, and he cannot correct them. It must be clear to the clinician and to the client that modification is not a general strategy of speech. Modification focuses on

227

words that are stuttered and on words that might be stuttered. There is no need to modify words that are not stuttered, so the client must be able to identify the specific targets of his modification techniques.

Although I have suggested that desensitization might be completed simultaneously with modification, I would never assert that desensitization is expendable. It is certainly not expendable, especially for the adult client. By the time the stutterer becomes an adult, fear is the single most significant factor in the total problem. Ignoring the fear and anxiety and dealing only with the motor aspects of stuttering is tantamount to treating the symptoms and ignoring the maintaining causes, or as Joseph Sheehan might note, it is tantamount to assuming that the portion of the stuttering iceberg one sees above the surface is all there is. "What you see is what you get" might accurately describe some things in life, but it does not even come close to describing stuttering. Stuttering is a multifaceted and multilayered problem that demands a multidimensional treatment. This is a multidimensional therapy— a totally integrated, eclectic program designed to attack the stuttering problem at every level of its existence. This is why none of the major components of the program can be discarded without jeopardizing the overall effectiveness of treatment.

The steps in modification are relatively specific and should be followed in the order of their description. Furthermore, the clinician should not omit or skip steps. Employed as presented, the steps will systematically move the client toward a comfortable and controlled style of speech that will hold up under the most stressful of speaking conditions. If the client achieves early success in this stage, there is sometimes a strong temptation to move forward too quickly. The clinician should resist the temptation. What comes easily in therapy relative to modification is often extremely difficult to incorporate into real-life speaking, without weeks and months of practice. If we move too quickly, the client can become discouraged and give up, and we will have learned the lesson in Benjamin Franklin's observation that "Haste makes waste."

Breaking the Shackles of Habitual Patterns of Behavior

The first step in modification is *variation*. The purpose of this step is to change, to break the client's habitual patterns of behavior. As I have already noted and emphasized a number of times, the stutterer often feels controlled by his behaviors. We want to show him once again that regardless of what he might believe, he *controls* the behaviors he produces. He has many options, even though he might believe he has no options. For the client who seems particularly reluctant to believe he is in control, we might begin by asking him to take inventory of his life. We ask him to examine every aspect of his life—what he thinks, what he believes, his opinions, prejudices, political and ethical convictions, his body image, hair style, his style of dress, personal habits, hobbies, his taste in music, etc.

The purpose of this exercise is not to suggest *good, better,* and *best* about the choices he has made in his life, but to make the client aware of all the things about his life he can vary if he chooses to do so. After he has made the inventory, and after he and the clinician have talked about all the choices represented in this inventory, the clinician might ask the client to experiment with changes. If he is clean-shaven, for example, he might grow a beard or a mustache. If he wears neckties, he might wear bow ties or no ties. He might use new gestures when he talks, make new friends, eat new foods, or change his moods at will. If he likes rock music, he might try listening to country music for a week, or he might try listening to opera or the stylings of the world's great polka artists. The purpose is not to discover better choices, but to demonstrate in a concrete way that change is possible. In fact, change is easy, sometimes frighteningly easy.

Even though this extreme demonstration of variation can be entertaining for both clinician and client, it is seldom necessary. Most clients have already been convinced about the control they have over their lives, and particularly over their speech, by the time they complete the identification and desensitization phases of therapy.

All clients, however, should spend some time varying their stuttering behaviors because these behaviors are at the crux of the problem we are trying to solve. The stutterer might be easily convinced that he chooses his brand of toothpaste and what movies he likes, but he might remain convinced that when he stutters, the devil, or his designated earthly representative, made him do it. The clinician might begin her persuasion campaign by targeting the anticipatory behaviors for variation because they are highly conscious behaviors, because the client typically perceives greater control over them than over the core behaviors, and because they are, by their nature, highly variable. The process of varying stuttering behaviors is quite simple. If the client avoids a particular word by substituting a synonym, the clinician instructs him to avoid in a different way, perhaps by substituting a different synonym or by circumlocuting. If he postpones by interjecting "uh," he might try a different interjection, or he might postpone in silence, or he might use an avoidance behavior. The client quickly discovers that he really does have options. He chooses to use anticipatory behaviors, and he can choose from quite an impressive menu.

The clinician then asks the client to vary his core behaviors and the behaviors superimposed on the core behaviors. The client might find this variation task more difficult because he tends to produce these behaviors at a fairly low level of consciousness, because he tends to produce them when he is a panic state, and because he feels controlled by them even IF he under-stands intellectually that he is the controller, not the *controllee*. If the client seems unable to vary these behaviors on his own, the clinician should offer to help by stuttering in unison with the client and then introducing a change in the behavior, which the client imitates. The client should then be instruct-ed to repeat the original behavior and create the change on his own. Eventually, if the client is to learn the lesson inherent in variation, he must be able to make changes in these behaviors on his own, without any prompt-ing from the clinician.

The variation step is very brief, usually not more than one or two ses-sions and sometimes only a portion of a session. Remember that the purpose is *to convince the client that change is possible.* We do not want to risk giving the client too many options for abnormality because he might decide he really likes some of these options. We want to move quickly from variation, during which we convince the client he has choices, to modification, during which we teach him that there are *better* choices for speech production, options that will facilitate fluency as the product of genuine control.

Training the Client to "Feel" Speech

The next step is to clarify the motor model of fluent speech. Specifically, we must help the client recognize precisely what adjustments he makes in his speech mechanism that result in nonfluency, and we ask him to compare those adjustments to what he feels in these same speech structures when he makes a fluent production of the same target word. Obviously, we laid the foundation for this step in identification. At this point, our goal is to extend the client's identification skills so they can be used, not only to recognize maladjustments in his speech mechanism, but to recognize the physiological modifications he must make to facilitate fluency. Toward this end, we want to heighten the client's proprioceptive awareness.

Several activities can be used to accomplish greater proprioceptive sen-sitivity. When the client speaks under some form of *masking* (e.g., white noise, recorded "cocktail party" noise, recorded laughter, or an electrolarynx held against one ear with the other occluded), he must attend to the propriocep-tive cues in his speech production in order to maintain normal articulation and prosody. While the client is engaged in some form of continuous talking, the clinician applies the masking noise and then fades it out as the client con-tinues to talk. The client's task is to concentrate on *feeling* articulatory move-ments and contacts in both fluent and nonfluent speech. Because stutterers tend to become more fluent under masking, the client might have to pseu-dostutter in order to make proprioceptive contrasts between stuttered and fluent speech, but both client and clinician should keep in mind that pseudostuttering is quite real in the sense that the client always makes the physiological decisions that result in nonfluency. The *only* difference is that in pseudostuttering, the decisions are more conscious, and they are made on demand.

Delayed auditory feedback (DAF) can also be used to enhance proprioceptive awareness. The application of DAF is the same as the application of masking. The clinician fades it in and out while the client talks continuously. The client tries to ignore the effects of DAF, which he will be able to do if he monitors his speech proprioceptively. Whether she is using masking or DAF, the clinician will know that the client is attending to proprioception if he speaks more slowly than usual, with articulatory movements that are exaggerated and precise.

Although it is best to begin with masking or DAF because they result in immediate and dramatic increases in proprioceptive awareness, the client also needs to practice attending to the motor cues of his speech without benefit of an artificial device. It is not likely, and it is certainly not recommended by most clinicians, that the client will use masking or DAF in his everyday life. *Pantomime* is an effective and natural activity for heightening proprioceptive awareness. In pantomime, the client moves his articulators in the pattern he would use for producing a specific word or phrase, but he does not produce voice or whisper. The client should stutter in pantomime 10 to 30 times on a feared word and then pantomime the same word another 10 to 30 times fluently. His task is to attend to the motor patterns of both stuttered and fluent productions and to compare them. The clinician will notice two things when the stutterer pantomimes speech: (1) His speech will be quite slow, and his movements will be greatly exaggerated, even without instructions. (2) He will have to pseudostutter because it is highly unlikely he will stutter *naturally* when he pantomimes, and if he does stutter, it will be easy, struggle-free stuttering.

Another technique that helps to lay the foundation for modification is *scaling.* I have belabored the point that stuttering behavior is *decided* or *volitional* behavior. The stutterer decides *when* he will stutter. He also decides *what* behaviors he will use when he stutters, how *severe* his stuttering will be, and even *how long* his moments will last. Scaling helps the client feel exactly how much control he has over all these decisions. The clinician begins by instructing the client to stutter as severely as he can on a specified word. If the client is typical, he will NOT stutter as severely as he can on the first attempt, so the clinician instructs him to stutter again, but with greater muscular tension and more struggle. Once the clinician is satisfied that the stuttering is *very severe,* she says, "Think of that production as a *10* on a 10-point scale. Now produce what you think would be a *1.*" This production should be made with muscular tension that is far below normal–much like the effort of someone who is absolutely, totally exhausted, with barely enough energy to speak. It might take several trials to get a true *1*. The clinician then asks the client to produce what he believes would be a *5*. If at any point, the client is not able to hit the targeted scale number, the clinician should demonstrate the production she wants to hear before asking the client to try again. After the client gets the idea that productions can range up and down the scale, varying widely in terms of muscular tension, duration of struggle, and degree of articulatory accuracy, the clinician gives him another word to scale. She instructs him to produce a *7* or a *3* or a *9,* etc. On each word produced, the client should be able to move up and down the scale and make physiological adjustments that fit the targeted scale number. Scaling helps the client understand the degree to which he controls his struggle, but there is an added benefit. In the process of purposely hitting the numbers on the scale, he begins to discover the kinds of adjustments he needs to make to facilitate fluency control when he has made maladaptive physiological decisions.

The client is now prepared to learn how to modify his stuttering behaviors. If the client has successfully navigated the identification phase of therapy, he recognizes all the behaviors that make up his particular pattern of stuttering. He knows *when* he produces these behaviors. He knows *what* they are, and he understands *why* he produces them. Most importantly, he understands that he does produce them. They do not simply happen. He has also developed a motoric sensitivity to the physiological differences between stuttered speech and fluent speech, and he knows that he controls the physiological variables that determine whether speech will be stuttered or fluent. He is now ready to learn HOW to adjust or modify these physiological variables when he stutters or when he expects to stutter.

The Nature of Modification

Before the client learns the mechanics of modifying, the clinician must give him a detailed word picture of modification, and she must demonstrate modification in a wide variety of phonetic contexts so the client can grasp the essential principles involved in this technique, principles that must be applied no matter what word is being targeted, no matter whether the word is targeted after, during, or prior to a fluency failure.

A modification possesses the following characteristics: (1) It is a **highly conscious** motor act. (2) The client articulates very **deliberately.** Synonyms for the word *deliberate* include *intentional, premeditated,* or *voluntary,* all of which convey the appropriate idea here. When the client says the word, he has a plan, and that plan is the modification. (3) The production, or at least that part of the production that focuses on the feared sound, should be in **slow motion,** not because there is something inherently valuable about slow motion itself, but because slow motion makes it easier for the client to feel his abnormality and to feel the adjustments he must make to facilitate fluency. (4) The client must begin with the **correct articulatory position,** and he must **shift gradually** to successive movements. (5) The articulatory contacts must be **easy and loose.** (6) Although the movements should be slow, the client must **follow through** on these movements. Following through is the end part of making the plan.

Sometimes when people learn new motor skills, whether it is in sports or in playing musical instruments or in modifying speech, they do not understand that any motor skill involves three parts: *preparation, execution,* and *follow through.* No part is more important than the others. If I do not prepare properly for a motor act, I will NOT execute it properly. If I prepare well, but make mistakes in the execution, my preparation has been for naught. Failure to follow through is usually evidence that the execution has been faulty, and it's usually faulty in this case because the movement was not made with purpose and with confidence. It was tentative. The tentative execution of any motor skill is failed execution, so . . . all three elements are crucial—*preparation, execution, follow through.*

The description of modification should be repeated to the client over and over again. A good golfer attends to certain keys before he swings a golf club to assure that the swing will be correct. The description of modification includes the keys that will assure that the stutterer will modify correctly and successfully. These keys must be understood, and they must be remembered.

I want to emphasize and expand upon my earlier caution about rate. Clients often fail to understand the purpose of slow rate in modification, and when they do not understand, they either do not slow down when they should, or they believe a slow rate alone is enough to achieve fluency control. If the client only slows his rate of speech, and makes no other adjustments in the way he articulates difficult sounds and words, the impact on speech will be minimal. The most significant value of slow rate during modification is that proprioceptive monitoring is easier and more effective when rate is reduced. A slowed rate also affords the client the time he needs to make the necessary facilitating adjustments. A return to the golf analogy will help make the necessary point here. A competent golfer makes his grip deliberately and moves the club head away from the ball slowly so he can effectively control his swing. In like manner, the stutterer will find making modifications easier and more effective if he approaches target words and sounds slowly and deliberately. This is part of the *preparation* for modification.

It should also be emphasized at this point that since the vast majority of moments occur on the first phoneme or syllable of words, the modification should be made at the beginning of words. Even if the client stutters on the first sound of a second syllable of a word, modification will still be effective if it is executed on the first sound or syllable of the word because in the process of modifying, he will create the relaxed, controlled articulatory set that promotes fluency throughout production of the word.

I need to insert a word of caution here about what needs to be modified and what should be left alone. There is a natural tendency for clients, after modifying the first sound or syllable, to produce the entire word in a slow, deliberate manner. This is not necessary, and it is not desirable. The idea underlying the motor modification approach is that the client fixes what he has broken and only what he has broken. This means that if stuttering occurs on the first sound of a word, the client should modify this sound and produce the remainder of the word normally. Applied this way, the modification will only minimally disrupt the normal flow of speech, and as the stutterer becomes more skilled in modifying, these adjustments will become virtually unnoticeable.

It is most effective to teach the modification in three steps, each step moving the modification forward in time: (1) **cancellation,** (2) **pull-out,** and (3) **preparatory set.** The rationale for teaching the client to modify in three steps rather than just teaching him the end behavior is two-fold. First, this is a difficult skill to master. Just as the piano student learns to play scales before he learns to play real music and he learns to play simple music before learning to play complex music, so the stutterer needs to move slowly from simple to more difficult. Second, when a person learns any new motor skill, he will always find it easier to monitor his mistakes after he makes the attempt than while he is making the attempt. He will also find it easier to catch his mistakes as he is making them than to anticipate that he might make a specific mistake and make anticipatory adjustments that will prevent the mistake from occurring at all.

Consider two examples in which this kind of progressive learning is involved. When a child learns to tie his shoes, an unbelievably painful and frustrating experience for both teacher and learner, he typically does not know he has made a mistake until he lets his loops go and the knot falls apart. As his shoe tying skills increase, he will recognize that he is making a mistake, perhaps making his loops too big or too small, as he is in the process of tying his shoe. He stops, adjusts his loops, and continues. After many hours of practice, he knows the kinds of mistakes he is most likely to make, and he makes preparatory adjustments that prevent the mistakes. Older humans, learning to keyboard, also understand this sequence of learning, monitoring, and adjusting. When we first learn to keyboard, we typically recognize our mistakes only after the deed is done. If I try to process the word, "encyclopedia," and I look at the monitor and see, "rmvuvp[fos," I know I have made a mistake, and I may or may not know how I did it. See if you can figure it out. . . . As I become a more competent keyboarder, I can *feel* my mistakes as I am making them, and as I become even more competent, I know the mistakes I most often make. When I am processing a word containing a letter or sequence of letters with which I tend to have difficulty, I slow up, make sure I use the right keystrokes and prevent the mistake from being made. In sequencing the application of modifications through cancellation, pull-out, and preparatory set, we take into account this human tendency to move mistake correcting forward in time as our skill level increases.

Modifying After the Moment

In *cancellation,* the stutterer modifies a moment of stuttering *after* it has occurred. That is, the client completes the stuttered word, pauses, and then repeats the word using the modification. The pause, like slow rate, is sometimes misunderstood by clients and is not used properly. While the pause alone will not dramatically improve the client's ability to modify, it does serve several important purposes, all of which are crucial to successful modification: (1) It is a form of operant punishment in the sense that it prevents continued communication contingent upon the occurrence of a moment of stuttering. (2) The pause allows the client time to prepare the speech mechanism for modification by reducing muscular tension and by returning the articulators to a neutral position. (3) During the pause, the client should covertly duplicate the stuttering so he knows exactly what maladaptive physiological adjustments he made that resulted in fluency failure, and what adaptive adjustments he must make to facilitate fluency control. (4) Finally, the client should use this time to rehearse the modification. In order that all of these purposes might be met, the pause, at least in the beginning, should be at least three seconds long, and it will probably be much longer.

The clinician should be aware that the client might use the pause as a silent postponement, a use that should be strongly discouraged. When the pause is used as a postponement, the client typically maintains excessive muscular tension, holds onto the inappropriate articulatory position, and by doing these things, he effectively prepares for another moment of stuttering rather than preparing for modification. The clinician will have no difficulty discerning the differences between correct and incorrect uses of the pause. When the pause is used incorrectly, the client's speech mechanism will reflect the excessive muscular tension, and the inappropriate articulatory position will be apparent, if only because the mouth area will be rigid.

The clinician must insist on the correct use of the pause. Even though the client might be able to say the target word fluently without performing the cancellation correctly, the client should be reminded that a short-circuited version of modification will not hold up consistently in normal conversation.

The client should be discouraged from taking short cuts while he is learning to modify. The modification must be correctly applied, every time, from the very beginning.

Modifying During Stuttering

Once the client can cancel successfully on the majority of his moments, we move modification one step forward in time to *pull-out*. Clinicians sometimes wonder if there is a magic criterion level for moving to this next step. There is not. Some clients, who are extraordinarily sensitive to the productions of their moments and who are more than usually insightful, may be able to cancel 95 percent or more of their moments. Others, even though they seem to concentrate as hard as they can, may be able to cancel only 70 percent of their moments. The number is not as important as effort. If a client gives his best effort and plateaus for several sessions at 70 percent, he is ready to move on. Neither he nor the clinician should be discouraged, however, because most clients improve their modification success rates as they move the modification forward in time, so the client who cancels successfully on 65 or 70 percent of his moments might pull out of moments with a success rate of 85 or 90 percent.

In the pull-out, the client makes the modification *during* the moment. Most clients find that they need to use the same kind of pause during pull-outs that they used during cancellation, at least at the beginning. The sequence of production unfolds as follows: The client attempts to say a target word, but stutters on the first sound. As soon as he feels the stuttering, he stops, pauses, releases the excessive muscular tension, plans the modification, and completes the word using the modification. As the client becomes more adept at using pull-outs, he will probably shorten the pause or even omit it altogether so that he stutters, interrupts the moment, and makes the modification immediately. In the absence of a calculated pause, the client should hold onto the inappropriate articulatory position until he is highly aware of what he is doing motorically before slowly and deliberately adjusting to the appropriate contact and movement. Whether or not the client uses a pause before modifying, it is absolutely essential that the modification be done correctly because, as I noted earlier, short-circuited modifications may work in the security of the therapy room, but they will not hold up in the real world of communicative pressures. If the client has difficulty mastering pull-outs after proper instructions and demonstrations have been given, the clinician might teach pull-outs while stuttering in unison with the client. When the client stutters, the clinician joins him. The clinician pulls out of the moment, and the client follows her lead. After doing this several times on a given target word, the clinician should ask the client to stutter and pull out on his own. The end emphasis should always be on teaching the client to be independent, but the clinician should never hesitate to share in the struggle and demonstrate how to get out of the struggle as a step toward the confidence and competence the client will need to become independent.

Modifying When Stuttering Is Anticipated

The final step in modification is the *preparatory set*. In the preparatory set, the client plans the modification when he *anticipates* a moment of stuttering. For the vast majority of adult stutterers, it is highly unlikely that they will ever experience speech without anticipating fluency failures. These anticipations are products of fear, and no matter how irrational that fear might be, it will persist. It can be controlled to some extent. We can certainly teach the stutterer how to cope with the fear, and we can definitely teach him better ways to respond to that fear, but the fear will persist. Consider people who are afraid to fly. By giving these people good information, we can convince most of them that their fear is irrational. Through counseling, many of these people can learn to cope with their fear effectively enough that they will actually fly in airplanes, but most of these people will continue to fear flying, no matter how much information they are given, no matter how much counseling they receive. Stutterers too can learn that their fears are irrational, but dealing with these fears at an intellectual level is not the same thing as eradicating the fears at a visceral level. The stutterer will continue to fear, and he will continue to anticipate fluency failure. In the preparatory set stage, we essentially concede that fear and anticipation, hopefully at greatly reduced levels, will continue to be factors in the client's struggle with stuttering. The client may not be able to choose whether or not he will fear and anticipate, but he can choose how he will respond to anticipations of fluency failure.

Consider that prior to therapy, the adult client anticipates and covertly rehearses stuttering. In this stage, we teach him that when he anticipates stuttering, he should *prepare for the modification* rather than preparing for abnormality and failure. The client's first attempts at using preparatory sets should be on nonfeared words so he can concentrate on mastering the skill without the disruptive influences of word-related anxiety. At this point, we tell the client that if he ever fails to use a preparatory set successfully, he should pull out of the moment. If his pull-out fails, he should cancel the moment, but he should never, ever allow a moment to go uncorrected. While the client must become tolerant of his own nonstuttering fluency failures, the kind of failures all speakers experience from time to time, he must become absolutely intolerant of fluency failures that result from fear, misperception, and from the decided physiological maladjustments that make stuttering inevitable. In other words, he should never give in to his fear, and he should not allow himself to become a victim of the motoric self-fulfilling prophecy that sets the stage for stuttering.

Even when the client masters the preparatory set, he must not abandon the pull-out and cancellation because his reactions to anticipation will not always be perfect. Sometimes he will be so absorbed in his message that he will ignore the warning inherent in an anticipation. Sometimes he will simply be speaking too quickly, and sometimes he will not be as attentive to what he is thinking and feeling as he needs to be. Whatever the reasons, the client will sometimes find himself producing a moment. When he does, he should pull out. Sometimes he will find that he has moved so quickly that the stuttered word is completed. When this happens, he should pause, plan the modification and cancel the stuttering in a second, controlled production of the target word.

When the client has mastered the technique of preparatory set, he should begin to attack his feared words, proceeding through the following substeps: (1) In the first substep, as the client is preparing for the modification, he pantomimes the old stuttering, pantomimes the modification, and produces a modified production of the target word. (2) In the next substep, the client covertly rehearses the old stuttering, pantomimes the modification, and produces a modified production of the target word. (3) In the third substep, he covertly rehearses both the old stuttering and the modification before producing the modification aloud. (4) In the final substep, the client omits any rehearsal of the old stuttering. He covertly rehearses the modification and says it aloud. This is the form of preparatory set the client will try to use in all speaking situations whenever he anticipates stuttering. The rationale for proceeding through these four substeps is similar to the rationale for moving from cancellation to pull-out to preparatory set. We move from relatively easy to more difficult. We also move from equal attention to stuttering and modification to less attention to stuttering. By the time we get to the fourth substep, the client acknowledges his anticipation of stuttering, but having done that, he gives his complete attention to making good articulatory decisions that will result in controlled, fluent speech.

Practice Makes Comfortable

When the client is first learning to modify his stuttering, his concentration is so intense he may become fatigued, and he will certainly become frustrated. This is quite normal. What he is doing is so far removed from his old habitual speech patterns that he must be more conscious of the act of speaking than he has ever been. When the client modifies, he is making the relatively unconscious act of speaking extraordinarily conscious. If you have ever watched someone who, because of an accident, has lost the ability to walk and is learning to walk all over again, you will have some sense of what the stutterer experiences when he modifies stuttered words. Just as the accident victim takes small, labored steps that seem to demand every ounce of his concentration and energy, so does the stutterer move through the production of a target word in a series of deliberate, labored articulatory adjustments. This is amazingly hard work. It is not surprising that the client might wonder if the effort is worthwhile. Even at its worst, he believes, stuttering was never this exhausting, and even if he could not speak fluently, he could at least get by. The clinician should reassure the client that his reactions are normal, but she should also assure him that these conditions will change. The hardships associated with making modifications will diminish. The more the client practices his modification techniques, the more habitual they will become. All aspects of modification, from anticipation to planning for fluency to making the adjustments that facilitate fluency will, as the result of practice, practice, and more practice, become as relatively subconscious as his old stuttering patterns once were. As a long-time practitioner of these techniques, I can attest that modification has become so habitual and so natural for me that I must now make a conscious attempt not to modify. What I still find frightening, however, is how easy it is, when I do not modify, to fall back into the old motoric patterns by which I squeeze my lips together, lock my tongue onto my alveolar ridge, and force my vocal folds into a state of hypertense medial compression. Modification is an effective strategy for controlling the nonfluencies of stuttering. It is not a cure.

Chapter 19

STABILIZATION

Is Stabilization Really Necessary?

Very often the clinician's first task in the stabilization phase is to convince the client that stabilization is necessary. After all, the client now knows what he must do to maintain fluency. He has learned to identify his moments. He has learned how to modify these moments using preparatory sets that, when used properly, make it difficult for most listeners to know that a problem has occurred. The client seems justified in wondering why we just do not turn him loose at this point to enjoy his newfound fluency? Even if he understands that stabilization is necessary, he may wonder why this phase requires so much time–approximately two years if administered properly. These are reasonable concerns, and the clinician is obligated to address them.

As to why stabilization is necessary, there are a number of important reasons. The stutterer's old avoidance and struggle behaviors are extremely resistant to extinction. These behaviors have been developed, reinforced, and habitualized over a period of many years. There have become firmly entrenched in the client's repertoire of speaking behaviors, and as unnatural and bizarre as they might seem to listeners, they are quite natural to the stutterer. The client might have no trouble modifying these behaviors in therapy, in the presence of a clinician he knows is supportive and understanding and who can provide him appropriate feedback when he makes mistakes, but the world of communication outside the therapy room is a much different place. It is not controlled. It is not always patient and supportive. Sometimes it is demanding, critical, and even hostile. In the *real world* communication environment, the client will be more vulnerable to his old fears, and much more likely to retrieve his old anticipatory and struggle behaviors which, while they have not produced normal fluency, have helped him muddle through. Sometimes muddling through can be comfortable even if self-esteem takes a hit in the process.

The stabilization phase allows the stutterer time to introduce his modification skills into the outside world gradually, under the guidance of the clinician who will watch carefully for mistakes in modification and for tendencies to slip back into old, comfortable patterns. At this point, the clinician is no longer teaching a novice. The basic learning has been done. The clinician now becomes the critical coach who points out flaws in the client's modification techniques and reminds him about what he already knows. Over the course of stabilization, the client will become his own clinician. When he reaches the point where he is better able to recognize his own errors than the clinician and to make the necessary adjustments on his own without reminders, he is nearing the end of his need for formal therapy.

Stabilization is also necessary for some psychological reasons. It is highly probable there will be changes in the client's self-image as a direct result of increased fluency. These adjustments are often problematic. Prior to therapy, the client might have been somewhat withdrawn, especially in speaking situations he found particularly threatening. Even with increased fluency, he might need to have his confidence bolstered so he can enter these situations willingly. Another client might overcompensate when he becomes fluent. He might become overbearing and obnoxious because he falls in love with the idea of talking. The clinician, as a friend and counselor, can help this client enjoy his fluency without losing friends in the process. She may be able to help him recognize undesirable social tendencies he simply cannot see because he is too absorbed in the joys of talking.

Yet another client might be overwhelmed by the new social demands that are made when he becomes fluent. He is now expected to participate and contribute in social situations that in the past were handled by people who could talk without stuttering. He might be asked to answer the phone, make reports, give speeches, and entertain guests of the company, whereas in the past, he was always excused from these responsibilities because he was a stutterer. The clinician must help the client view these activities, not as *punishments* for being fluent, not even as responsibilities, but as exciting challenges to put his fluency to the test. The clinician must persuade the client that the more challenges he accepts and meets successfully, the greater his confidence will become, and the greater his confidence as a speaker, the more fluency he will gain. In this sense, stuttering goes out the same door it entered. In the beginning, as stuttering develops, stuttering begets anxiety about speaking which begets more stuttering, and a vicious cycle begins. When stuttering comes under the client's control, the cycle reverses itself. As he learns to modify his stuttering, he becomes more fluent and more confident, and as he becomes more confident, his tendency to stutter is reduced.

We now have a wonderful cycle of improvement driven by increased fluency and increased confidence.

A final purpose served by stabilization is to help the client develop, or regain, what Van Riper calls *sentence-mindedness*. This rather strange term accurately describes something the stutterer loses when his nonfluencies fracture speech. Prior to therapy, the client developed the habit of focusing on the initial phonemes or syllables of specific words. His speech often advanced one word at a time, sometimes even one syllable at a time. In the process of attacking speech word by word, the client becomes less competent in the art of stringing words together into fluent, rhythmic sentences. The client in stabilization needs to practice speaking in longer, more fully integrated units of speech, with attention given to rhythm, rate adjustments, stress patterns, and intonational patterns.

It should be clear to the clinician that stabilization is an absolutely essential phase of therapy that cannot be omitted or rushed. Without careful and extended stabilization therapy, there is a high probability that the client will relapse quickly and extensively. Stabilization does not guarantee long-term fluency, but it increases the odds for continuing fluency by preparing the client to become his own clinician. The clinician will not always be available, but the client will be with himself for as long as there is a himself to be with.

The stabilization phase is usually introduced with a conference. During this conference, the client and clinician discuss the purposes of stabilization, assess what has been accomplished so far, and establish goals for the final phase of therapy. The clinician redefines her role as a consultant rather than teacher. The client is told that he must now assume even greater responsibility if his progress is to continue.

The Schedule Changes During Stabilization

Sessions are scheduled differently during the stabilization phase than during the first three phases. There will be fewer individual sessions, and group sessions will include visitors from the outside. During the first month or two, there is usually one session, either individual or group, each week. Sessions will then be spaced at increasingly longer intervals. Assuming the client is doing well after a month or two of weekly sessions, he and the clinician may agree to a one-month interval until the next session. If the client is still doing well, the next appointment may be in three months, then in six months, and then one year later. The entire process usually covers about two years. If the client shows signs of regression at any time, an appointment will be made for the following week and weekly sessions will continue until he is back on track. If the client maintains fluency throughout the stabilization phase, the prognosis for continued success is excellent. Even when the client is dismissed, however, the clinician should advise him that if he begins to experience a relapse, he should schedule an appointment with the clinician immediately. It is much easier to repair damage as soon as it occurs than it is to wait until fluency control falls completely apart. Early in relapse, the client can usually regain control in just a few sessions.

What happens during stabilization sessions? Obviously, this depends to a large extent on the client's specific needs at the time, but there are some relatively common needs for which there are reliable activities.

Making Modifications Automatic and Developing Speaking Continuity

Probably the most common needs are to make the modification automatic and to develop continuity in the client's speech. Van Riper suggests a number of activities that will serve to simultaneously meet both of these needs:

1. **Shadowing.** The client repeats the words spoken by someone else immediately after they are spoken. Perhaps the best model for shadowing is a network news anchorperson who speaks in fluent, evenly paced, well-constructed sentences.

2. **Narration.** The client tells the same story to one person at a time until he can tell it fluently and smoothly. Many clients enjoy telling jokes in this exercise because stutterers have a notoriously difficult time telling jokes, especially the punch lines, because the propositionality is so great. His increased fluency provides the client an opportunity to tell a joke without *choking* on the punch line.

3. **Paraphrasing.** The client silently reads a newspaper article or a paragraph or two from a book and then expresses the content in his own words.

4. **Continuous Speaking.** The clinician develops a series of cue cards (3"x5"), upon each of which is written a topic of interest to the client. The clinician reveals the first card, and the client talks about that topic until he runs out of things to say. The clinician then reveals the next card, and the client continues to talk.

All four of these activities allow the client to practice his modification with minimal interruption from the clinician. They also challenge the client to speak in whole sentences rather than focusing on individual words.

The following are two activities designed especially for making preparatory sets more automatic:

1. **Increasing Rate.** The client repeats memorized material or repeatedly reads written sentences that are loaded with his feared words. Each

time he repeats, he increases his rate, but he makes sure he always uses proper preparatory sets. The idea is to develop as much speaking speed as possible without sacrificing modification accuracy.

2. **Cue Cards.** A series of cards upon which are written feared words and nonfeared words are flashed to the client. The client says only the feared words and must modify, using preparatory sets, each of these words. This exercise can be altered to make it more challenging by having the client say each of the nonfeared words normally and each of the feared words with preparatory sets.

These are excellent activities for outside assignments. The more the client practices his preparatory sets, the more automatic and the more natural they become. The client and clinician should carefully note that it is impossible to practice too much or too often.

Attacking Remaining Sound and Word Fears

With increased fluency and the concomitant increased confidence, the number of sound and word fears decreases significantly. The client has known for years that stuttering begets more stuttering. As noted early, he now needs to understand that fluency begets more fluency. Although one of the by-products of this increased fluency is a reduction in the number of sound and word fears, there will always be some of these fears to face.

One of the needs in stabilization is to identify and attack the client's remaining sound and word fears. Once identified, there is a simple but effective exercise for reducing the stimulus value of these sounds and words. It is an application of *massed practice.* As the word, "massed," suggests, the client repeats a feared word as many as 100 times. The first few productions of the word are stuttered, using all the client's old behaviors. Most of the productions, perhaps 80 or 90, employ the client's modification skills, and the last few productions are spoken normally. Will the client be able to produce the last few normally? Yes, he will. Remember the lessons of *nonreinforcement* in the desensitization chapter. This massed practice exercise is best used as a home assignment. Many clients, including the author of this book, continue to use this exercise as new word fears develop over the years, and clients can be virtually certain that new word fears will develop. For reasons that are not always clear, feared words become nonfeared words and new feared words emerge. This is one of the mysteries of stuttering. As long as the client accepts that discarding old word fears and creating new fears is typical in the stuttering experience, and as long as he does not react emotionally to these linguistic *comings* and *goings,* he will remain objective and in control. A new feared word is simply a new challenge to be met and won. Sound fears, by the way, can be mass practiced in nonsense syllables of varying phonetic contexts.

Coping with Communicative Stress

There may also be some communicative stresses that present special problems for the client. An exercise called *buffering* can be used to help the client deal more effectively with these stresses. In buffering, the clinician purposely exposes the client to the specific stresses that give him trouble. If the client is sensitive to interruption, for example, the clinician or members of his therapy group constantly interrupt him as he speaks. If he has trouble dealing with the stress of answering questions, especially unexpected and personally offensive questions, the clinician or group members bombard him with questions. The more practice he gets dealing with these stresses in therapy, the more prepared he will be to deal with them in the real world.

To Control or Be Controlled

In an exercise called *resistance therapy,* the client tries to fight off the temptation to revert to his old struggle behaviors. In resistance therapy, the client speaks in unison with the clinician who stutters as severely as she can, or the client enters a speaking situation after the clinician has given him a powerful negative suggestion, or the client talks under DAF while the clinician fades the DAF in and out. In each of these activities, the client is challenged to resist being manipulated into his old stuttering behaviors and to speak under control at all times, modifying as necessary to maintain fluency. This is a very difficult challenge for the stutterer. It is not unlike being told, "Do not think about a pink elephant!" Just as it is impossible to not think about a pink elephant, it is impossible for the stutterer to not think about stuttering under these conditions. His task is to maintain control, no matter how powerful the temptation is to give in to the stuttering. The client who successfully weathers resistance therapy will find the challenges of the real world easier to handle.

Preparation Through Practice

Finally, the client must continue to practice pull-outs and cancellations. He never knows when he might need to rely on these skills. The client's reactions to his anticipations will not be perfect. Most of the time, he will react with preparatory sets, but if he fails to do so and is able to use a pull-out or a cancellation to modify a moment of stuttering, he will still be in control of his behavior. The importance of this control, physiologically and psychologically, cannot be overstated.

Chapter 20

THERAPY FOR CHILDREN WHO STUTTER: AN INTRODUCTION

When Should Intervention Begin?

As has been noted several times in preceding chapters, one of the few things we accept as fact about stuttering is that it usually begins during childhood, and as has also been noted, it often ends during childhood by spontaneous recovery. Nevertheless, not all children who begin to stutter will recover without intervention.

Even if the clinician accepts the most liberal estimates of spontaneous recovery, she cannot or should not avoid treating the young stutterer because the longer the disorder persists, the less likely there will be a spontaneous recovery and the poorer the prognosis for successful treatment. The clinician should initiate a treatment program for any child whose nonfluencies exceed what she judges to be normal limits in terms of type and frequency of occurrence, keeping in mind that there are no absolute parameters for making these judgments. There is, of course, the real possibility that a young stutterer will recover without intervention. There is also the possibility that even with professional intervention, the child's improvement will be due to factors other than the treatment program. I would remind the clinician, however, that the goal in therapy with the young stutterer is the elimination of abnormal nonfluency. How that goal is achieved or who should receive credit for achieving it are far less important than meeting the goal. The clinician fulfills her professional obligation by enrolling the young stutterer in therapy and by implementing the most viable treatment program she can devise to meet the client's individual needs.

A Complex Problem That Evades Simplistic Solutions

We will return to the obvious focus of this chapter momentarily. For now, I want to divert your attention from therapy for children who stutter to a much larger issue–the complexity of the stuttering problem. It is my hope that parents and clinicians who pay attention to this section will become as committed as they need to be to treating stuttering in its early stages because, left to its own evolving devices, stuttering often becomes a behavioral monster out of control. That evolution, however, is not inevitable. In many cases, the metamorphosis from early and relatively simple stuttering to complex and life-altering can be stopped, but it will typically not be stopped unless parents and clinicians take specific and calculated actions to arrest the metamorphosis of stuttering and then reverse it.

In Charles Dickens' *A Christmas Carol,* Scrooge is visited by three ghosts– the ghosts of Christmas past, Christmas present, and Christmas future. The most frightening of these apparitions is the ghost of Christmas future. Why? Because Scrooge already knew what happened in his past, and he was mostly aware of what was happening in his present, but the future . . . oh, the future is somewhat frightening for all of us because we have no idea what the future will bring. In our most vulnerable moments, we imagine the future to be frightening, and we have every reason to believe–based on our experiences so far in life–that some of what will happen in the future WILL be frightening. So it is with the future of stuttering. This section addresses the story that might be told by the *ghost of stuttering future.* It is a future that young stutterers might face, but as Scrooge learned, the future need not unfold exactly as it appears to be scripted. How we conduct the present will affect what transpires in the future. The lesson for Scrooge, and the lesson for parents of stuttering children and the speech-language clinicians who treat them comes in the form of a warning: *If you continue the course you have currently charted, or if you choose to do nothing and take your chances, this is what you can expect.*

Few communication disorders challenge the speech-language pathologist more than stuttering. For this reason, many well-meaning people, including speech-language pathologists, as well as other professionals and laypersons, have attempted to make stuttering therapy easy. A few writers have managed to develop what might be called *easy to administer* therapies, and what knowledgeable critics would call *naive* and *simplistic* therapies. Those treatments that promise easy and painless solutions to the stuttering problem seldom work. The successes they can claim are limited in scope and are usually enjoyed by a small number of people who are uniquely suited, by reason of their specific behaviors and/or personality traits, to these treatments.

One of the facts we can assert about stuttering is that it is a complex problem that rarely responds to simple solutions. In this sense, stuttering is not unlike many other human problems. I want to focus on one of these problems to make a point, a problem I have used as an example throughout this book, weight loss and weight management. Weight control problems plague many of us, some of us from time to time, others for a lifetime. Over the years, there have been countless books and magazine articles devoted to the subject of weight loss and weight control. Many of these books and articles promise quick and easy programs for losing weight and for maintaining weight. We all know, probably from personal experience, that precious few people actually lose weight on these quick, easy programs, and even fewer people are able to prevent the pounds they do lose from finding their way back to the waists and hips from which they temporarily disappear. When one of these programs fails us, we look for another. The programs are much easier to find than the pounds are to lose. No matter how much we might want to believe otherwise, losing weight is not easy, and it is not painless, and it is not a problem that once solved, stays solved. Weight control is an extraordinarily difficult battle that requires much time, great effort, and supreme self-discipline. Even when using a rational, thoughtfully constructed weight control program, success does not come quickly, and it does not come easily.

What is the point? There are some meaningful and helpful comparisons between weight loss and stuttering. Like weight management, stuttering is a problem that is solved, if it is solved, over a long period of time. Success for the stutterer is the product of hard work, dedication, and self-discipline. Losing weight and stuttering have something else in common, and this commonality is crucial to an understanding about what must happen in stuttering therapy. It is also crucial to understanding why therapy should be initiated as early as possible in the stutterer's life, before he develops the fears, misperceptions, and motor habits that make solving the stuttering problem increasingly difficult. Despite the arguments I have been making, I want to point out that losing weight and stuttering are, at their base level, relatively simple problems to solve. In order to lose weight, all one must do is to consume fewer calories and/or burn more calories than are necessary to maintain one's current weight. It's just that simple. In order to stop stuttering, all one must do is stop anticipating that certain sounds and words are difficult and stop creating the excessive muscular tension and inappropriate articulatory positions that make fluency failures inevitable. It's just that simple.

Unfortunately, neither of these problems, for adults at least, operate at the base level. Excessive weight is a problem that is often connected to inappropriate eating habits, self-esteem issues, and other factors that may or may not be directly related to what one puts into one's mouth. The solution, therefore, is not as simple as reducing intake or increasing exercise, although these adjustments are necessary parts of the solution. In the same way, stuttering is more than anticipation and struggle. It too is connected to other factors, including *misperceptions* about the act of speaking and about the inherent challenges in producing certain sounds and words, *fears* tied to certain words, situations, and listeners, and even the same kinds of *self-esteem* issues that plague people with weight problems. While it is true that therapy must focus on anticipation and struggle, it must also address the other levels of the problem, and this can be very complicated business. It is difficult to conceive of any quick, easy approach that will deal effectively with such a multifaceted problem. As I have already acknowledged, one can find a few stutterers who have responded to *quick-fix* programs, but it is fair and accurate to conclude that the majority of stutterers, young and adult, need programs that offer more than *magic cure* treatment.

The reader may wonder why this discussion is included in a chapter intended to introduce therapy for youngsters, and this would be a fair and reasonable wonder. Clearly this discussion could have been included somewhere in the chapters on therapy for adult stutterers. It is included here in order to draw the reader's attention to the issue of complexity in stuttering because speech-language clinicians, parents, teachers, and anyone else who has responsibility for children who stutter should be sensitized to what lies down the road for young stutterers. Stuttering is complex enough when clients are young. When the disorder is carried into adulthood, there is considerable baggage dragged along with it. While it may be tempting to say: "Perhaps Johnny will outgrow this problem if we just let it lie for awhile," there is great risk in this waiting game. It is true, of course, that Johnny MIGHT spontaneously recover, and when he is very young, the odds for spontaneous recovery are favorable, but what if Johnny does not recover? The longer we wait before we intervene–if the problem continues to worsen, as is likely–the more difficult stuttering is to solve. What begins as a fairly straightforward speech problem becomes layered with many other issues that make it more and more complex and more and more resistant to change. The moral of this story will be repeated a number of times in the pages that follow; but in simple terms, if we err, we should err on the side of intervening too early as opposed to intervening too late.

Can the Youngster Endure Therapy?

Clinicians who work with children often question whether young stutterers will be able to tolerate anything but the most superficial treatment programs. Is the child too delicate? Will he give the necessary time, invest the necessary effort, and will he tolerate the frustrations inherent in a comprehensive therapy program? Fortunately, most children do not spend much time thinking about these things, and they do not get caught up in the cost-payoff dilemma that becomes a focal point in motivating adult clients. If the child is comfortable with the clinician, and if the clinician is reasonably creative, enthusiastic, and supportive, the child will do whatever is asked of him. Fortunately too, children tend to be quite resilient and will comfortably tolerate the frustrations that often arise in the therapy process, especially if the clinician is caring and encouraging. In my own clinical experiences, I have found that young stutterers handle the negative aspects of therapy with less trauma than most adult clients.

Why do children who stutter suffer the unpleasantness of stuttering with relative grace? Children who tolerate therapy well probably do so because they have already learned one of the most important lessons of life. That is, life is not always easy, and if human beings expect to survive, they must learn to relish the good times and gird themselves up for the bad times. Most of us are taught at a young age, either directly or by the examples of well-adjusted adults in our lives, that human beings grow through adversity, and most of us come to believe that the greater the adversity we battle and defeat, and the greater the effort expended in battling the adversity, the more we grow and the stronger we become. In short, young stutterers respond well to the challenges of therapy because it is human nature to find, meet, and win challenges. Even if the child does not understand exactly why he is in therapy or what "stuttering" is, he will find challenges to meet in the activities of therapy, and if he is a typical human youngster, he will respond enthusiastically to these challenges. The clinician's task is to identify the challenges that are appropriate for a given child, encourage him in his efforts, and praise him for his victories, no matter how small those victories may seem.

Those children who survive therapy with greater grace than adults probably do so because they have not yet reached the conclusion that stuttering is a permanent, awful state. One of the marvelous perspectives of childhood is that tomorrow is always better, always more promising. If I have problems today, the child believes, they will almost certainly be gone tomorrow. Adults tend to drag today's problems into tomorrow whether they belong there are not, and this is certainly true for adult stutterers. Children who stutter often do better than adults who stutter simply because they have a purer, more optimistic, less baggage-cluttered view of life.

Understanding Versus Experience

Clinicians are often reluctant to work with stutterers, especially young stutterers, because they believe nonstuttering clinicians do not or cannot understand the disorder. They assume that a normal-speaking clinician cannot understand or identify with the stutterer's experience. This concern is magnified by the fact that since stuttering is a low incidence communication disorder, many clinicians have little experience working with this population, so they worry that they do not know enough, and they worry that they cannot relate to these clients. I understand the concern, but it is a concern that is not proportional to reality. While it is true that most speech-language clinicians have not walked in the stutterer's shoes, we have all experienced frustration, anxiety, and embarrassment, and we have all been nonfluent. The fact is we have all experienced frustration, anxiety, and embarrassment in the act of speaking, and we have all had fluency failures that have been the direct products of these negative emotions. Nonstuttering clinicians may need to remind themselves from time to time, as Wendell Johnson noted, that there is nothing that the stutterer does that the nonstutterer does not also do at some times to some extent. Even if a nonstuttering clinician has not walked in the stutterer's shoes, she has tried them on occasionally.

It is important to have some empathy for what the stutterer is experiencing, and it is not difficult to find sources for that empathy in any ordinary life, but it is even more important that the clinician understands exactly what her stuttering client is doing motorically when he stutters. If the clinician expects to help her client eliminate or modify the physiological aspects of his stuttering, she must know precisely what he is doing that is abnormal, what maladaptive adjustments he is making that interfere with fluency. The best and easiest method for accomplishing this physiological understanding is for the clinician to repeat her client's moments of stuttering, not once or twice, but many times, and she should ask the client if he believes she is getting it right. A constructive by-product of this imitation is that it demonstrates the clinician's willingness to share her client's abnormality, which helps foster the open and supportive relationship so critical to therapeutic success. By imitating her client's moments in a businesslike manner, the clinician also models the objectivity that underlies long-term success.

It should be noted, for reasons that will be made very clear in the next chapter, that we do not imitate the moments of young beginning stutterers, but imitating the moments of young advanced stutterers who are old enough to understand their responsibility for their behaviors derives all the benefits identified in the preceding paragraph.

The Risk of Permanent Damage in Therapy Is Minimal

Another common concern expressed by clinicians is that they will do something in therapy that will result in permanent damage to the stuttering child. While such damage is possible, it is highly unlikely that any clinician with a modicum of talent, insight, and sensitivity will continue a procedure that is seriously harming a child. By way of trying to allay this concern, I will repeat an observation I made earlier. Children are naturally resilient. They are resilient because they are still naive and uninformed and have yet to discover how unfair and cruel life can be. Children are happy and optimistic by nature. They do get sad and angry, of course, but they seldom remain in these negative states for long. When two children argue, for example, they can be the worst of enemies, vowing eternal hatred and awful revenge, but they can become the best of friends again in mere minutes. Sometimes it is difficult to understand exactly what turns these situations around so quickly, but children do have greater capacities to forgive and forget than adults who can carry grudges for so many years they often forget the original source of their negativity. Children can be so disappointed it is heartbreaking to watch them suffer, but disappointment can be transformed into joy instantaneously by a smile, a hug, or a reassuring word. The point is, and it is an important point, even if the clinician does something in therapy that has a negative consequence, the effect will not last long. The clinician must simply be sensitive to what she does that makes the child stutter more, stutter harder, or suffer more intensely. When she observes these consequences, she should adjust. The doctor says to the patient, "Does it hurt when you hold your arm over your head?" The patient says, "Yes, Doc, it does." The doctor says, "Well, don't do that anymore. That'll be $75.00, thank you." If the clinician does something that increases the frequency and severity of stuttering, or that causes the stutterer to be more frustrated or embarrassed, she should hear a voice in her head that says, "Well, don't do that anymore!" The clinician should also find some comfort in the knowledge that if she is too insensitive to grasp what is happening, the child will probably adjust on his own.

There is another recognition that is difficult for some clinicians to accept, but accept it they must. The stuttering child might get worse, or he might get better, independent of anything the clinician does. The clinician simply cannot control all factors that might influence fluctuations in the child's fluency problem. She must guard against bludgeoning herself with guilt if stuttering is not quickly and smoothly resolved. She must not overreact if the child regresses after some obvious progress, nor should she consider herself a failure because her client never makes progress and gets worse. Consider that a coach sometimes instructs his players to do exactly the right things, but when players fail to execute perfect plans, the result is failure. The fault for the failure more often rests with the players who did not execute the perfect plans than with the coach who devised the plans. A speech-language clinician quite often develops the right goals and devises the perfect treatment to reach those goals, but if the client fails to execute, the results will be poor. I also want to emphasize that the clinician should be careful not to take too much credit when the client improves. The improvement MIGHT be the direct result of a beautifully designed and executed therapy plan, but improvement might also come from sources other than the clinician's remarkable talents.

Categorizing Young Stutterers: A Difficult and Imperfect Process

Before moving into the specifics of therapy for children who stutter, I need to emphasize the heterogeneity of these clients. *Young stutterers* can range in age from two years to 14 or 15 years. Not even the most single-minded clinician, using the simplest treatment program, would suggest that we should treat a teenage stutterer the same way we would treat a preschool stutterer. Age is clearly one factor that must be considered in selecting a therapy approach, but there are other factors that are just as important. These factors include the client's awareness of speaking difficulty, the frequency and severity of his nonfluencies, the presence and power of situational and linguistic cues, the level of the child's self-esteem, the influence of misperceptions about the act of speaking, and many others. The treatment program for a given client must be designed to address the specific problems and satisfy the special needs of that child.

For the sake of organizational convenience, I will describe therapy for the young beginning stutterer in Chapter 21 and therapy for the young advanced stutterer in Chapter 22, but the clinician should understand that many children who stutter do not fit neatly into either of these two categories. Many young stutterers will have characteristics of both categories and will need elements of both therapy programs. There is also the real possibility that a child as young as 12 years might be more suited for the adult program than for either of the approaches designed for stuttering children. In making decisions about the specific design of therapy for each individual client, the onus is on the clinician to follow the lead of Winnie the Pooh who said, "Think! Think! Think!"

Chapter 21

THERAPY FOR THE
YOUNG BEGINNING STUTTERER

A Profile of the Young Beginning Stutterer

The young beginning stutterer is usually between two and six years in age, but be aware that age is less important in determining the type of treatment to be used than the behaviors exhibited by a child, and to some extent, less important than the child's level of maturity, insight, and emotional reactions to his nonfluencies. A profile of a *typical* young beginning stutterer would include the following characteristics: The dominant speech symptom is excessive syllable repetition. The word, "excessive," is obviously problematic because it is a relative term, but since there are no hard and irrefutable data to demarcate between a *normal* frequency of nonfluency and an *abnormal* frequency, "excessive" is the best parameter we can establish. We need to remind ourselves that all children produce syllable repetitions. When these repetitions occur more frequently than expected, in the judgment of a speech-language clinician, this speech characteristic might signal the beginning of stuttering. A few young beginning stutterers produce closures and postural fixations, but these behaviors are rare in very young stutterers. The stuttering is cyclic or episodic. That is, there are periods of fluency that last for days, weeks, or months followed by periods of excessive nonfluency. During the periods of excessive nonfluency, the speech behaviors are highly inconsistent. Nonfluencies might range from easy repetitions to hard closures within hours or even minutes. In this client, there is typically little evidence of awareness, and little evidence of situation or linguistic fears. The child does not react with expectancy, and except for rare occasions when talking is complicated by emotions or unusual communicative pressures, he does not struggle when he stutters.

Rationale for Treatment: PREVENTION

With this description in mind, it should be easy to understand that the major rationale for the treatment program used with these clients is *prevention*. Specifically, treatment is designed to prevent any increase in the frequency or severity of the nonfluencies already present, and to prevent the development of new stuttering behaviors that emerge when struggle increases. We try to prevent an escalation in struggle by choking off those factors that feed struggle. That is, we try to prevent increased awareness of speech difficulty, and we try to prevent the development of misperceptions about speech, speaking situations, and listeners, perceptions that form the bases for linguistic and situation fears. These problems, incidentally, do not emerge in a particular order. If they did, we could stop stuttering in its tracks by attacking *the next step* in severity. In fact, the only way to effectively prevent stuttering from becoming worse is to effectively address all of these factors, more or less simultaneously.

In the most traditional treatment programs, prevention is attempted through parental and family counseling. In this program, parental counseling is an important part of the treatment package, but it is not the whole program. The wise clinician will work with the client's family because she understands that the child's stuttering cannot be isolated from his most important communicative relationships, but she will also work directly with the child because, if the disorder has progressed enough to be treated, the child has already established some degree of ownership for it, no matter how subconscious that ownership might be. It is vital, however, for the clinician to work directly with the child without working directly on the stuttering. How it is possible to work directly with the child and not focus directly on the stuttering will become clear as details of the program are described.

Treatment Should Be as Direct as Necessary

One of the general principles of this program is that therapy for young beginning stutterers should only be as direct as necessary. The clinician should begin conservatively and attack the stuttering as the child and his particular needs dictate. If, for example, it is possible to prevent fluency problems from escalating by counseling with the parents and by making minor, fluency-facilitating adjustments in the child's environment, that is the approach the clinician should take. If, however, environmental manipulation is not feasible to the extent necessary, or if the clinician believes the problem is substantially owned by the child, a more direct approach is appropriate.

The clinician should keep in mind that there are risks associated with direct therapy. As soon as we make therapy direct, the child knows there is problem, and he knows he bears some responsibility for it. After all, when the clinician uses a direct approach, she is saying to him, in essence: "You are having difficulty talking. I need to show you how to fix your problem." With direct therapy comes increased awareness, and there are two dangerous reactions to increased awareness: (1) trying hard to not make mistakes, and in the process, making the mistakes bigger and more frequently, and/or (2) avoiding words, or speaking situations, or avoiding talking altogether. When the conditions dictate, these are risks we must take, but until it becomes obvious we have no choice but to confront the problem head-on, we should try to be as indirect as possible. It should also be noted that it is always easier to make therapy more direct than to begin with a frontal attack and retreat to a more indirect approach.

Develop a Supportive Relationship

Assuming the clinician works directly with the child, her *preliminary* goal is to create an extremely supportive relationship with her client. Some clinicians worry that the child might become too dependent on his clinician. Dependence is rarely, if ever, a legitimate concern. The child at this age craves dependence and needs to be dependent on people who are bigger, stronger, and smarter than he is. Dependence on adults is part of the young child's normal life experience. The clinician may need to be reminded that the child will become independent as a natural consequence of maturity and increased confidence. In truth, the child will become more and more independent whether the clinician or his parents like it or not, so the clinician should not fret about dependence because it is a temporary condition. I would argue that it is especially important that the child with fluency problems be permitted to feel dependent on the speech-language clinician who may be the only adult in his life who understands the speech part of him and who can relate to him as a communicator without reacting emotionally or critically to his nonfluencies.

A Guiding Principle: Reduce Severity and Frequency Takes Care of Itself

The clinician should keep in mind that the primary focus of therapy with young clients is on reducing the severity of stuttering rather than on reducing the frequency of nonfluencies. Frequency of fluency failures can be a misleading measure of the disorder with clients of all ages, but it is particularly meaningless with young children because these failures are so common in their speech. If we can reduce the child's tendencies to make speech harder than it really is, there will be a natural return to normal speech, complete with normal nonfluencies, without regard to how many of these nonfluencies there might be. This is a common sense principle that can be applied to any problem in which the frequency of failure is linked to panic and struggle. If a basketball player has an abysmal free throw shooting percentage because he is an emotional wreck when he stands at the free-throw line, his coach will not help him by focusing his attention on the number of free throws he is missing. His coach will help him by finding ways to reduce the panic and struggle that result in the misses. In the same way, the speech-language clinician does not focus on fluency misses. She focuses on the panic and struggle that give birth to the fluency misses. The calm and relaxed basketball player will miss fewer free throws. The calm, struggle-free child will produce fewer nonfluencies.

We will now review six specific goals that can be addressed in the therapy process. The clinician should remember that a supportive client-clinician relationship underlies all else she may attempt to achieve in therapy. In other words, these six goals will be difficult, perhaps impossible, to attain unless the client trusts the clinician and feels comfortable with her. As with any multifaceted treatment program, the clinician might not include all six of these goals in the therapy designed for a particular client. Not all clients will need all of the experiences that are incorporated into the six goals. The clinician should select the goals and the experiences within these goals she believes will best meet the needs of her client.

GOAL ONE: Make Speech Pleasant

The first, and probably the most basic goal, is to *make speech pleasant*. In order to appreciate the importance of this goal, the clinician must be sensitive to the fact that even though the young child is not as aware of his stuttering as the older client, he often experiences frustration as a result of his stuttering. He might not make the connection between his frustration and the stuttering because "stuttering" is probably not a word he uses, and even if he does use it, we can be confident he does not understand what it means. The child might not even link the frustration with speech. Keep in mind that children in the age range of the typical young beginning stutterer are not particularly introspective or analytical. If the child is excessively nonfluent, he might experience frustration without identifying at any level of consciousness what he is feeling, even if the frustration is obvious to the external observer. After a period of nonfluency, the child's frustration might manifest itself in temporary irritability, silence, or rapid, compulsive speech, but if you ask this child what he just experienced, it is highly unlikely he will have an answer for you. Even adults, in certain circumstances, can experience negative emotionality without being able to identify what it is or even why it is occurring. That children are often clueless about similar experiences should not be surprising. From the stuttering perspective, it is most important to understand how these experiences might impact the child's speech over the long term. If the experience of speech-related frustration occurs repeatedly, speech can become a negative stimulus for the child, and we want to do everything we can to prevent that from happening.

If the clinician senses that speech has become unpleasant for the client, she must reestablish speech as a positive experience, and we should not overlook the fact that speech is a naturally positive experience for human beings. People of all ages love to talk. We begin early in life to make noises even when the noises are meaningless. By the end of our first year on earth, we are producing meaningful words. Within three years, we have mastered most of the basic words we need to communicate our needs and desires, and we never stop talking, even when we have absolutely nothing to say. When the stuttering child stops talking, he is retreating from one of the activities he loves most. The clinician must reestablish the pleasantness of talking, a fairly simple task in most cases.

The general approach we use to make speech pleasant is to engage the child in free and directed play. We choose this avenue for three reasons: (1) children enjoy play, (2) children are play experts, and (3) talking is easily and naturally incorporated into play. Play is the means by which we attempt to accomplish the end of making speech more pleasant, and it is ideally suited for our purpose. Our job is to channel or direct play so that speech becomes the primary *toy* or tool. In this way, we can begin to make speech as much fun as any popular toy. This might seem an ambitious goal, but it can be achieved if the clinician is energetic, creative, and uninhibited.

Because the child may be reluctant to talk, especially to a stranger, the clinician must be careful about how she initiates play therapy. The opening move in this little drama depends on the child. If he is active, outgoing, and highly verbal, the clinician might need to do no more than get acquainted with him, introduce him to the therapy environment, and enjoy the verbal onslaught. If the child is passive, fearful, and withdrawn, the clinician might begin with an enjoyable nonspeech activity such as drawing, molding clay, or desecrating a perfectly tidy coloring book with crayons. If the activity is nonthreatening, the child will feel increasingly comfortable with the clinician, his fear will dissipate, and he will become more verbal.

Another popular approach for reaching the passive, reticent child involves two boxes of toys, one box for the client and one for the clinician. Play proceeds through a series of three predictable stages: (1) *solo play* during which the client and the clinician play with their own toys in their own space in relative silence, (2) *tangential play* during which the clinician makes occasional contact with the child or his toys while there is intermittent sharing of toys and limited interpersonal and intrapersonal communication, and (3) *cooperative play* during which the client and the clinician play with the same toys while engaging in mostly interpersonal communication. The progression from solo to cooperative play is seldom linear. The passive child might let his barrier down for brief periods of time while he is trying to discover if the clinician is really trustworthy and really as fun as her publicist claims she is. If the child begins to withdraw, the clinician should not press him to engage beyond his comfort level. She should return to a lower, less threatening level of interaction until the child is ready to move forward again. The clinician's patience, sensitivity, and understanding may be tested during this process.

Since the goal is to make speech pleasant, the clinician systematically introduces talking into the play activities. During the earliest stages of solo play, the clinician and the client play in relative silence. The clinician then introduces nonspeech noises, including mechanical noises and animal noises, into play. During tangential play activities, the clinician makes single-word commentaries on her own toys, activities, thoughts, and feelings. As play moves into the cooperative stage, the clinician introduces short phrases and sentences. The overall object in this progression, as has already been noted, is to make speech itself the primary vehicle of play.

I want to emphasize that the goal of making speech pleasant, as well as the other goals I will identify and describe, are accomplished within the context of play therapy. The clinician must always operate with specific goals in mind, and she must manipulate the child's speech behaviors so that fluency is facilitated, but the child's attention, if the clinician is competent and successful, will always be on the play. In other words, the child will become more fluent in spite of himself, and he will become more fluent while he is having a good time.

GOAL TWO: Fluency Through Modeling

The second goal is to *create appropriate fluency models*. When any young child, whether or not he has a fluency problem, is presented with speech models that are long, complex, and hurried, he is likely to become silent, hesitant, or nonfluent. Since the clinician is dealing with a child who is unusually vulnerable to factors that can disrupt fluency, she must take great care to use models that are natural and linguistically correct, but are also simplified and unhurried.

As play shifts from solo to tangential to cooperative, the clinician and the client will shift from self-talk to parallel-talk to social-talk, but at every level the clinician's models should be simple, brief, unhurried, and fluent. The clinician should use mostly simple declarative sentences, imperative sentences, and basic question forms, avoiding complicated embedded forms and even compound sentences if they are too long. Her models should be expressed within the child's linguistic abilities, and most importantly, her speech should be delivered in a slow, relaxed, comforting style. She should try to accomplish this style, however, without unduly distorting prosody. Sometimes in attempting to produce this kind of speech, the clinician will produce a mechanical, robot-like style of speech, and that is not what we are looking for here. What is called for is a calmer, quieter, more controlled form of normal speech, the style of speech one might use to put a child to sleep or to settle him down when he is upset. It is, in fact, the kind of speech adults instinctively use with one another when they are upset. If you are dealing with someone who is hysterical, you will certainly not yell and scream at a frenetic pace. You will lower your pitch, slow your pace, and speak in a calm, reassuring manner. This is the kind of fluency model we try to create for the excessively nonfluent child when he is being excessively nonfluent.

In my own clinical experience, I have found fluency modeling to be the single most effective method for facilitating fluency in young beginning stutterers. If fluency modeling is executed properly, most children with fluency problems will adopt this style of speaking, with no direct prompting from the clinician. Remember that children are great imitators. In fluency modeling, we are giving the young client a style of speaking to imitate that will greatly reduce his tendency to make speech difficult and, therefore, his tendency to become nonfluent.

Many of the methods we use with young beginning stutterers should not be attempted by their caregivers, but fluency modeling is an exception. The clinician can teach caregivers how to make these changes in their own speech, practice with them to make sure they are making the proper adjustments, and provide specific guidelines about when fluency modeling should be used. If, for example, the child is having a good fluency day, caregivers should be instructed to use normal speech. The child must eventually learn how to cope with the communicative stresses that are inherent in rushed, highly intense interpersonal exchanges because most people talk this way most of the time. When he is not having a problem, therefore, we should let him experience the normal chaos of routine talking, but if he is having a difficult fluency day, caregivers can use fluency modeling to take the pressure off, to give him greater success in his communicative attempts, and not coincidentally, to make speech more pleasant.

GOAL THREE: Reducing the Vulnerability to Breakdown

The third goal is to *integrate and facilitate fluency*. With the older stutterer, the primary goal of therapy is to eliminate or reduce abnormality by attacking specific moments of stuttering. This goal delineates one of the critical differences between therapy with young beginning stutterers and therapy with adults. With the adult stutterer, the primary goal of therapy is to eliminate or reduce abnormality by directly attacking specific moments of stuttering. The client and the clinician work together to identify maladjustments that result in nonfluencies, and they focus on making better adjustments that will result in fluency. The focus with young beginning stutterers is radically different. No direct attention is given to the child's fluency failures. Instead, the clinician attempts to facilitate fluency and to extend the child's experiences in being fluent. The young client is unusually vulnerable to fluency disruption. The clinician's task, in reference to this goal, is to do whatever she can to stabilize the child's motor speech, to make it less susceptible to breakdown.

One method that can be used to facilitate fluency involves the use of *rhythm methods*. We have known for centuries that rhythm methods can produce fluency quickly and easily, but we also know that they are seldom effective in producing long-term fluency in adult stutterers who struggle and avoid and have developed entrenched motor habits. Recognizing the limitations, we also know that rhythm methods, used properly in the correct context, can be effective with young stutterers who do not show fear or awareness and who have not yet developed strongly established struggle habits. Rhythm methods can be used to indirectly suggest to the child that he can speak fluently, that he is not the victim of a physical problem that makes stuttering happen.

More importantly, rhythm provides the child an opportunity to experience and feel fluency in a way that is inherently pleasurable for all human beings. Young children are soothed by lullabies, delight in nursery rhymes, and love to play on swings, teeter-totters, rocking horses, and other toys that create rhythmic movement. Most adults enjoy rhythm-based activities such as dancing or rocking in rocking chairs and porch swings. Adults who are emotionally anguished or mentally disturbed will often wrap their arms around themselves and rock back and forth. When babies cry or adults are upset, we hold them, pat them and sway in a gentle rhythm. There is no denying that human beings of all ages enjoy rhythm and are comforted by rhythm.

Many clinicians, including Charles Van Riper, argue that all many young stutterers need in order to gain or regain normal fluency is vivid experience in being fluent. Rhythm is one simple way to provide this experience. Rhythm activities that can be used in therapy with young stutterers include syllable-timed speech, chanting, nursery rhymes, or even singing. While the child is vocalizing, the experience can be intensified by adding foot tapping or hand movements.

Two important cautions must be made at this point: (1) The clinician should use a variety of rhythm activities so the child does not become dependent on a particular activity for facilitating fluency, and so he does not conclude, consciously or unconsciously, that this activity is the solution to a problem. (2) Rhythm methods should never be applied as forms of direct therapy but always within the context of play therapy. If the child concludes anything about these activities, it should be that they are play activities, just some of the things he might do in the course of a therapy session.

A second method that can be used to facilitate fluency is **unison speech.** By reading, reciting memorized material, or repeating previously formulating sentences in unison with the clinician, the child will experience a high degree of fluency. This activity allows the child to be directly influenced by the clinician's fluency and prosody models. Unison speaking also reduces the child's communicative responsibility and therefore reduces the communicative pressure he might feel. Most importantly, children enjoy unison speaking as a kind of playing together exercise so we are, once again, providing a fluency experience within an activity that is fun and pleasant. As with any activity we might use to facilitate fluency in a young beginning stutterer, this one should be used in moderation. Unison speech is not a cure, and it is not a therapy. It is one of many means to a common end, *experienced fluency.*

A third method we can use to facilitate fluency involves activities that will indirectly and subtly **heighten tactile-proprioceptive feedback.** We often instruct the adult client to pay greater attention to tactile-proprioceptive feedback and to rely less on auditory feedback. The primary rationale for this monitoring adjustment is that, at its most basic level, stuttering is disturbed motor speech. By training the stutterer to attend to his tactile-proprioceptive feedback, we make him more sensitive to the physiological conditions that result in nonfluency and to those physiological adjustments that will facilitate fluency. Unless he is aware of these maladaptive and adaptive adjustments, the reasoning goes, he will not be able to choose between them. For obvious reasons, we are much less direct in developing tactile-proprioceptive sensitivity in young stutterers than in adult stutterers. I would also emphasize that not all children who stutter will profit from heightened tactile-proprioceptive awareness. For those who might benefit from this sensory shift, the clinician can accomplish it by using a number of simple activities.

For example, if the client and clinician play and talk while wearing Halloween masks, the child's attention will automatically focus on the mouth because the mouth will be the most mobile stimulus in the mask's otherwise static visual field. In the course of playing with a magnifying glass, the clinician can hold it in front of her mouth as she talks, drawing the child's attention to the motor aspects of speech in a very entertaining manner. Well, it might not entertain you, but trust me, small children find visually distorted mouths quite amusing. Masking with white noise or with an audiotape of laughter while the child is talking will force him to attend to tactile-proprioceptive feedback. If the clinician has access to an electrolarynx, she might find this the most interesting way to heighten a child's tactile-proprioceptive sensitivity. The clinician instructs the child to use the electrolarynx exactly as a laryngectomee would. The child will find that he must slightly exaggerate his articulation and reduce his rate in order to use the instrument effectively. The combination of a slower rate and more precise articulation works well to make the child more aware of the motor aspects of his speech. No explanation for any of these activities is necessary. Remember that everything we do with the young beginning stutterer is done in the context of play. The clinician should simply introduce them as play activities. They are different and fun, and most children love to do them.

GOAL FOUR: Reinforcing Fluency

The fourth goal in this program is to *reinforce fluency*. The most general approach for reinforcing fluency, an approach we can use in therapy as well as in the child's home environment, is to take advantage of days when he is particularly fluent by evoking as much speech as possible. No matter what the clinician might have planned for a particular session, if the child arrives and is wallowing in fluency, the clinician should set her plans aside and spend as much of their scheduled time as possible just talking to the child. Spontaneous fluency is the best possible fluency for the child to experience. When it occurs, the clinician should take advantage of it. We advise the child's caregivers to be alert to these good fluency days at home. When he has them, his caregivers should give him every opportunity to talk. When the child is having a difficult day, the clinician and caregivers should decrease communication opportunities and remove communicative pressures. Whether we increase or decrease talking time, we should always make the adjustment subtly. In the therapy room, since the general format is play therapy, the clinician can simply direct play into speech or nonspeech activities as the child's needs dictate.

What is the reinforcement the child receives when he is fluent? One can correctly assume that the fluency itself, the freedom to talk without stumbling and hesitating, has the potential to be positively reinforcing, but the clinician's responses and the caregivers' responses can also be powerfully reinforcing. The clinician and the child's caregivers can reinforce fluency by subtly showing more attention and appreciation for what he is saying when he is fluent and by offering only ordinary responses to nonfluent speech. Under no circumstances should the clinician or the caregivers react with criticism or judgment when the child is nonfluent. This kind of reaction can increase the child's awareness of his speech difficulty and lead to the escalation of the struggle and avoidance we are trying to prevent.

In the therapy room, the clinician can use therapy games to reinforce fluency, but caregivers should not attempt to engage the child in these games at home because too many clinical judgments are involved, judgments best supported by the clinician's knowledge and objectivity. Van Riper has described a number of such games I have found useful in reinforcing fluency. One of these games is called *Boss Me*. The child gives commands to the clinician such as, "Stand up," "Sit down," or "Put the pencil in the box." When the child gives the command fluently, the clinician obeys immediately. If he is nonfluent when giving the command, the clinician resists in a friendly, playful manner. Obviously, if a game such as *Boss Me* precipitates an increase in nonfluency, the clinician should abandon it, but if it is played in the spirit of fun, that is not likely to happen.

Another game that can be used to reinforce fluency is called *Escape*. The child and the clinician take turns pleading to be released from an imaginary jail or some other place of confinement. When the captive asks to be released, the captor asks, "Why should I let you go?" The captive must then plead his or her case. When the child is the captive and his pleading is fluent, the clinician releases him immediately, but if he is nonfluent, she hesitates and requires further explanation. Ideally, the explanations and pleadings continue until the child is fluent.

My personal favorite among these games is called *Say the Magic Word*. The clinician and the client talk about a picture, book, movie, television program, or any topic of interest. The clinician begins by announcing that if the child says the *magic word,* he will win a prize. The clinician has no specific word in mind, of course, but when the child has been fluent for a time, she selects any word he has said as the *magic word*. She then rings a bell, blows a whistle, or in some other way signals that the child has won. The clinician announces the *magic word* and rewards the child with his prize. The younger clients especially enjoy this activity, particularly when the celebration is huge.

The activities designed to accomplish this goal should make it clear that the goals in this program are very much interrelated. Although the primary goal of these games is to reinforce fluency, we are also making speech pleasant, and the clinician has many opportunities to model appropriate fluency. The lesson to be stressed is that no matter what activity the clinician is using in therapy at any given time, she should consider all the goals that can or should be met in that activity. Considering all the possible benefits of an activity should prompt the clinician to plan carefully and to execute precisely.

GOAL FIVE: Increasing Tolerance for Communicative Stress

The fifth goal is *desensitization*. Communicative pressure or stress is a major component in the stuttering problem, regardless of the client's age. The adult stutterer is affected by many of the same stresses that affect the young stutterer, but the adult's disorder is compounded by anticipation of fluency failure, specific linguistic and situation fears, and by habituated motor responses that trigger nonfluencies. Dealing with the communicative stresses that affect the stuttering youngster is extremely important because these stresses can lead directly to the development of the compounding problems surrounding advanced stuttering. In other words, we must help the young beginning stutterer deal with his communicative stresses so we can prevent escalation of the severity and complexity of his behaviors. This gets us directly to the essence of desensitization. Desensitization therapy is designed to increase the child's tolerance for stress in speaking situations.

It should be clearly understood that desensitization therapy does not call for the removal of stress. On the contrary, the clinician deliberately injects stress into the therapy situation, but she controls the type and degree of stress that will be injected. She decides when the stress will be injected and when it will be withdrawn. There are very tight controls in this therapy, and because desensitization exercises have the potential to evoke considerable frustration and increased nonfluency, the clinician should not attempt this therapy until she has established a warm, friendly, trusting relationship with the client.

Clinicians are sometimes reluctant to administer desensitization therapy because they are afraid they will make the child's stuttering worse. While there are no guarantees, the clinician should remember that most children who stutter are pretty tough and will tolerate stress, especially when the stress is controlled by people they like and trust. The sensitive clinician will discover what her client's level of tolerance is for communicative stress and will increase that tolerance without damaging the child in any way. The child will actually become stronger, tougher, and more confident.

One obvious way we can attack communicative pressures is through environmental therapy. The clinician and the child's caregivers can identify and eliminate those factors that precipitate frustration and subsequent stuttering in the child. If we take only this approach, however, we make a serious miscalculation about real life. The child must learn how to handle stress because stress is a natural part of life at all ages. No human being can expect to live a life free of communicative pressures and frustrations. A person can-not choose to live in a stress-free bubble. The choice he can and must make is whether he will control and tolerate the pressures in his life or be manip-ulated by them. Desensitization therapy allows the client to see that he does have a choice, and even though the young client will not see this option as clearly as the adult, his reaction to the therapy will indicate that he does or does not understand the option.

The technical aspects of desensitization will be described in the follow-ing paragraph, but I want to emphasize that desensitization is as much art as it is technique. The clinician must be sensitive to the smallest changes in the child's behavior that signal frustration and impending stuttering. She must be skillful in manipulating the child's behaviors so that frustration tolerance is increased and stuttering is thwarted. The greatest challenge is that she must be able to do all this without focusing the child's attention on what is hap-pening. As I have stressed throughout this chapter, this means that the clini-cian must desensitize the young beginning stutterer within the context of play therapy.

The desensitization procedure follows four steps: (1) Create basal fluen-cy by any appropriate means, including the techniques described relative to the four preceding goals. Basal fluency is the best fluency the child can achieve. The young beginning stutterer, whose behaviors are still extremely variable, will be capable of producing speech that is free of any abnormal nonfluencies. (2) Once basal fluency has been established and maintained for approximately five minutes, the clinician should gradually introduce a flu-ency disruptor (e.g., questioning, challenging, interrupting). She should take care to use just one disruptor at a time so she knows exactly what causes flu-ency to break down. (3) When nonfluency begins or when the clinician sens-es it is imminent because of nonverbal indicators, she should withdraw the disruptor. (4) Return to basal fluency and maintain it for another five minutes before beginning the next cycle.

The goal is to increase the time lapse between the introduction of the dis-ruptor (Step 2) and the beginning of fluency breakdown (Step 3). Eventually, assuming the client responds well to desensitization therapy, he will tolerate any kind or degree of disruption without any unusual reaction. In the early stages of this therapy, each cycle will require about 15 to 20 minutes. It is probably not wise to subject the child to more than three or four consecutive cycles within a single session, assuming you have time for that many, because there is some accumulation of stress, and it becomes more and more difficult to return to basal fluency.

Even though most children do not understand what is happening during desensitization therapy, there are exceptions. I experienced a classic excep-tion some years ago with a four-year-old stutterer who was the most severe preschool stutterer I have ever seen. He was also the most intelligent, most energetic young stutterer with whom I have ever worked. He loved dinosaurs, and regaled his clinicians with detailed lectures about dinosaurs during every therapy session. Desensitization was an important component in this client's program, and he endured the procedure often during the one year he was in our clinic. Toward the end of that year, during which he made remarkable progress, he was sitting on the floor telling us more stories about dinosaurs when the clinicians began a cycle of desensitization. This child was particularly vulnerable to interruption, and that was the disruptor the clinicians were using during this session. After about two minutes of interruptions, this bright little boy, this courageous young stutterer who had improved dramatically over a period of about nine months, stood up, put his hands on his hips, looked directly at his clinicians and proclaimed in a calm, confident, controlled voice, "I know what you are trying to do, and it won't work!" He was absolutely right. No matter what the clinicians tried to do, they could not induce nonfluency. The harder they pushed, the more controlled he became, and the bigger and brighter was the smile on his face. This was an incredible turning point for this client. We learned that day that he was making the same kind of adjustment at home. Whenever he felt pressure, he collected himself, slowed his rate slightly and continued to talk with confident fluency. This child was dismissed from therapy one month later. We followed his progress for two years after termination to make sure there would be no relapse. There was not even the hint of relapse. Not all young stutterers will respond this well to desensitization therapy, of course, and some do not respond to it at all, but for the young client whose stuttering is significantly affected by communicative stress, it may be the most important therapy the clinician can offer.

GOAL SIX: Prevent Increased Awareness

The sixth goal in the program for young beginning stutterers is to *prevent increased awareness*. As the reader will undoubtedly note, this goal has been indirectly included in other parts of the program, but it is a goal that also needs direct attention.

It is probably not correct to say that the young beginning stutterer is unaware of his fluency problems. It is more accurate to acknowledge that his initial awareness is intermittent, not particularly focused, and does not seem to reflect any serious concern on the child's part about speaking. After he produces a moment of stuttering, the child might widen his eyes and look startled. He might take a quick inhalation, or he might pause for a few seconds, but he does not give up on talking. He continues to talk because he is more interested in communicating his messages than he is upset about his fluency failures.

As the stuttering screw turns, we see changes in awareness, changes that should cause concern. When the child shows signs of awareness *during* stuttering as opposed to *after* stuttering, there is danger of escalating severity. When the child becomes aware of fluency difficulty to the extent that he avoids and struggles, he is entering a critical period in the development of the disorder. If we can prevent the child from reaching that level of awareness that produces struggle and avoidance, the stuttering will tend to disappear, but if the awareness dam breaks, the young beginning stutterer will likely become a young advanced stutterer, and we will be forced to draw new battle lines.

I want to suggest three specific strategies the clinician and the child's caregivers can employ to help prevent increased awareness: (1) As mentioned earlier in this chapter, when the child is having a noticeably difficult time maintaining fluency, *reduce talking time and talking demands*. During these nonfluent periods, the clinician should step up her efforts to accomplish the first four goals in the program. If those goals are met, it is highly unlikely that awareness will increase. (2) When the child is in the midst of a particularly nonfluent period, *distract him from the stuttering* by changing the subject or directing him to another activity. This needs to be done subtly, of course, but if his attention is redirected, he will be less preoccupied with his speaking problems. At this juncture in the book, the reader should clearly understand why this is so important. Stuttering is as much about what the stutterer, even the young stutterer, thinks and perceives as about what he does physically when he creates fluency failures. Anything the clinician and the child's caregivers can do, therefore, to direct his thinking to something other than stuttering or the possibility of stuttering will have a decidedly positive influence on his speech. (3) A simple but effective technique for defusing awareness is called *restimulation*. In this technique, after the child produces a moment to which he reacts, and after the child has completed the thought he was trying to express, the clinician calmly reflects the child's message and expands upon it. Calm restimulation helps the child forget the unpleasantness of the stuttering because he has been reassured that the listener was attending to his message. Restimulation, like fluency modeling, can be effectively used by caregivers, but they must be given precise instructions about how and when it should be used.

Chapter 22

THERAPY FOR THE
YOUNG ADVANCED STUTTERER

Fit the Program to the Client

Most of the children in this category are seven to 14 years old, but I want to reiterate that age is not the most important criterion in determining the type of therapy that is appropriate for a given child. It is true that the young advanced stutterer shares many of the later developing behaviors we see in adult stutterers, BUT he is still a child in most respects, and he cannot be treated as an adult in therapy. The clinician should note that the young advanced stutterer presents some special problems that are common to neither adult stutterers nor to young beginning stutterers. Depending on the needs and problems of a given client, the clinician must develop a therapy program that includes elements of the therapy used with young beginning stutterers and elements of the therapy we use with adults.

The clinician should be forewarned that the variability of symptomotology, maturity, sensitivity, insight, and every other factor that might impact the efficacy of treatment is tremendous within this group of stutterers. It will become quickly and abundantly clear that no one-dimensional or simply designed program will meet the needs of these clients. We should be reminded that one of the classic principles of speech remediation is that the clinician should fit the program to the client rather than trying to fit the client to the program. The need for applying this principle will be no more apparent than when the clinician works with young advanced stutterers.

Special Problems Demand Special Solutions

Charles Van Riper has identified a number of important differences between the therapy experiences of children and the therapy experiences of adults. I want to emphasize several of these differences: (1) Whereas most adult clients are self-referrals, the child is usually brought or referred to therapy by an adult, typically his caregiver. This means we cannot assume the child will be motivated in therapy. At the very least, we can assume that the adult who refers himself *wants* to stop stuttering, even if it would be naive to assume he is willing to invest the time, effort, and pain required for therapy success. We can assume nothing about the child's level of motivation. He is often not motivated to be present, let alone motivated to do the work of therapy. (2) With the adult stutterer, we discuss the idea that the client must accept some temporary unpleasantness in order to achieve future payoff in the form of increased fluency. We cannot expect the child to accept unpleasantness in the present in exchange for future fluency. For a child, even a child in adolescence, a semester or a year is a long time, and unpleasantness is not something he willingly embraces for even the briefest moment. Children want and expect immediate results, and they want those results without pain. These are children reared on television and video games. In their world, there are definite beginnings, clearly and simply drawn plots, and at the end of the program or the game, the good guys always win. Sometimes bad guys with endearing traits win too, but they also win at the end of short scripts. Children who stutter are products of this immediacy culture, and the wise clinician will take this into account when she charts her therapy course. (3) Whereas the clinician might spend considerable time explaining the rationale for therapy procedures to the adult client, she will probably waste her time if she tries to explain rationale to the young advanced stutterer because it is not likely he will understand, and it is highly unlikely he will care. If the clinician insists on trying to explain rationale, she should be alert for signs that she is not making contact, signs such as rolling eyes or a blank stare. (4) The clinician insists that the adult client be responsible for his own therapy progress. The child cannot, or will not, accept much responsibility for implementing therapy; and, I would hasten to point out, in the case of adolescent children, there is virtually no difference between *cannot* and *will not*. (5) To a greater extent than the adult client, the young advanced stutterer does not want to observe his stuttering, experience it on purpose, or do much to change it because he finds the act of stuttering unbearably embarrassing and uncomfortable. The adult does not like to stutter on demand either, and he certainly does not enjoy the physical, emotional, and perceptual aspects of stuttering, but he is usually willing to stutter and to analyze his moments because he understands how this experience advances him toward the goal of increased fluency. The child prefers to ignore the stuttering, or to dismiss it as an insignificant nuisance, because he believes, or wants to believe, that all this stuttering nonsense will go away when he grows up. In the child's view of life, all bad things will disappear when he becomes an adult. He will no longer be afraid of the dark. He will not be physically and socially awkward. He will not suck his thumb, and he will not stutter. From an adult perspective, this is not a realistic belief, but one of the advantages of being a child is that inside your own head and heart, you can make up your own rules. By the time you figure out that your childhood hopes and beliefs were bogus, you are an adult, and you find it somewhat easier to accept life as it really is.

Motivating the Young Advanced Stutterer

An even casual reading of the preceding section suggests that *motivation* is a serious problem for the young advanced stutterer, and so it is. Motivation is a major problem for the adult stutterer too, but at least with the adult, we can confront motivation problems head on. The child's sensitivity is usually too great, and he is too immature to handle direct confrontations on issues of motivation. We cannot ignore motivation, however, because the stuttering is too far along in development for there to be a reasonable hope for spontaneous recovery. It is also highly unlikely, at this stage in development, that environmental manipulation alone will recover lost fluency. So how does the clinician handle a child whose problem cannot be solved indirectly, who needs to accept some responsibility for his disorder and for its treatment, who is not as motivated as he needs to be, but who cannot cope with direct confrontation? Obviously, the problem as I have described it, is not simple, and the questions surrounding it are difficult to address. There are no easy answers to the motivation problems of the young advanced stutterer, but I will offer a few suggestions:

1. This child needs someone who understands his problem and who accepts him as he is–a person who stutters, not a figure to be pitied or ridiculed. The clinician may be the only person in his life who can relate to him in this way. As a speech-language pathologist, she understands what stuttering is, how it develops, how it affects people who stutter, and what must be done to treat it. She also understands how truly difficult the treatment process is, and she knows how to help her client through the process. Knowing that the clinician is a knowledgeable professional who understands the disorder and who cares about the client can, in itself, be powerfully motivating.
2. The clinician can be a fair, compassionate listener, offering neither judgment nor solicitude. Through the technique of reflection, the clinician can help her client develop a healthy objectivity about himself, his stuttering, and his listeners. As the client talks about his problem, the clinician will say, "What I hear you saying is that your jaw got locked. Is

that really what happened? Did your jaw involuntarily slam shut, or did you in the course of struggle force your mouth shut?" At another point, she might say, "What I hear you saying is that whenever you stutter on the telephone, people are rude and hang up? Is this what really happens? Do people really hang up every time you stutter?" As the client listens to his own statements being reflected by the clinician, he will realize that much of what he says about his stuttering experience has little or no basis in reality. Any reasonably intelligent adolescent stutterer knows that his jaw does not *involuntarily* lock. His lips do not *get stuck*. His tongue does not *freeze to the roof of his mouth*. No matter how much trouble he has talking on the telephone, he knows that *not every person he talks to hangs up* when he stutters. If this happens at all, it happens rarely, but the trauma of the one time or even the thought that it might happen has blown his perception out of line with reality. He only needs to hear his own perceptions filtered through an understanding, knowledgeable clinician to realize that not only are these assertions not true, they get in the way of progress. Once the child no longer reacts emotionally to every aspect of his stuttering, he can face it, and once he can face his stuttering objectively, he is in a much stronger position to engage in the therapeutic process that will help him deal with it more effectively.

3. The clinician can allow the child to feel dependent on her. The young advanced stutterer often feels very alone in his struggle with this disorder. If he believes he can share the burden with the clinician, he will feel greater courage to attack his stuttering. With courage comes commitment, and with commitment comes motivation. The clinician should be assured that no matter how much the young client leans on her in the beginning, his dependence will not last long. As the child gains fluency, he will gain confidence, and he will become progressively independent.

4. As with the adult client, the clinician can require the child to observe normal speakers in order to discover that normal speech is not perfect speech. Once the child understands that the goal of fluency is attainable, he will be more motivated to work for it. The idea here is simple but important. No one is motivated to work for a goal that is impossible. I stand barely six feet tall but would love to be six feet, five inches tall. No matter how much you might encourage me to engage in exercises that are advertised to make me six feet, five inches tall, I will not be motivated to engage in these exercises because I know they will not work. If the stutterer believes that fluent speech is impossible, he will not be motivated to work toward that goal. The clinician must convince him that fluency can be achieved, and it can.

5. The clinician can use analogies to help the child better understand the nature of stuttering. Ignorance is perhaps the greatest obstacle to moti-

vation. The child will probably not be receptive to academic lectures about stuttering, but he will be receptive to lessons to which he can personally relate. Carefully crafted analogies are very effective tools for teaching these lessons. A commonly used example will help make this point. Clients often believe that certain words are inherently difficult, and it is this inherent difficulty that causes them to stutter. The following analogy might be used to attack this misperception:

> "If I place a plank of wood about six inches wide on the floor here and asked you to walk across it, do you think you could do that? Of course, you could, but if I put that same plank of wood 200 feet in the air–without a safety net–and asked you to walk across it, suddenly it would be *very difficult*. In fact, there is an excellent chance you would fall off. Why? It's the same plank whether it's on the ground or 200 feet in the air. The act of walking across the plank does not change just because it's elevated. The only thing that actually changes is the way you *think* about walking across the plank. The potential danger changes your perception of the task, and because you think about the consequences of failure, you believe it is a difficult task, and you *make* it a difficult task. Speaking for you is very much like walking across that plank. Alone in your room, you can probably say any words you want to say without stuttering because you do not perceive any risks, but in the presence of a threatening listener, you might stutter on those words. Why? Because of the threatening listener, you think about failure, and you think about the consequences of failure. You *think* that speaking is going to be difficult, so just as you would do if you were walking on that plank 200 feet in the air, you tense up, you panic, and you *make* speaking difficult."

I have found analogies to be very helpful in creating understanding in young advanced stutterers, as well as adult stutterers. As I have noted repeatedly in this book, and as I will note again before all the pages have been flipped, a client who understands his disorder is far less intimidated by it and is, therefore, more motivated to do what needs to be done in therapy.

6. The clinician can use high fluency activities (e.g., choral reading, rhythmic speaking, whispering, speaking under masking) to help convince her client that there is nothing physically wrong that prevents him from speaking fluently. If the client is persuaded that his behavior is within his control, he will be more motivated to do what he needs to do to exercise the control he wants. As long as he believes that stuttering is permanent and unmanageable, there is no reason for him to do anything to try to change it. He will simply resign himself to his fate.

THE PHASES OF THERAPY

The therapy program for young advanced stutterers proceeds through the same four phases used with adult clients: **Identification, Desensitization, Modification,** and **Stabilization.** The expectations and procedures within each phase are adapted to meet the needs and abilities of younger stutterers.

Identification

As with the adult stutterer, the young advanced stutterer *must* be able to identify his stuttering behaviors if he is to change or eliminate them, but we do not expect the child to identify as accurately or as fastidiously as the adult.

The young advanced stutterer will have little difficulty identifying avoidance behaviors, postponements, and starters because these are relatively conscious behaviors, and he is already aware of them, even if he is not aware that other people notice them. Since these behaviors, when they first emerge, are used consciously and since they have yet to develop great habit strength in the young stutterer, the clinician's task is to simply increase the client's awareness of their occurrences, help him understand their purposes, and persuade him to surrender these behaviors. The clinician must convince the client that, while these behaviors might seem to help the client cope in the short-term, they actually add to the fear and struggle components of stuttering and threaten to complicate the disorder in the long-term.

Van Riper recommended a game called *Catch Me* to help young clients identify avoidance, postponement, and starting behaviors. The clinician begins by describing the behaviors targeted for this exercise. In the course of conversation, the clinician and client take turns trying to catch one another producing these behaviors. Most clients find this game less threatening if the client is first allowed to catch the clinician as she talks and purposely includes avoidance behaviors, postponements, and starters in her speech. After the client is comfortable with the idea that this really is a friendly and enjoyable game and sees that the clinician is uninhibited in producing these behaviors, he will be more inclined to stutter openly and will be less embarrassed when the clinician catches him in the act of producing the targeted behaviors.

It is much more difficult to identify the core behaviors (repetitions, closures, and postural fixations) and interrupters because these behaviors are more habitual and are produced at a much lower level of consciousness. The young advanced stutterer might never reach the point where he identifies these behaviors consistently. If he can consistently differentiate between *hard* moments and *easy* moments, however, he is doing quite well because this differentiation includes an awareness of degrees of excessive muscular tension and inappropriate articulatory positions. These maladjustments are the pillars upon which the core behaviors are built. If the child can find and identify these pillars, he will know what to attack when it is time to modify his moments of stuttering. It is noteworthy that even if the child cannot accurately explain the differences between hard and easy moments, once he knows he has a choice, he eventually learns to choose the easier way.

As a general rule, the clinician should not ask the young advanced stutterer to identify word and sound difficulties. There is no doubt that he has linguistic fears, but they tend to be unstable and inconsistent, and nothing is gained by fixing these fears in the child's awareness. There may be, of course, the exceptional young client who will profit from detailed analyses of his linguistic fears, and the clinician should offer that opportunity. The clinician must *always* be prepared to adjust to the special needs and abilities of her young stutterers, whether that means more direct or less direct, more specific or less specific, more challenging or less challenging.

The young advanced stutterer will usually have little difficulty identifying his situation fears, at least the most intense of them. One of the positive consequences of identifying the child's situation fears is that just talking about these fears often helps to diminish them. There is a catharsis in this exercise similar to what we all feel when we talk aloud about something that has burdened us. The child usually cannot discuss the fear aspects of stuttering with anyone who understands them as well as the clinician. An important purpose is served, therefore, by letting the child talk through his fears of listeners and situations. In some cases, we can also test the child's situation fears to help him understand that the perception of difficulty or penalty is probably greater than the reality. If he claims, for example, that store clerks are rude to him when he stutters, the clinician can accompany him to a few stores, have him talk to store clerks and then talk about what happened. Were the clerks rude? Were they more rude to the client than they were to their non-stuttering customers? When the young advanced stutterer learns that his fears are out of proportion to the reality, his fears will usually begin to subside, and if he discovers that some of these fears are completely unfounded, they may fade away completely.

Desensitization

In most cases, we cannot use the systematic desensitization procedure with young advanced stutterers that we use with adult clients because children usually cannot develop accurate hierarchies of anxiety-evoking situations, and they rarely possess the insights to benefit from this form of therapy. Instead, we use the same desensitization procedure we use with young beginning stutterers, with a few important adaptations. For example, basal fluency for the young beginning stutterer will be speech with no stutterings at all. Basal fluency for the advanced stutterer will probably not reach this level. It might be *easy* stuttering, at least in the beginning. That is, he will still stutter, but he will stutter without struggle and without avoiding. As therapy progresses, however, he may very well achieve total fluency as his basal level. Depending on the age of the young advanced stutterer, desensitization therapy may be done in the context of play, as with the young beginning stutterer, or it may be done within the context of conversation. Especially with older clients in this category, desensitization can be presented more directly. The clinician begins by explaining exactly what is going to happen and with what purpose, and she provides generous encouragement and praise as the therapy moves forward. She might say, for example, "Today we are going to do something called 'desensitization therapy.' We will talk for a few minutes, very calmly, until you are doing very well with your speech. Then I am going to try to make you stutter. I might ask you a lot of questions, or I might interrupt you, or I might try to make you hurry, but whatever I do, you try to continue to talk as calmly as possible. Don't let the way I talk influence the way you talk. Do you have any questions?" Because the child is likely to forget what he is supposed to do, or because he allows himself to be unduly influenced by the clinician's disruption tactics, the clinician might have to repeat this explanation a number of times.

A common problem for the young advanced stutterer that can be addressed in desensitization therapy is the mocking and teasing he might receive from his peers. In some cases, talking directly to the offending child can solve this problem. Most children will stop teasing the stutterer if they are helped to understand what stuttering is, and if they are helped to appreciate the pain they are inflicting. Contrary to what we are commonly taught, I have not found that children are naturally cruel. I have found that children tend to be naturally compassionate, but also naturally ignorant. The best way to combat the perceived cruelty then is to give them good information. Whether or not the clinician can confront the offending child or children, she should also counsel the stutterer. I have found that the best counsel is to advise the client to react with good-natured humor. The person who is able to laugh at himself is rarely the target of cruel mocking and teasing. Consider that people tease in order to get a reaction. If the reaction the teaser gets is self-acceptance and laughter, the game is no longer fun. We can also counsel stutterers to be more assertive, although not necessarily aggressive. Assertive, confident, self-assured people find ways to compensate for their liabilities. An assertive, confident stutterer will probably not be viewed by other people as a *stutterer*. He will be valued for his worth as a person, and his stuttering will be no more a target for ridicule than shortness or freckles are for other people.

The clinician and the child's caregivers should make a concerted effort to improve the child's self-image because, as I have noted repeatedly, how the stutterer feels about himself will have a significant impact on his speech. We established early in this book that when the stutterer is confident, when he feels good about himself, when he feels equal or superior to the people to whom he is talking, he tends to do very well with his speech. The child's significant others, including his speech-language clinician, can bolster his self-image by being supportive and encouraging and by appreciating all of the client's talents, positive personal traits, and achievements. When the stutterer perceives himself in positive ways, others will begin to focus more on who he is as a person, and they will pay less attention to his stuttering and to his eleventh toe.

Modification

Most young advanced stutterers find it difficult to attend to specific moments of stuttering, so we do not attack specific moments, nor do we concentrate on the specific behaviors that comprise their moments of stuttering. Furthermore, most of these youngsters do not have the patience or the insight to handle the detailed instructions involved in teaching the modification, and they cannot endure the tedious drill work involved in the progressive application of the modification through cancellations, pull-outs, and preparatory sets. Instead of teaching the modification and then moving it forward through this sequence, therefore, we work for the immediate replacement of moments of stuttering with modified productions of stuttered words or words that might be stuttered.

The clinician says to the child, "I want you to speak in this new way whenever you stutter or whenever you think you might stutter." Instead of *describing* the characteristics of the modification, the "new way of speaking," the clinician *demonstrates* it. She fills her own speech will examples of the modification, allowing her examples to model the highly conscious and deliberate articulation, the light and easy contacts, and the slow, calculated movements that characterize modifications. The clinician's models should emphasize the modification of the first sound or syllable of words since these are the loci of most moments of stuttering, and she should blend the sound or syllable as smoothly as possible into the remainder of each word. She should make an effort to demonstrate modification on the full range of phonemes, although she should give special attention to those phonemes and words that are most often stuttered by her client.

In addition to flooding her own speech with examples of modifications in a wide range of phonetic contexts, the clinician should intermittently stop the child after he produces a hard moment of stuttering and instruct him to say the word again in the "new way," first in isolation and then in the original sentence. If the client produces a long, complicated moment, the clinician might stutter in unison with him and then model the modification while the client follows her lead. After a number of trials, perhaps over several sessions, the child will readily follow the clinician's model, without constant reminders. Remember that we have a natural advantage here. Children learn quickly and easily, and they love to imitate. Children are far less reluctant and inhibited about trying new skills than the typical adult. Watch a youngster sit down at a computer keyboard for the first time, and then watch an adult do the same thing. The differences are startling. Adults tend to be intimidated and fearful about this new experience. Children are excited and do not have to be prompted to explore this new technology. They are far less concerned than adults about failing. They truly live the maxim adults preach to them: "If at first you don't succeed, try, try again." I recently watched my four-year-old grandson playing with his new **Game Boy** for the first time. He was the model of concentration. His eyes never left the screen. He pushed the arrow buttons in every direction. The more he pushed, the faster his fingers flew. After watching him for at least five minutes, I asked, "Peyton, do you know what you're doing?" Without looking up and while still maintaining his digital frenzy, he calmly replied, "No." It did not matter that he had not mastered the game he was playing or all the technological details of the instrument with which he was playing the game. He was willing to try and fail, try and fail, and try and fail until something–anything–good happened. The young advanced stutterer learning to modify is very much like Peyton. He is more than willing to try, try again, and if he fails, he will try, try again some more.

Once the modification is identified and understood, the client and clinician should use it constantly, and the clinician should provide generous praise, not just for successful modifications, but for good efforts to modify. In the beginning, reinforcement should be continuous, but as the child becomes more proficient in using the "new way of speaking" to deal with his actual and anticipated fluency failures, the clinician should use a more intermittent reinforcement schedule. The eventual and best reinforcements for appropriate modifications are fluency and successfully completed communications. It must be unmistakably noted that the clinician should not, under any circumstances, punish the child's nonfluencies. The young advanced stutterer's sensitivity is too great, his psyche too unstable, and the critical client-clinician relationship too fragile to risk the consequences of punishment, even if it is administered properly and gently.

Although we do not generally teach young advanced stutterers to move the modification forward in time through cancellations, pull-outs, and preparatory sets, we usually observe a natural tendency for the child to use modifications in a forward-moving manner. That is, he first modifies *after* he produces moments of stuttering, but as he becomes accustomed to the new way of speaking, he will modify as he is producing moments, and eventually he will plan modifications when he thinks he might have trouble with a word. Only rarely will a young advanced stutterer need any specific instructions to help him move the modification forward in time. Even then, instructions are far less helpful and far less effective than the clinician's demonstrations. In case the clinician is inclined to forget this point, she should remember the proverb I mentioned earlier in this book: *A good example is worth twice as much as good advice.* This truth is applicable in an infinite number of situations involving interactions between children and adults, and it is certainly applicable in the clinician's treatment of the young advanced stutterer.

Stabilization

In contrast to the adult client who usually needs an extensive period of stabilization, the young advanced stutterer rarely needs much time in this final phase of therapy. Once the client begins to use the modification and feels comfortable with it, the disorder dissolves fairly quickly. During the brief stabilization period that is necessary, the clinician should provide as much practice as possible within and outside the therapy room. To repeat the advice of Wendell Johnson, the client should talk as much as possible, to as many different people as possible, in as many different situations as possible.

Following the formal stabilization period, the clinician should maintain some contact with the client for a period of 12 to 24 months because relapse is a common occurrence in advanced stutterers of all ages. If the client shows any signs of relapse, formal therapy should be resumed for as many weeks or months as necessary to reestablish fluency control. If the client can maintain fluency control for a year or two, the chances for long-term success are excellent.

Chapter 23

INTERVIEWING AND COUNSELING

Those of us who teach students how to be speech-language pathologists are often guilty of assuming that students will instinctively know how to interview and how to counsel. People who routinely interview and counsel will know that this is a terribly naive assumption. These skills are not instinctive in most clinicians, and all clinicians quickly learn that interviews and counseling sessions handled badly can destroy the efficacy of treatment. I cannot and will not pretend that this chapter will contain everything the clinician needs to know about how to conduct an interview and how to counsel, but it is my intention to identify the basics of these processes, especially as they relate to stutterers.

CONDUCTING AN INTERVIEW

If the clinician skillfully handles the interview portion of the evaluation session with the informant, either the client himself or the client's caregiver, it will be a comfortable experience for both parties. Without question, the level of comfort depends on the opening of the interview. It is the clinician's responsibility to set the tone. This is not an interrogation, and it is not a casual conversation. It is something in between. The clinician is a professional seeking information about a person who has a problem the clinician knows and understands, but the tone must go beyond this. The clinician must let the informant know, by what she says and by her general demeanor, that she genuinely cares about the client and about the informant, if the informant is not the client. In addition, she must convey the message that she will respect the informant no matter what he says. If the clinician indicates, verbally or nonverbally, that she disapproves of the informant or what he is saying, or if she indicates that the informant is making her feel uneasy, the interview is not likely to yield much substance. The informant must trust the clinician, and the clinician must engender this trust.

One simple way to engender trust during an interview is to maintain an appropriate visual relationship with the informant. This does not mean the interviewer should stare at the informant. Uninterrupted visual contact is uncomfortable, and it is unnatural. It does mean that whether or not the interviewer maintains eye contact when she is asking questions, she should certainly maintain eye contact when she is listening to the informant's responses. Even then, however, it should be natural eye contact, in combination with nods of the head and appropriate facial expressions. A glazed stare might work in a horror movie, but it is not what we want in an interview. The clinician should be as natural as possible, remembering the old admonition: "If you can't be sincere, fake it!"

The information obtained during an interview will be useful only if it is retained. Unless the clinician has an extraordinary memory, this means that the interview should be recorded. If the informant grants permission, the best way to preserve the interview is by tape recording it. If it is not possible to tape record, the interviewer should take notes. In fact, even if the interview is being recorded on tape, the interviewer should take written notes. Most informants find note-taking reassuring because it suggests the interviewer is really listening and that she finds what the informant is saying important enough to be noted. The interviewer should be careful, however, to use some kind of shorthand version of note-taking so that long silences are avoided.

The clinician will get off to a good start by explaining the purpose of the interview–that she is gathering information that will help her make a proper diagnosis, information that will help her design a remediation program that will be best for the client. She must make sure the informant knows how the information he reveals will be used, with whom this information will be shared, and from whom this information will be kept confidential. If the informant is assured that the information being sought is relevant and will be revealed only to professionals who need to review it, he will be more open and honest in his responses. We should not assume that informants will lie, but we should assume that informants will be careful about what they say to strangers. If the interviewer expects good and complete information, she will give the informant all the guarantees she can regarding relevance and confidence.

It is interesting that when one person identifies another person as a *good conversationalist,* he usually means that the other person is a good listener. A good interviewer is very much the good conversationalist. She listens attentively, and she listens with interest. Among other things, this means that the interviewer does not ask questions twice. When an informant is asked the same question two or three times, he is likely to conclude that the interviewer was not paying attention the first time, that the interviewer does not care enough to listen intently, that the interviewer did not approve the first answer, or that the interviewer asked the question a second time because she thought the informant was not telling the truth the first time. None of these conclusions will advance the interviewer-informant relationship. When the interviewer asks a question, she *should* be interested in the answer. Otherwise, why did she ask the question?

A good interview is characterized by a certain communicative energy. It is not a frenetic exchange, but it is certainly a lively exchange of information in which the interviewer is genuinely interested. A simple strategy the interviewer can use to make sure she is listening as intently as required is to allow adequate time for an answer. That is, she should not be in a hurry to get to the next question. She should ask a question and wait. Sometimes informants need time to formulate their answers. It really is not terribly difficult to determine if the informant is thinking about what he wants to say or if he is finished. If the nonverbal signs indicate *still in progress,* the clinician should be patient. The goal is to obtain information, not to obtain information *quickly.*

How the interviewer constructs her questions will have a definite impact on the nature of the interview and on the quality of the information she elicits. Questions should be clearly and economically structured, and they should be devoid of words that suggest an expected answer. As I indicated, the interviewer should know why she is asking each question, and if she does not know why a question is posed, she should not ask it. There is nothing wrong with using technical terms in these questions because they are sometimes the best words to frame the question and because they suggest the interviewer is knowledgeable and professional, but technical terms should always be defined, especially if the informant seems to be unsure about them. Examples may be useful in helping the informant understand terms. Avoid questions that can be answered with "yes" or "no," and avoid wording that might bias the response. If, for example, the clinician wants to know something about how a parent manages her child's behavior, she should not ask, "You don't beat your child, do you?" A better, more neutral question would be, "What strategies do you employ to manage your child's behavior?" With some questions, it may be necessary to provide answer options or a scale because the informant may not know enough about the topic to provide a good answer. For example, the clinician might want to know the informant's judgment regarding the severity of a child's stuttering. By way of assisting the informant, the interviewer might ask: "On a scale of 1–7, on which '1' represents 'no stuttering' and '7' represents 'very severe stuttering,' how would you rate Johnny's stuttering?" She might also ask, "In your judgment, is Johnny's stuttering mild, moderate, or severe?"

During the course of an interview, especially an interview concerning a problem like stuttering, it is highly likely that there will be some sensitive subjects to discuss. The interviewer should arrange topics and questions in an order that takes into account the informant's potential anxiety and sensitivity levels. That is, she should begin with easy, nonthreatening questions. After some rapport has been established, and the interviewer has established some trust, she should move into the more sensitive topics. If the clinician is interviewing a recently divorced mother, for example, and if she suspects that the trauma of the divorce is affecting the speech of a stuttering child, she should not begin with the question: "How do you think your divorce is affecting Johnny's stuttering?" This does not mean that this question should not be asked. If the interviewer believes the divorce is a relevant issue, she should ask the informant about it, but after the informant is comfortable. Even then, however, the question should be sensitively framed. The interviewer might say, "I understand that you are recently divorced, and I want you to know that my heart goes out to you and your children. I know this can be very difficult for everyone concerned. Do you think this change in your life has affected Johnny' speech in any way?" This example affords an excellent opportunity to establish another rule of interviewing: The interviewer must not hedge on difficult questions. An evasive question is a clear invitation to an evasive answer, and most evasive answers are worthless.

If, in the process of talking about an emotional issue, the informant becomes upset, the interviewer must be prepared to deal with the emotionality. It is always a good idea to have facial tissues handy. In most cases, the informant will simply need a little time to regain composure. The interviewer should be quiet and allow the time required. In some cases, it is appropriate to express understanding, but if the emotionality is over an issue such as divorce in which there are two sides to be considered, the interviewer should be very careful not to take sides. It's one thing to say, "Yes, that had to be very painful for all of you." It's quite another to say, "Yes, he was a real jerk. I'm surprised you stayed with him as long as you did." If the emotionality is the fault of the interviewer, intentionally or unintentionally, she should apologize. In a worst case scenario, the interviewer might have to excuse herself from the room while the informant tries to regain control. This is a perfectly acceptable response to extreme emotionality. Some people find it difficult to regain composure in the presence of others. As a general rule, the interviewer should be empathic. If she were in the informant's position, how would she feel, and how would she want the interviewer to behave? More often than not, following empathy's lead will put the interviewer in a pretty good position to do the right thing and say the right words.

Inexperienced interviewers often find that they are halfway through their questions when the time allotted for the interview has expired. The clinician must allow enough time for the informant to answer her questions, but she also needs to keep the interview moving forward. She should not spend too much time on any single topic, and above all else, she should avoid talking about things that are not relevant. As a general rule, if the interviewer finds herself talking to the informant about recipes, summer vacations, or favorite movies, the interview has strayed off course.

Sometimes the interviewer is faced with a very different problem. She moves through the interview too quickly. All the questions are asked, but because of her rush to cross the finish line, the answers she elicits from the informant are brief and superficial. The clinician must make sure the information she is getting is complete enough to be useful. She must make sure the informant gets dates and names straight, that events are in the right sequence, that real or perceived cause-effect relationships are clearly described. If the interviewer senses that information is incomplete, she may ask the informant to fill in the missing details. If she senses that there are discrepancies in the informant's story, she should point out the apparent contradictions, but in a constructive, nonaccusatory manner. She might say, for example, "Earlier you indicated that Johnny began to stutter when he was about four years old, and just now you indicated that the problem started when he entered school. Could you clarify this for me? Was he doing something at four that was different from what he was doing at six?"

The informant should be encouraged to express his interpretation of the events about which he talks. He should be encouraged to offer his opinions, and he should be allowed to express his emotions. Assume that the interviewer asks, "What do you think caused you to stutter?" The informant could simply answer, "It was my father's fault," but that is not enough information. The interviewer should ask the informant to elaborate by posing a follow-up question such as, "In what sense was it your father's fault? What did he do to make you stutter?" As long as the interviewer recognizes that there are differences among facts, interpretations, and opinions, all of these responses are potentially useful. After all information is gathered, the clinician might conclude that the informant's father was not responsible for the onset of stuttering, but she might also conclude that the informant's feelings about his father have contributed to the development and maintenance of his stuttering and that the informant's opinions about these matters have helped shape his perceptions of the people and situations that affect his stuttering.

Throughout the interview, but certainly near the end of the interview, the clinician should be prepared for questions from the informant. She should anticipate questions the informant is likely to ask, and she should make sure she knows how to answer these questions. Many informants want to know what causes stuttering, how it develops, why it is more common in boys than girls, what they can do to help, and what the future holds. The clinician should make sure she knows how to respond to these questions, but she should also be prepared to say, "I don't know the answer to that question, but I will find out and get back to you." It is not wrong to be ignorant, but it is wrong, and it is professionally irresponsible to provide answers that are grounded in reckless guesses and speculation. If someone other than the person conducting the interview will make the final decision about whether therapy is indicated or not, she should defer questions about therapy to that person.

Finally, the clinician should close the interview as gracefully as possible. She should thank the informant for his time and cooperation, and assure him that the information he has given will be helpful. She should indicate by her nonverbal behavior that the interview has ended. She can turn off the tape recorder, put her pen and paper away, stand up, and move toward the door. If all else fails, she can gently nudge the informant into the elevator and push **G.**

COUNSELING THE CAREGIVERS OF YOUNG STUTTERERS

The therapies for young beginning and young advanced stutterers described in the preceding two chapters involve direct intervention with clients, but they do not exclude environmental therapy, or counseling. It is imperative that the clinician involves caregivers, teachers, and other significant adults in the treatment of the youngster who stutters. Not only does the child spend most of his time with these adults, he is also significantly affected by their behaviors and attitudes. If we hope to accomplish the ultimate goals of treatment, we must enlist the aid of those people who are most important in the child's life.

I have organized this section on counseling around questions I have been asked about counseling, questions posed by students in training, clinicians in practice, and by caregivers themselves.

Before we proceed, I want to remind the reader that many of the topics discussed in this section have already been addressed in Chapter 9 (*Helping the Stuttering Child*). The difference between that chapter and this is one is largely a matter of *audience*. The information included in Chapter 9 is addressed primarily to caregivers, with speech-language clinicians listening in. The information in this chapter is addressed to speech-language clinicians, with caregivers listening in. If you read both chapters, you will notice the differences and the similarities, but I trust you will recognize that the overall message about what caregivers, parents, and other significant adults need to do to help the stuttering child is very consistent.

Is Caregiver Counseling Really Necessary?

Yes, it is, and for a number of interrelated reasons. A human child is not reared in a vacuum. He is the product of his genes, of course, but he is also dramatically affected by his environment, and he is especially affected by his caregivers. His caregivers give him his values. They help shape his dreams, and they chart the direction of his early life. The attitudes of the child's caregivers determine the family's communicative style. The rules and strategies in this communicative style may contribute to the young stutterer's speaking problems. Whether they like it or not, whether they choose to believe it or not, whether they are comfortable with it or not, the child's caregivers are such powerful influences in his life that they *must* be brought into the treatment process. They need to understand that this is not a matter of blame or fault. They are, in fact, probably blameless. No matter how much or how little the child's caregivers are contributing to the problem, however, it is absolutely essential that we enlist their help in solving the problem. It is important to acknowledge that the vast majority of caregivers *want* to help their stuttering children, and they are willing participants in the counseling portion of the treatment program.

Will Caregiver Counseling Work?

Anyone who works with human problems for any length of time will attest that there are never guarantees in treatment programs for these problems. Does incarceration rehabilitate criminals? Are drug treatment programs effective in getting addicts clean and sober? Does Alcoholic Anonymous work, or Gamblers Anonymous, or Weight Watchers, or . . . ? Well, you get the picture. Any program designed to change human behavior *can* be effective, and anyone who implements this kind of program can trot out success cases to show just how wonderful the program is, but human behavior can be a monstrous enemy. For every success, there is a failure, and in many cases, for every success, there are three or four or more failures. Will caregiver counseling work? Given a legitimate chance, it *can* work, but the counselor and the person being counseled must approach the process with realistic expectations.

The clinician should approach counseling with the attitude that changes in the attitudes and behaviors of caregivers are difficult, but these changes *are* possible. She should remember that the purpose of counseling is not to directly change attitudes and behaviors, but to lead caregivers to the insights and knowledge that will allow them to make changes on their own. To paraphrase an old adage, *You can lead caregivers to the possibility of change, but you cannot make changes for them.*

The two primary goals of counseling are (1) to alter the child's environment so that fluency can be more easily facilitated, and (2) to help caregivers understand the child's fluency problem and his reactions to it. Caregivers often fail to understand how they influence the way their child talks. The clinician must cultivate this understanding by pointing out some of the more obvious ways that caregivers affect the speech of their children. Why does the child speak American English, for example? Why does he produce the dialect he uses? Who shaped his vocabulary and his conversational style? The child's caregivers provide him models for every aspect of speech and language. By their models, they determine the child's native language, his dialect, his prosodic patterns, his vocabulary, his grammatical competence, and his pragmatic skills. His caregivers also establish the rules and procedures for family interactions, including speech and language interactions, for good or ill. After establishing the power of their models, the clinician counsels the caregivers to understand that, if they choose to do so, they can directly modify the child's speech. They can modify vocabulary, conversational courtesy, grammar, prosody, and they can, if they choose to do so, influence the child's fluency. Will caregiver counseling work? The answer is now a little clearer. It will work if caregivers will it to work, and if they work to make it work.

How Should the Clinician Approach Caregiver Counseling?

This is a more important question than you might imagine because the counselor is in a difficult position. Going into the process, she knows that she will probably ask, and perhaps demand, that caregivers make fundamental changes in their communicative lives. She knows that, despite their best intentions, caregivers often interact with their stuttering children in ways that are harmful. She also knows that many caregivers, no matter how well-educated and intelligent they might be, are ignorant about speech and language development in general and about stuttering specifically. How she approaches the caregivers, therefore, and her attitude toward them will impact the efficacy of counseling.

The counselor cannot be timid. She cannot evade difficult issues. There are times when she must make critical judgments about the attitudes and behaviors of the child's caregivers, but she must do so in a consistently constructive, supportive, and empathic manner. This becomes problematic because so many of the issues that are discussed during counseling are emotional in nature. Caregivers are often frightened and confused. They often feel guilty. Sometimes they are angry about what is happening to their child, and they want someone or something to blame. Almost always, they feel a kind of helplessness. Caregivers' emotions tend to come tumbling out during counseling sessions, and the counselor must know how to deal with them.

First and foremost, she should not try to contain these emotions. Caregivers should be allowed, even encouraged, to release them, and the counselor must provide caregivers opportunities to talk about their feelings openly and objectively. The counselor should understand that much of the emotional load associated with stuttering is the product of misunderstanding and ignorance. This means that the counselor can help caregivers deal with their emotionality by giving them information about the disorder and by answering their questions. Knowledge can be a great emotional healer, especially if it is offered by someone who is supportive and understanding. In the process of providing information, the counselor may have to point out mistakes caregivers have made in dealing with the child's stuttering; but whenever possible, the *blame* for these mistakes should be laid at the feet of well-intentioned ignorance, not bad or insensitive parenting. The counselor should provide information and answer questions at a level appropriate to the caregivers' ability to understand. It is obviously a mistake to talk down to caregivers, but it is also a mistake to talk up if this means that communication fails. The counselor should try to avoid theorizing, and she must avoid pontificating. She should stay within the limits of what we really know about stuttering, and she should always allow her approach to be dictated by compassion for the caregivers and their child.

The technique I have found to be most effective in helping caregivers understand stuttering is to relate what the stutterer experiences to what the caregivers themselves experience. For example, the young advanced stutterer has developed fears about certain words and certain speaking situations. The counselor should remind caregivers that all speakers fear certain speaking situations. Most people would rather have their nostril hairs plucked with tweezers than to speak to large audiences. Many people find it intimidating to talk to authority figures, and many people are fearful of talking when there is a possibility they will be criticized or rejected. Many people can also identify words they would rather not say. Words such as "statistics," "aluminum," or "linoleum" are viewed by many adults as *hard to say*. Caregivers will find it much easier to understand their child's situation and linguistic fears when they realize that all people have these fears, at some times to some extent. I have found few, if any, aspects of stuttering to which nonstuttering people cannot relate. More importantly, I have found that when nonstuttering people do relate to the disorder, their understanding and their tolerance increase dramatically.

What Attitude Toward the Child Should the Counselor Cultivate in the Caregivers?

In my view, this the most crucial question we must answer about counseling caregivers for reasons I hope will be clear by the time I reach the end of my answer. The counselor should begin by reminding the caregivers that how the child feels about himself *will* influence what happens with his stuttering. She should then remind the caregivers that they are largely responsible for how the child feels about himself. If their attitudes about life, about themselves, and about the child are positive, the child will generally feel pretty good about himself. If their approach to life is pessimistic, if they do not like themselves very much, and if their attitudes toward the child are critical and judgmental, the child's self-image will tend to be poor. The counselor should stress the powerful connections that exist between attitudes and behaviors, and she should trace these connections to their ultimate conclusions. That is, if a growing child is told every day, in verbal and nonverbal messages, that he is a worthless, irresponsible bum, it is highly likely he will become a worthless, irresponsible bum—a classic and tragic example of self-fulfilling prophesy. The counselor should then turn the coin over. If a child hears truthful praise and encouragement every day of his life, if he is told that he is bright and capable and delightful, he has a good chance of growing up to be a bright, capable, delightful, and I might add, productive and well-adjusted adult. The lesson should be obvious, but in case it is not obvious, I will state it clearly. The counselor should cultivate in the caregivers an attitude toward their child that resonates with **acceptance** and **appreciation.**

How does the counselor cultivate this attitude? She begins by listening to what the caregivers are saying about their child in order to gauge how they feel about him in the present. She should listen to what they say about his friends, about his performance in school, about how he relates to members of the family, and about his fluency problem. It will not take the counselor long to determine how much or little the caregivers *understand* their child, how much they *accept* him, and how much they *appreciate* him.

The next step is critical but delicate. The counselor must discuss the caregivers' attitudes and feelings toward the child. The counselor should approach this step with great caution, remembering that there is sometimes a wide gap between what caregivers *should* do and what they actually do. It is universally accepted that caregivers should love their child and that they should accept him unconditionally. In reality, even the most loving caregivers do not have absolutely positive feelings about their child all the time. Even the best child is flawed in ways that cause caregivers to have some reservations about the child, at least some of the time. Any caregiver who says otherwise is not being truthful. What caregivers must understand is that ambivalence about their child is normal and understandable because there are times when any child is absolutely lovable, and there are times when that same child is at the other end of the *lovable* continuum. The counselor must help the caregivers recognize their child's positive and negative traits in order to facilitate an objective attitude about the child that will lead them to the next step.

Caregivers take the next step when they learn to accept their child in spite of perceived or real weaknesses, faults, and failures. Acceptance, after all, is not predicated on perfection. I have found it useful to point out to caregivers that their child accepts them, usually without reservation when he is young, in spite of their flaws. In a good marriage, the partners accept one another and love one another in spite of their flaws. What we are asking the caregivers to do, therefore, is not extraordinary, and it is not extraordinarily difficult. We are asking them to accept their child as he is—smiles, frowns, charm, tantrums, good deeds, warts, and all. The counselor might call the caregivers' attention to the affection and appreciation shown the child by his teachers, peers, and other significant people in his life. Sometimes caregivers are so close to the child, so caught up in his problems, so influenced by a few, usually minor flaws, that they cannot see the child's *big picture,* a picture filled with more beauty than ugliness, more accomplishment than failure, more promises than promises broken. The counselor should also remember the power of examples. She might find that the most effective way to teach caregivers to be accepting and appreciative is to model these attitudes toward the child and toward the child's caregivers in her interactions with them.

Do Caregivers Influence the Development of Fluency?

To some extent, this question was addressed in the answer to the first question. Caregivers do influence, *heavily influence,* virtually every aspect of the child's communicative system. This being true, there is no doubt that they influence the development of fluency.

For example, caregivers influence the child's attitudes about time pressure in speaking. We should be clear about the fact that time pressure in speaking is neither good nor bad. It simply is. There is always a sense of time pressure in interpersonal communication. We cannot wait forever to respond when someone speaks to us. If we wait too long, we lose our listeners. If time pressure becomes urgent, however, there develops a communicative stress that can lead directly to nonfluency. When caregivers talk to one another and when they talk to the child, they model a certain level of conversational time pressure. If the counselor determines that the time pressure the child's caregivers are modeling is too great for him to handle, she might suggest that they reduce time pressure to a more manageable level. They can do this by talking more slowly, by talking at an even pace, and by using an unhurried turn-taking style. If caregivers talk quickly, use an uneven pace, and engage in rapid turn-taking, the child learns to expect the transfer of information at a rapid rate, and while that can happen, it is not a prerequisite of effective interpersonal communication. Common sense suggests that a slower pace and casual, relaxed turn-taking place an emphasis on exchanging the contents of messages, not on the speed of their delivery.

The child also learns how to interrupt by observing his caregivers in conversation. In fact, he learns that interruption is necessary if one is to become a conversationalist. That is not a lesson most caregivers intend to teach, but it is a lesson they do teach and the child learns. Imagine the child's confusion when he learns this lesson and is then criticized for learning it. How does this happen? Consider that a competitive, highly verbal, hectic-paced style of conversation is very common in many American homes, especially when there are several children. The young stutterer wants to get into the conversation because what one says in this kind of environment is very important, but he finds it extremely difficult to get in. He quickly discovers, in fact, that if he waits his turn, if he waits until everyone stops talking, he never gets into the conversation. He observes that the next participant in the conversation begins his utterance before the speaker is finished, trying to time the beginning of his utterance on the final few words of the speaker. This is not easy to do, and when the next participant improperly times the beginning of his utterance, he might say, "I'm sorry. I thought you were finished," when it is clear to everyone that the speaker was not finished. He might have been *almost finished,* but in a normal conversation, a speaker is seldom completely finished before someone else begins to talk. What I am saying here is that interruption is not just an acceptable conversational strategy, it is a conversational necessity. The stuttering child, after observing this apparently conventional strategy being applied countless times, tries to get into the conversational fray. His interruption must be precisely timed, and when it is his turn to speak, he is under considerable pressure to speak before someone else interrupts him. It is not surprising that under these conditions, he often succumbs to the communicative pressure and stutters. The counselor, therefore, must help caregivers understand that it is not only inappropriate to interrupt the stutterer—a rule everyone seems to understand—it is also inappropriate to require him to interrupt in order to be a conversational participant.

Should the Clinician Attempt to Change the Caregivers' Speech?

After everything you have read to this point, this might seem a silly question. I have tried to establish, successfully I hope, that caregivers powerfully influence every aspect of the child's communication system. If this is so, and if the caregivers are engaging in communication practices that are adversely affecting the child's communication practices, the clinician should indeed try to change the caregivers' offending speech habits. This will NOT be easy. It is amazingly difficult to change caregivers' speaking habits, but if the counselor determines that their rate of speech is excessive, that their turn-taking is too rapid, that their speech is too nonfluent, etc., she should try to help them adjust their speech in ways that will facilitate fluency in their child. Several strategies can be employed. First, the counselor should try to help the caregivers understand how their speech is affecting the child. Understanding often leads to change. Second, she can direct the caregivers to more appropriate speech models and suggest they try to adopt the more desirable features of these models. It helps, of course, if these models are people the caregivers like and respect. Third, the counselor can try to take a more indirect approach by changing the caregivers' attitudes about speech and nonfluency. If she can help them acquire objective, forgiving attitudes about speech and speech failures, they may become more relaxed speakers, which translates into slower rate, less hurried exchanges, and more tolerance of their own mistakes and the mistakes of others.

How Should the Counselor Deal with the Caregivers' Reactions to their Child's Stuttering?

The counselor should begin with the understanding that when caregivers react to their child's nonfluencies, they do so because they are genuinely concerned, because they love their child, and because they are doing what they honestly believe is best for him. Unfortunately, most of these reactions will cause the counselor to cringe, because even though they seem reasonable and appropriate to the typical layperson, they will not have the positive effect caregivers intend. No matter what the counselor says to the caregivers about these reactions, however, she must ensure that they do not feel guilty about what they have done or said relative to the child's fluency failures.

I have found it best to approach this part of counseling by first talking about young stutterers in general. The counselor might point out, for example, that young stutterers tend to be adversely affected by a wide range of natural, well-intentioned reactions including sympathy, finishing sentences, and advice about how to talk including, "Slow down," and "Take a deep breath before you say that word."

She might then invite the caregivers to think of other ways that adults might react to a child's stuttering, realizing that they may or may not identify their own reactions to their child's stuttering in the examples she provided. She should then ask them to consider the possible effects of these reactions, gently and objectively correcting any misperceptions they might have. Caregivers, for example, often fail to understand how advice can be harmful. The counselor might point out that the message underlying advice such as "Slow down" is that the child has failed to talk in a manner that is correct or acceptable. While an adult might perceive finishing a sentence to be *helpful*, the child might be receiving a number of negative messages, including the following: (1) My caregiver thinks I am incapable of finishing sentences on my own, (2) My caregiver is impatient and wants me to talk faster than I can, (3) I can never do anything right. The counselor should emphasize that most caregivers intend none of these messages, but in communication, the sender of a message cannot be guaranteed that the intended message will be received.

After some discussion of reactions in general, the counselor should focus the caregivers' attentions on what they do when their child stutters. It may be helpful to videotape the caregivers interacting with the child and then discuss their reactions during playback. The counselor should not be surprised if the caregivers try to justify their reactions. This is natural. She should support and accept their motives even if she advises them to reject their reactions. The counselor should be reassured by the fact that most caregivers discover for themselves, in the context of these discussions about reactions to nonfluencies, that their reactions do not have the effects they intended. Their self-discoveries lead to understandings, which lead to change.

Just as there are no guarantees in therapy, there are no guarantees in counseling. If caregivers are open to the process, however, and if the counselor is sensitive to their needs, counseling can help caregivers better understand their child and his disorder. The caregivers' understanding, in combination with an effective therapy program implemented by a competent speech-language clinician, provide the child an excellent chance for either regaining fluency lost or developing fluency he never had.

Chapter 24

EVALUATING PEOPLE WHO STUTTER

One of the guiding principles of speech-language pathology is that therapy should fit the diagnosis, and I accept that principle. I would take it a step further in the context of stuttering. If therapy does not fit the assessment data, the diagnosis, and the conclusions drawn about the client's disorder, it is highly unlikely that the therapy will be effective, unless by dumb luck.

The problem with assessing stuttering is that it is extraordinarily difficult to know what to measure, how to quantify, and what the numbers really mean once they are generated. I would argue that much of what makes stuttering *stuttering* is not observable and is not quantifiable. When we count behaviors and apply scales, we assume that we have assessed and that we have the information we need to draw conclusions about whether or not a person is a stutterer and about where that person's aggregate of stuttering behaviors should be placed on a continuum of severity, but that assumption is dangerously untethered to what we actually know about stuttering.

Consider again that ALL people are nonfluent at times, and consider again that some people experts agree are stutterers are more fluent than people those same experts would agree are nonstutterers. Consider that one stutterer might produce very few moments of stuttering, but the moments he does produce are long and involved, whereas another stutterer produces many moments, but his moments are relatively simple and brief. Consider that one stutterer's disorder might be quite overt, whereas another stutterer navigates the communication trails so carefully that he seldom stutters openly because he is so skilled in the art of avoidance. No matter what instruments we use, direct comparisons among stutterers are difficult at best, and none of them is able to tap into the machine that drives stuttering–the stutterer's belief system as it relates to speech, to stuttering, to listeners, and to himself. The instruments that have been developed to assess stuttering are mostly designed to give us a view of the end product, the results of the disorder. By comparison, if a physician wants to assess an illness for the purpose of finding an effective treatment, he or she is much more interested in finding and assessing the factors that are driving the disease than in simply measuring the patient's temperature, heart rate, and blood pressure. These need to be measured, of course, but the physician recognizes that changes in these measures reveal little or nothing about *why* the changes are occurring. In the same way, it is helpful to determine the frequency of stuttering, the length of moments, the degree of anxiety associated with stuttering, the frequency of anticipatory behaviors produced, etc., etc.; but these numbers reveal little about the true nature of the disorder for a given stutterer, and they provide little guidance to effective treatments.

Another compelling problem in assessing stuttering is that it is a *moving target* disorder. Whatever numbers an instrument generates today are not likely to match the numbers generated a week later or a week earlier. In fact, stuttering is so variable in its presentation that measures in the morning of a given day may not match measures generated in the evening of that same day.

Finally, we need to remind ourselves that there is much in the stuttering problem we simply cannot see, and if we cannot see it, we cannot be confident that we can measure it. The stuttering complex includes attitudes, perceptions, beliefs, and fears, as well as visible behaviors. The stutterer's self-image, his overall level of self-confidence, and his general assertiveness impact the nature and severity of his stuttering. There are instruments that purport to assess these hidden dimensions of the disorder, but any time we try to tap into the covert bases of human behavior, we are on shaky ground. The problem is complicated by the fact that these factors are not in a steady state. The stutterer's self-image and his level of confidence might be high one day and low the next. All reasonably introspective adult stutterers know when some days will be *bad* and some *good* in terms of speech, just because they know that when they are in a good place emotionally, speech is likely to be good, and when they are in a bad place emotionally, fluency will suffer. Whether or not this is self-fulfilling prophecy does not matter because the point to be made here is that assessing stuttering in its overt, and especially in its covert, dimensions is risky business precisely because stuttering is such a variable disorder.

Why then assess at all? I would argue that there are at least two excellent reasons to assess: (1) The exercise of assessment gives the clinician an opportunity to learn something about the client as a person, to understand how he views himself and his disorder. Even if frequencies are subject to change from time to time, we can usually get a pretty good idea about the range of behaviors a client might produce during the time we spend in evaluation. We can discover how the client responds to his nonfluencies and how he responds to speaking conditions we would expect to influence frequency and severity. We can often learn a great deal about the client's willingness to accept responsibility for his disorder, about his level of motivation and commitment to the therapy process. There are certainly opportunities during the evaluation to instruct and counsel, to challenge and encourage. No matter the numbers, we should end the evaluation with some sense about prognosis, based on how the client conducts himself and how well he understands and accepts what must be done to deal effectively with his stuttering. (2) If we gather numbers over several sessions, spaced generously apart and at different times of the day, there is a good chance we will get a *baseline picture* of the client's disorder. That is, we can use the numbers to establish a starting point against which to assess progress in therapy.

I want to offer what I believe is a reasonable evaluation protocol for evaluating the stutterer, but I first want to include a review of some of the evaluation tools that have been developed over the past several decades. The purpose of this review is to give the reader a sense of the kinds of tools that might be used to assess stuttering without promoting one, two, or three as *better* than the others. Each tool has been developed with the best of intentions. The author or authors of each instrument had their eyes wide open about the problems inherent in this kind of assessment, but they were not afraid to try, and they deserve considerable credit for that courage.

A Review of Available Tools

According to the common expression, "What you see is what you get." While that may be true for some things in life, it is definitely not true for stuttering. What you see and/or hear in stuttering is only what lies on the surface of a very complex, multifaceted, and multilayered disorder. Another common expression might be better suited to stuttering: "You can't judge a book by its cover." The repetitions, closures, postural fixations, all the overlaid behaviors, as well as the facial grimaces and other bodily evidences of struggle are features of stuttering that are hard to miss, but they tell only part of the stutterer's story. People who have developed tools for assessing stuttering either understand that this true, or they should understand. For that reason, no single instrument has yet been devised for evaluating stuttering that can possibly tap into every dimension of the disorder.

Severity Rating Scales

When we evaluate stuttering using rating scales, we are making *global* and *subjective* judgments. This is the same kind of scaling used by people who judge figure skating, gymnastics, diving, or dancing. Any activity in which winning and losing cannot be determined by time or by points scored, lends itself to rating judgments. When a judge gives a figure skater a rating, he or she takes into account athleticism, technical skills, artistic expression, and factors that are even less tangible than these. When a diagnostician rates a stutterer, she takes into account the frequency of stuttering, duration of moments, secondary features, emotional reactions, the intensity of the struggle, and other factors that may be even less obvious than these. A rating is a global judgment about how severe that stutterer seems to that judge at that moment in time.

When a clinician uses words such as *mild, moderate,* and *severe,* she is applying a rating. The most commonly used ratings are anchored by numbers in what are called *equal-appearing interval scales.* If the clinician uses a 7-point scale, for example, "0" represents "no stuttering" and "7" represents "very severe stuttering." The psychological distance between each number on the scale should be the same. That is, the distance between "1" and "2" should be the same as the distance between "6" and "7." In actual practice, people tend to use the central number on the scale and the anchor numbers more often than they use the other numbers. That means that even with 7 numbers or 9 numbers, most stutterers are clustered at the numbers that suggest "mild," "moderate," and "severe."

One of the first rating scales devised for evaluating stuttering was the **Scale for Rating the Severity of Stuttering,** also known as the **Iowa Scale,** because it was developed by Johnson, Darley, and Spriestersbach (1963) at the University of Iowa. The authors intended that the scale be used, not just by clinicians, but also by the client, members of the client's family, and even by friends of the client. If used by all these people, the clinician would presumably gain a wider, and hopefully more accurate, perspective on how the client's stuttering severity varies over time and with different audiences. This presumption depends, of course, on the accuracy of the judgments. Even though the authors used a 7-point equal-appearing interval scale, they did provide some guidance. They suggested that the number assigned should be affected by the frequency of stuttering, the degree of muscular tension observed, the duration of the moments, the complexity of the behaviors produced, and by the presence of associated behaviors that tend to make the stuttering more noticeable. The authors also provided numbers and standards to guide the evaluator. For example, if the client stuttered on fewer than 2 percent of the words in the sample of speech being judged, if muscle tension was barely noticeable, if the patterns were *simple,* and if there were no associated behaviors, the number selected should be at the *mild* end of the scale. In addition to the usual problems associated with scaling, including the tendencies to use the middle and ends to the exclusion of the intermediate numbers, there was the problem that one has to assume that factors such as frequency, duration, and muscle tension move up and down the severity scale together, and that is clearly not true in all clients. One client might have a high frequency of stuttering, but his moments might be brief, and there might be only moderate muscular tension. Another client might produce relatively few moments, but when he produces them, they are long, complicated, and noticeable to everyone. One could make the argument that if one is using a rating scale, he or she should not be restricted to pre-established criteria, that the judgment should allow for interpretation of how all the relevant factors—as determined by the judge—interact to result in a global judgment of severity. This freedom will result in sometimes widely disparate judgments, but subjectivity is inherent in the process. We see that in the ratings of figure skating, diving, and gymnastics judges at times, even when we are assured that they are all competent and unbiased. We should not be surprised that those who rate the severity of stuttering are often in profound disagreement about what they hear and see.

The rating scale most often used today is the **Stuttering Severity Instrument for Children and Adults–3rd Edition (SSI–3),** developed by Riley (1994). The author's intention was to develop a scale that would be simple enough to be used in a wide variety of settings, objective, and sensitive enough to identify changes in severity over time. He also believed it was important to establish normative data and that the scale should be applicable to children as well as adults. The SSI, through all three versions, assesses severity by considering the frequency of stuttering, the duration of moments, and by taking into account physical behaviors produced during stuttering. Numbers are assigned to each of these three dimensions. The numbers are added, resulting in a total overall score that ranges from 0–45. The total overall score establishes a judgment of severity, and it also establishes a baseline against which therapy progress can be measured. The original SSI used the word as the unit of speech by which frequency was measured. The SSI–3 uses the syllable. The argument for using the word is that it allows for consideration of linguistic factors that might affect stuttering. Using the syllable, according to some experts, places the focus on the motoric aspects of stuttering. What is important, I believe, is to understand that stuttering is a disorder that cannot be limited to either linguistic considerations or to its motoric characteristics. It is all that and more. When we evaluate, we need to be certain that our appraisal tools allow the broadest possible view of the disorder.

Attitude Scales

Attitude scales are designed, or at least are intended to be designed, to examine the unseen aspects of stuttering—feelings, attitudes, and perceptions. I would certainly make the argument that it is important to try to assess the hidden, or covert, features of stuttering because they contribute to the impact of the disorder, and they serve to maintain it. The covert features shape the quality of the stutterer's life, and in a very real sense, the unseen aspects of stuttering are the nuts and bolts that hold the disorder together. If we could somehow eliminate all the fears, if we could make the stutterer's attitudes about speech and himself and his listeners uniformly positive, if we could reshape his perceptions about the challenges of communication so they reflect the true nature of speech and speech failures, stuttering would dissolve. Unfortunately, it is extremely difficult to make these changes. It is much easier to change behaviors than it is to change attitudes, feelings, and beliefs. In spite of the difficulties, the clinician must examine this part of the disorder because the motoric aspects of stuttering do not exist in a vacuum. They exist within the context of a person's whole life, complete with the feelings, attitudes, and beliefs that chart his course toward success or failure, happiness or despair.

One of the first tools devised to assess the covert components of stuttering was developed by Johnson, Darley, and Spriestersbach (1963). It is called **The Iowa Scale of Attitudes Toward Stuttering.** It was designed to assess the attitudes of the stutterer and the important people in his life. The instrument includes 45 statements about what a stutterer should or should not feel or do in specified situations. The first statement on the scale will serve as an example: *If a person at the family dinner table is about to stutter on a word, he should substitute another word for it and go on.* The respondent is asked to indicate, using a scale from 0–4, the extent to which he agrees with each statement. A rating of "4" indicates "strong agreement." A rating of "1" represents "strong disagreement," and a rating of "0" indicates "undecided." Excluding the items that generated a rating of "0," an average of the ratings is calculated. The lower the average, the better is the individual's attitude. According to the authors, an average between 1.0 and 1.4 represents "very good attitudes, considerable tolerance of stuttering," whereas an average above 2.2 represents "poor attitudes, considerable intolerance of stuttering." The authors acknowledge that the score itself does not reveal much because the respondent might quickly figure out the responses that are expected or would be most favored. This instrument can be used, however, to guide the clinician to issues that should be addressed in counseling.

Others have tried to build upon and expand the intent of the **Iowa Scale of Attitudes Toward Stuttering.** Erickson (1969) developed **The Scale of**

Communication Attitudes, later revised into what is called the **S–24** or **The Modified Erickson Scale of Communication Attitudes** (Andrews & Cutler, 1974). The original instrument consisted of 39 statements to which the stutterer responded *true* or *false*. Since 15 of these statements did not effectively differentiate the speech-related attitudes of stutterers and nonstutterers, the list was reduced to 24, resulting in the shortened name, **S–24.** One of the statements included on the **S–24,** offered here as an example, follows: "I find it easy to talk to almost anyone." If a person responds to a particular statement as the authors predict a stutterer would respond, he is given one point for that item. The score is the total number of statements to which the responses are parallel to those the authors assumed would be given by stutterers.

A somewhat different approach to assessing attitudes was taken by Ornstein and Manning (1985) who developed **The Self-Efficacy Scale for Adult Stutterers.** This instrument was designed to gauge the level of confidence a person feels when he approaches designated speaking situations. The scale has two parts. In the first part, the *Approach Attitude Scale,* the respondent indicates how likely it is that he would enter each of 50 speaking situations. In the second part, the *Fluency Performance Scale,* he indicates how confident he is that he would be able to maintain a level of fluency he believes is satisfactory. This kind of assessment might be useful in evaluating progress in therapy. That is, as the client improves, we would expect that he would be more likely to enter speaking situations and to feel confident in his ability to maintain a satisfactory level of fluency.

Evaluating the attitudes of children who stutter is particularly challenging because introspection does not typically emerge at a young age. It is important, however, to try to gauge the attitudes of a young stutterer because how he feels about his speech, himself, and others, will affect the course of his disorder's development. Brutten and Dunham (1989) developed a tool, **The Communication Attitude Test (CAT),** which is designed to assess the beliefs a child might hold about speech. The **CAT** consists of 35 declarative statements. The child responds to each statement as *true* or *false*. A *true* response means that the statement is consistent with the child's attitude regarding that topic. A *false* response means, of course, that it is not consistent with what the child believes. The **CAT** was designed so that 19 statements reflect negative attitudes about speech, and 16 reflect positive attitudes about speech. The score is the total number of responses that are negative. Since the authors' own research has established normative data, it is possible to look at a young stutterer's score to determine if his attitudes toward speech are predominantly negative in comparison to the attitudes of children who do not stutter. At the least, **CAT** results may help the clinician decide if she needs to address attitudes, beliefs, and misperceptions in therapy with a youngster who stutters, or if she can focus exclusively on the behaviors of stuttering.

A Recommended Evaluation Protocol

Anyone who has wrestled with stuttering as a clinician for an extended period of time knows that there is NOT a single avenue of treatment that is right for every client. The most bizarre of therapies, a treatment approach that is not at all grounded in reason or research, will produce—or seem to produce—good results in some clients. Other therapies, widely viewed as rational and consistent with the best research data available to us, will be largely ineffectual with some clients. Just as there are many, quite different, roads to therapy success, so are there many ways to evaluate people who stutter. I do not claim to offer the one and only evaluation protocol, the approach handed down to me from the St. Sinai of stuttering expertise. I claim only to offer the protocol with which I am most comfortable. It has evolved over the years of my career, and in truth, it has become simplified because I have come to believe that there is absolutely no way to objectify a disorder whose boundaries for a given individual change constantly. That is, what you see, hear, and measure today will not necessarily, or even usually, be what you see, hear, and measure tomorrow.

The truth about diagnosis, as I see it, is this: The *diagnosis* of stuttering, with adults and with most children, is not the product of numbers generated by paper and pencil tests. The diagnosis is usually made within the first few minutes of a clinician's contact with a person who stutters. If I ask a person his name, and he responds with four or five repetitions of the first sound of the first syllable, characterized by excessive struggle and muscular tension, in combination with a closure that lasts for five seconds, in combination with a facial grimace, followed by a head jerk and forceful expulsion of air as he finally manages to get the sound, syllable, and word out, I do not need a test or scale to determine that he is stuttering. On the other hand, I might listen to a person who is *normally nonfluent* who fills his speech with so many pauses and interjections that I lose track of his message, BUT if his speech is produced without struggle, with no hint that he is anticipating difficulty, no suggestion of avoidance and postponement, and no evidence of a level of muscular tension beyond what I consider to be normal, I will not identify him as a stutterer no matter how many benign nonfluencies he produces.

We come back to a problem we have addressed a number of times in this book. ALL speakers are nonfluent at times. The difference between a *stutterer* and a *nonstutterer* is not that one has perfect speech and the other has broken speech. The difference is not that the *stutterer* produces many fluency failures, and the *nonstutterer* produces few fluency failures. The difference is not that the *stutterer* produces certain categories of fluency failures, and the *nonstutterer* produces other categories of fluency failures. The difference is not that the *stutterer* produces speech that is significantly slower than the speech of the *nonstutterer*. No matter the measure of fluency we use, there is considerable overlapping when we evaluate people who stutter and people who do not stutter.

Assuming there are differences between people who stutter and people who do not, what are those differences? No matter what I suggest here, I want to make clear that the differences are not tidy and beyond debate, that the differences are shades of gray, not black versus white. I also want to make clear that not all differences I will identify will be true for all people who stutter, and some differences that might be true for some people who stutter, I will fail to identify. I will answer the question with which I opened this paragraph in the context of my own experience as a stutterer because that is the most complete and honest perspective I can offer you. Does it represent the *truth* about stuttering? It represents the *truth* about MY stuttering, and in four decades of clinical experience, I have found that my journey with stuttering has been remarkably similar to the journeys of the clients with whom I have interacted.

First and foremost, when I stutter, I know it–absolutely, positively for sure. When I produce normal nonfluencies–and I produce many normal nonfluencies–I know that too, and I know it absolutely, positively for sure. This gets at the first difference, and I believe the most fundamental difference between a *stuttering* and a *normal fluency failure*. When I stutter, I stutter because I anticipate that I am going to stutter, because I predict that I am going to stutter, because in response to my prediction, I create the physiological conditions, including excessive muscular tension and inappropriate articulatory adjustments, that make fluency failure inevitable. When I stutter, I *feel* the failure before it occurs. Anticipations of stuttering are linked to perceptions of difficulty, and I have a mental catalog of those perceptions, a catalog that is updated on a regular basis. When I speak, the words formulated in the planning stages of speech are processed through that catalog. Every word I am about to speak that matches a word in my catalog is marked by a mental red flag, and those words/red flags become my cues for stuttering. When I produce normal fluency failures, none of this processing occurs, and here's the tricky part. Sometimes when I formulate messages containing some of those words that I perceive as difficult, the words are not processed through my *catalog of difficulty*. That happens when my focus on message is so intense that I am thinking more about communicating than I am about failing. Sometimes the emotionality of communicating is so powerful that I do not process words through my *catalog of difficulty*. Sometimes I am so confident or so relaxed or so angry that I bypass my *catalog of difficulty*. I may, in these circumstances, be nonfluent, but if I am, the nonfluencies are *normal,* and how do I know they are *normal?* They are normal because they are not anticipated, they are not produced with excessive muscular tension, they are not produced with inappropriate articulatory adjustments, because I either ignore them or pay them scant attention, and because the forward flow of my speech is not interrupted at all. Now, reader, consider this. How does ANY standardized test of stuttering tap any of this? I will repeat for emphasis that stuttering is not about frequency of fluency failures, not about duration of moments, not about categories of fluency failure. It is about all the hidden platforms, the mental operations, the emotional springboards that set the stage for fluency failures, failures that are recognized by nearly every listener as *abnormal.*

There are other problems with common evaluative instruments that need to be mentioned here. Some stutterers are very skilled avoiders. Some produce postponements that sound very natural and are not at all intrusive. Some stutterers know how to reduce the propositionality of speech by speaking words without paying conscious attention to what those words mean or how important some words are in comparison to others. Some stutterers know how to manipulate prosody so that propositionality is reduced, or they create prosodic variations so consciously that they are sufficiently distracted by their attention to these details of speech that they do not respond to their cues for stuttering. In other words, some stutterers are clever enough that they can–in the short term, at least–find ways to not stutter. This kind of stutterer could go through a screening undetected. This kind of stutterer could respond to any of the instruments I have described above or to any other instrument that is commercially available and deceive the evaluator by manipulating his speech so that it is artificially fluent and by choosing answers that reflect healthier attitudes about speech, himself, and listeners than he really possesses.

I would add that the problems I am describing here are not unique to people who stutter. There are alcoholics who manage to not only delude themselves about their problem, but who are also able to fool significant people in their lives, sometimes for many years. Some people who are depressed are able to disguise their depression. Some people who are truly psychotic are able to fool people into believing that they are normal, healthy, productive citizens. There are, in short, some human conditions, that just do not lend themselves to paper and pencil measures, and I believe that stuttering is one of those conditions.

Does all this mean that we should not *measure* stuttering? Actually, I think it is important that we calculate frequency of stuttering and the duration of moments and that we develop a list of the behaviors a given client produces, but I do not believe these measures do much to advance us to diagnosis.

Instead, they help us to establish baselines against which we can measure progress in treatment. Even when they are used for this purpose, however, it is important to obtain data several times over a reasonable period of time, perhaps a month or two. A *snapshot* of a stutterer's speech might provide an accurate picture if we happen to obtain data on his prototypical average day. We are more likely to get an accurate assessment, however, if we take measures on several days spread out over a period of 30 to 60 days and if we take those measures on different days of the week at different times of the day.

Case History

The evaluation of any client with any kind of communication disorder must include a case history, of course, but the case history is particularly important in the evaluation of a stutterer because stuttering is as much about *history* as it is about the *present*. We cannot rewrite the client's history, but if we pay close attention to what happened on his journey from the time he began to stutter to the present day, we will learn a great deal about his understanding, his perceptions and misperceptions, and his attitudes. We will learn something about the important people in his life and the kinds of influences they have had, and continue to have, on his behaviors, his life choices, and his beliefs system. We will very likely come away from the case history with some idea about the client's level of motivation and about whether or not he is willing to endure the costs of therapy in order to gain the payoffs.

It is not my intention to persuade the clinician to use any particular case history, but I will emphasize those elements I consider to be most important. If the client is an adult, we should begin by asking something like this: "Why are you here today? How would you identify and describe your speech problem?" Even if we know exactly why the client has come to the evaluation, it is important to hear him explain the problem in his own words because we may learn something about his attitude toward the disorder in his description. Some clients, for example, abdicate responsibility from the very beginning. They might describe the problem as something someone else caused, or they might indicate that they have come to the evaluation because someone else required it or recommended it. Even if the client's words seem to embrace personal responsibility, however, the clinician should be aware that there is a difference between saying, "This is my problem," and "This is my problem to solve." There is also a difference between "I am motivated to having my problem solved," and "I am willing to do whatever is required to solve my problem." There are many ways to abdicate responsibility, and there are many steps on the journey to personal responsibility.

I am not suggesting that if the clinician hears language that reflects abdication of responsibility, she should immediately show the client the door.

Many clients, in the beginning, truly do not grasp what it means to *own* their stuttering. The clinician must guide the typical client to that understanding, but the very first words out of the client's mouth may help the clinician gauge how difficult it will be to facilitate understanding of ownership, and the clinician should not wait to begin that aspect of counseling. We make a mistake when we think of evaluation, therapy, and counseling as separate processes. They are not, especially when we work with stutterers. If the client says something during the evaluation that indicates an unhealthy attitude or makes a statement that is based on faulty logic or that is simply baseless, the clinician should address the attitude or the misinformation immediately–in a calm, reassuring manner, of course.

The clinician will ask questions about the client's developmental, academic, social, vocational, medical, and family histories, but she should be guided by this basic principle–Do not ask a question unless you know why you are asking it. While it might be appropriate to ask the mother of a young stutterer about "toilet training issues," that is not an appropriate area of questioning for the adult who stutters. Even IF problems related to toilet training were involved in the adult's early stuttering history, the connection is speculative at best, and the events are so distant in time that nothing is gained by talking about them now. On the other hand, the clinician will ask about the informant's relationships with his parents, siblings, other relatives, and peers during his growing up years because those answers may shed light on how he interacts with people today and how much or how little responsibility he takes for making relationships work. In asking questions about the client's relationships with other people, the clinician may learn a great deal about how assertive the client is, how much he depends on other people, how affected he is by the judgments and criticisms of other people. Anything that helps the clinician understand the kind of person the client is will be useful because stuttering is a problem born within the context of a person's whole life, and it is a problem that will be solved, if it's solved, within the context of a person's whole life.

Knowing the kind of student an adult client was is important for many of the same reasons we want to know what kind of family member he was and is. A person who was cavalier about academic responsibilities, who did not invest the necessary time to be successful in the classroom, and who blamed teachers for his failures is likely to be exactly that kind of client. A stutterer who was a good and conscientious student, who never had to be told to do his homework but did it because he knew it was his responsibility to do it, who took pride in not just meeting academic standards but exceeding them, who was proud of his accomplishments but also took full responsibilities for his failures, who invested more time and energy than was required–that stutterer will almost certainly be the kind of client who will make great progress in therapy. He will be the kind of client who owns his disorder, who is committed to the therapy process, who demands more of himself than even the clinician requires, who accepts his failures as his responsibility but is absolutely determined to move beyond the failures, who understands that success is measured not just by the final outcome but by all the small victories along the way, victories that may be as much about facing fear and embracing challenge as about fluency. The clinician wants to know what kind of student he was because the *student* reflects the *person.*

If the client is an adult who works, the clinician will want to ask the same kinds of questions about work as she would ask a student about school. Why did the client choose this job? Where did he begin, where is he now, and what does he hope for the future? What obstacles lay in the path of ultimate success on the job, and what is the client going to do to overcome those obstacles? How does he interact with his boss, with his subordinates, with his peers? How does he account for his progress on the job or for his lack of progress? Again, in exploring the *person* subsumed within the *worker,* the clinician might learn a great deal about what kind of client he is likely to be.

The point to be made and emphasized with all the energy I can muster is that you cannot separate *client* from *person.* I have never known a person who is unmotivated in his personal and professional life who is motivated in stuttering therapy. I have never known a person who blames other people and circumstances for all his personal and professional problems who accepts personal responsibility for his stuttering. I have never known a person who is not committed and determined in his personal life who IS committed and determined in stuttering therapy. The clinician needs to examine the informant as a person before she can assess his potential as a client because what she sees in him as a person is exactly what she will get from him as a client.

I recommend asking questions about overall development and general questions about a potential client's medical history in order to determine if this person's stuttering might be a neuromotor problem. I also want to know if there are other stutterers in the extended family in order to have some sense about a possible genetic connection. The clinician should not assume that just because there are other stutterers in the extended family that this client's problem is genetically based because it is impossible, given present technology, to prove a genetic connection, but it is useful to know if there might be some general familial vulnerability to fluency problems. If this is a possibility, it would be just as important to explore the possibility of a family environment conducive to the development of stuttering that is handed down from generation to generation, as well as looking for possible medical clues to a familial history. Any information of this nature the clinician can gather might be useful in developing a more complete picture of the client's problem, even if the information is mostly speculative. Keep in mind that when detectives solve crimes, they begin with speculations based on the evidence available. Sometimes that evidence is thin. Some evidence turns out to be irrelevant, but if enough pieces of the puzzle fall into place, it becomes possible to determine how a crime unfolded. In the same way, the diagnostician considers all leads and all evidence, no matter how insignificant some of the information may seem. She then tries to connect as many dots as she can in order to develop a reasonable hypothesis to explain a given client's problem. The diagnostic picture, even if it is not complete and even if it is not entirely accurate, might provide some direction for therapy. If the outcomes of therapy are positive, the clinician assumes—even if she is not correct in her assumption—that the diagnostic picture was correct, and she stays the course. If the outcomes are less than expected, she looks for more clues, connects more dots, develops a new or revised hypothesis and begins again.

Without question, the most important part of the case history is the *History of the Speech Problem*. The clinician wants to know when the problem was first noticed. Who noticed it? How did that person react? With what results? What were the circumstances of the client's life at the time the problem was first noticed? When did he first become aware of the problem and under what circumstances? How did he react? How has the problem changed over time? How has the client's attitude toward the problem changed over time, IF it has changed? Have there been attempts to treat the problem? By whom? With what results? How have the client's *significant others* reacted to his problem? Have they tried to help? How? With what results?

These are just sample questions, but they will suffice to identify the kind of information we are seeking. We are asking, in reference to the client's stuttering, the basic journalistic questions—Who? Where? What? When? How? Why? The responses from the client or from his significant others may provide no solid answers to questions about the origin of the client's stuttering, but embedded within the responses the clinician might uncover attitudes, beliefs, and perceptions. She might discover something about the stutterer as a person that will help her determine what kind of client he might be. In his history, she might find guidance for therapy in the present, and she might find hints about what the client's stuttering future holds. As long as every question can be justified, the clinician wants to cast the widest possible net in taking the case history because she cannot know when she begins what she might discover that will be relevant and useful as she moves from *information intake* to *appraisal* to *diagnosis* to *therapy*.

The Speech Examination

I recommend taking samples of speech that range from *highly structured* to *unstructured*. Although it is always risky to talk about the "typical" stutterer, I think it is fair to say that most stutterers will stutter more when there is less structure. When reading aloud, for example, there is no language formulation because it has already been done. There is no pressure to decide what to say or how to say it. The reader does not have to select vocabulary or create sentences or fret about the rules of grammar. That work has already been done. This is a highly structured form of speech. In this kind of speaking, the stutterer can—if he chooses to do so—say the words without really processing what they mean. That is, he can suppress propositionality. This is the easiest speaking situation for most stutterers. Keep in mind, however, that stuttering is a fickle and unpredictable disorder. What is *most comfortable* for some stutterers may be *most uncomfortable* for others. Reading aloud may be very difficult for the stutterer who has trouble reading, and it may be more difficult for the stutterer who embraces avoidance as his best hope for coping. The clinician should also be sensitive to the fact that the style of language in the reading passage might be quite different from the style the client naturally uses, and that would make it more difficult than it needs to be. If the client is a child, the clinician should choose a reading passage that is one grade level below the reading level for that child so that reading competency does not become an issue in evaluating speech. If the client is an adult who reads at an adult level, the clinician might choose something from a newspaper because most articles are written at about an eighth-grade reading level, and the style could be described as *journalistically generic*. The clinician would be wise to avoid editorials, especially nationally syndicated columns because these writers sometimes have styles that are more difficult to read.

At the next level, somewhat less structured than reading aloud, we ask the client to tell a well-established children's story, such as **The Three Bears.** No matter who tells the story, the language is fairly universal: "Once upon a time, there were three Bears—a Papa Bear, a Mama Bear, and a Baby Bear. . . ." The client is not reading already established sentences, but he is following a predetermined pattern. When Goldilocks gets to the porridge, for example, the client is likely to say, "This porridge is too hot. This porridge is too cold. This porridge is just right." Clearly, the structure is not mandated word for word or detail for detail, but as the client tells the story, he follows a well-established narrative path.

We then ask the client to read a printed story and paraphrase it, or tell it in his own words. In this case, the client is not responsible for all the language formulation, but he must decide how he will tell the story, and he must choose the words and sentences by which his version will be told. That is, there is far less structure than in oral reading or in **The Three Bears,** but there is more structure than in freewheeling spontaneous speech.

Finally, we collect a sample of spontaneous speech. Ideally, this sample will be in the form of a monologue, not a give-and-take conversation. We might ask the client to talk about his hobbies, a recent vacation, a favorite television show or book, or a recently viewed film. We might ask him to describe what he does in his job, or we might ask him to give us his autobiography. Whatever he talks about, we want him to talk for several minutes without interruption. In this sample, all of the communicative responsibility rests on the client. If he is talking about a television show, a book, or a movie, some of the content is predetermined, but the pressure is on the client to explain this content clearly to someone who, presumably, knows nothing about the show, book, or movie. There is even less structure if he talks about a hobby, a vacation, his job, or his life's story.

Each of these four samples should contain about 400 words. That's about two minutes worth of talking, a little more if there is significant stuttering. Since we are not drawing research-like conclusions, however, if the samples are smaller—even if they are about 100 words each—that still allows us to take some basic measurements.

On each sample, the clinician should calculate frequency of stuttering (percentage of words stuttered), speaking rate (words per minute), mean duration of moments, and frequency of anticipatory behaviors (percentage of words on which postponement/avoidance occurred). In addition, the clinician should make note of the kinds of overt behaviors the client produced. All of the samples should be tape recorded, and the clinician should transcribe each sample to facilitate analysis.

The easiest way to determine speaking rate is to play the tape about 30 seconds and stop. Mark the transcribed copy at that point. Play the tape for 60 seconds and mark the last word spoken. Count the words between the two marks. If the clinician thinks that 60-second sample is not representative of the whole sample, she should count all the words in the sample and divide by the total time in minute units. If the total talking time was 4 minutes, 20 seconds, the divisor would be 4.33.

The mean duration of moments in a sample can be determined by using a stop watch and simple math. Measure the durations of 10 moments, randomly selected. Add the times and divide by 10 to determine the mean duration of moments. It is also useful to make note of the moment of longest duration in each sample.

Determining the frequency of anticipatory behaviors is a difficult task and certainly an inexact science. On the transcribed copy, the clinician will circle the words on which she THINKS the stutterer used postponements and/or avoidances. The clinician might want to adopt the rule I use: If I am not sure, I count it as an anticipatory behavior. At the evaluative stage of treatment, I would rather err on the side of identifying something as a problem when it is not a problem than to ignore a behavior that really is a problem. Over time, the clinician will determine which of the client's behaviors are *abnormal nonfluencies* and which behaviors are *normal nonfluencies*. In the beginning, I would argue, it's best for the clinician to have her evaluative antennae fully extended. Whatever standards the clinician uses, she counts the total number of words circled and divides that number by the total number of words in the sample to determine *frequency of anticipatory behaviors*.

The clinician will want to make a list of all the overt behaviors the client used in each sample for two reasons: (1) She will want as complete an inventory of these behaviors as possible in order to have a complete view of the client's problem; and (2) The client might produce just core behaviors in oral reading, whereas he might produce superimposed behaviors in samples with less structure. That information will help the clinician understand some of the variables that affect severity for that client. We know that stuttering is an extremely variable disorder for all people who own it. The clinician will be in a stronger position to help her client if she understands the factors that shape variability for her client. Not only should she share that information with her client to promote his understanding about what he does in certain circumstances to make his stuttering worse, but she should use that information to select the tasks she will incorporate into therapy, using the principle of working from least difficult to most difficult and the principle of *optimal match*, whereby the client can take what he learns at a manageable level of communication and apply those lessons to the challenges of the next, and more difficult, level of communication.

Variations of Speech and Communicative Stresses

One of the ways we can identify factors that affect the severity of stuttering for a given client is to put him in a variety of speaking situations that are purposely manipulated to take one factor at a time into account. It is likely that some of these adjustments will have no impact at all on the client's stuttering. Others may have dramatic effects. It is as important to know the adjustments that have no impact, as it is to know those that have negative consequences. It should also be noted that in the process of this exercise, the client might discover the kinds of adjustments he can deliberately make that will facilitate fluency. In fact, that is our hope. It must be emphasized that we subject only ADULT clients to these variations and stresses.

In terms of speech variations, we require the client to speak softer than normal, louder than normal, slower than normal, and faster than normal.

Most clients discover that *loud* and *fast* make it more likely they will make maladaptive physiological adjustments, resulting in more stuttering. Conversely, they discover that *soft* and *slow* make it easier to maintain physiological adjustments that promote fluency. If, however, the client's fluency is unaffected by these adjustments for good or ill, that is important to know as well, especially if this tendency is confirmed by future experiences with the same adjustments. At the least, this would suggest that *soft* and *slow* are not among the paths that will lead to fluency control for this particular client.

We also need to identify the communicative stresses that negatively affect a client, and we need to identify those stresses to which he seems to be–at least for the present–immune. In the course of conversation, the clinician might *challenge, question,* and *interrupt.* She might increase the *rate* of her speech, and she might *speed up turn-taking.* All of these stresses have the potential to precipitate an increase in stuttering. The clinician not only measures changes in behavior, but she notes how the client seems to react to each form of stress. If he seems to collect himself before continuing to speak, for example, that is a positive prognostic indicator. It means that he understands he is in control of his share of the communicative process. If, however, he allows his speech to be manipulated by changes in the clinician's speech, and if he gives in to her manipulations with no attempt to maintain or regain control, it is clear that he needs to learn the lesson that he is the master of his own mouth, no matter what his conversational partner might do.

Trial Therapy

If the clinician intends to use the motor modification therapy described in this book, she should set aside some time at the end of the evaluation for trial therapy, to determine if the client is a good candidate for this kind of treatment.

As I tried to establish and emphasize repeatedly in the chapters devoted to therapy for the adult stutterer, the client cannot modify behaviors he cannot identify. The short version of what is required is that the client must be able to identify the *when, what,* and *why* of his moments. That is, he must know *when* he produces his moments. He must have some understanding about *what* the behaviors are he is producing, and eventually he must understand *why* he produces the behaviors he produces when he produces them and in the order in which he produces them. We would certainly not expect the client during the evaluation session to identify as well as the client who has been in therapy for weeks or months, but we want to know if–under direct instruction–he can identify at least the *when* of his moments. If he can, that is a positive prognostic indicator. If he demonstrates even a rudimentary understanding of the *what* and the *why,* we have every reason to believe this client is an excellent candidate for motor modification therapy.

The clinician begins then by explaining to the client that she is going to do some trial therapy to determine how well he responds to the kind of therapy the clinician advocates. The clinician says, "I'm going to ask you some questions. Whenever you produce something you believe is *stuttering,* raise your hand." It does not matter, of course, what questions are posed, but they are usually questions about name, address, occupation, family, and interests. If the client is catching few of his moments, the clinician might stop the tape recorder, rewind it, and ask him to identify moments while he listens to himself. If the client is able to identify 50 percent or more of his moments, the clinician should then say, "We're going to make the task a little more difficult. Now when you produce a moment, I want you to stop and tell me what you did." If the client stops after half or more of his moments, even if he is not able to provide accurate descriptions of his moments, that is an excellent sign. One of the most difficult things for a stutterer to do is abandon the moment, to stop the struggle while he is producing it. Keep in mind that during the modification stage of therapy, the client must be able to abandon struggle in order to *pull out* of moments, and eventually, he must, in a very real sense, abandon the struggle before he produces it, when he uses *preparatory sets.* If the client, during evaluation, demonstrates that he is able to put the brakes on struggle, that is another very positive prognostic indicator. Assuming he is able to identify the *when* and the *what* about 50 percent of the time, the clinician raises the bar one more notch. Now when he stops and identifies what he did, she asks, "Why do you think you pressed your tongue against the roof of your mouth?" or "Why do you think you said 'Uh, uh, uh' before you finished that sentence?" If the client responds with insights, no matter how incomplete they may be, the clinician should praise his understanding, and she should allow herself a ration of professional giddiness. This client is well suited for motor modification.

If the client has struggled with the identification tasks, that should be the end of trial therapy. If he has done well, or even reasonably well, in the clinician's judgment, she should challenge the client to modify. After a difficult moment and the client's attempt to describe it, the clinician will say, "I want to see if you can produce that word using what we call a *modification.* Instead of pressing your lips together on the 'b' in 'Bob,' try it like this." She then demonstrates a slow, calculated approach to the first sound, with a slow, deliberate bilabial closure, characterized by light contact and an easy release. She does not explain it. She just demonstrates it, and asks the client to try it. If his attempt is anything less than excellent, the clinician should demonstrate again and have him try it again. If he shows improvement over three or four trials, the clinician has gathered yet another positive prognostic indicator. This client, if he is willing to invest the necessary time and effort, if he is self-disciplined and motivated, will do well in motor modification therapy.

A Little Persuasion

It is not unusual for an adult client to believe that stuttering is beyond his control. In my experience, this belief is the norm, not the exception. If the client's statements and behaviors during the evaluation suggest that he believes stuttering is not within his control, the clinician should use a little persuasion therapy.

Assume, for example, that the client stutters when he reads. After stuttering during the reading of a short passage, the clinician asks him to read it again, but this time he should read with a whisper or with rhythmic speech or with nasal speech, or he should read in unison with the clinician. If there is no reduction in frequency and/or severity of stuttering under any of these speaking conditions, that should be the end of the exercise. If, however, as is likely, the client's stuttering is reduced or eliminated under one or more of these conditions, the clinician asks, "What does this exercise prove to you?" The client might respond, "I don't know." If he does, the clinician should say, "When you spoke nasally, when you whispered, and when you read in unison with me, you did not stutter. What does that indicate about your ability to speak fluently?" At this point, the client must acknowledge that he spoke fluently even if he is still not convinced that he can be fluent when he wants to be. He might conclude, not incorrectly, that the fluency under these speaking situations was contrived. The clinician, therefore, needs to continue the persuasion by saying something like this: "Even though these were unusual speaking conditions that produced what you might believe is contrived fluency, this exercise should convince you that you have the physical ability to produce speech without stuttering. The fact is, you produce the conditions that make stuttering happen, and you can produce the conditions that will make fluency happen. You will learn techniques in therapy that will help you make better decisions about the adjustments in your speech mechanism, adjustments that will facilitate fluency."

The clinician should be forthright with the client about the challenges inherent in therapy. The road to fluency control is not easy, and the journey is not brief, but there is a map. We know how to get from where the client is to where he wants to go. It is important that the client leaves the evaluation session believing there is hope, that stuttering is a problem that can be managed, that he has the power to change his life by learning how to control his speech.

If the Client Is a Child . . .

Most of what has been included in this chapter has been directed at the adult or adolescent stutterer. If the client is a child, the clinician should complete a case history, of course. She should also collect samples of the child's speech, ranging from structured to unstructured, and she should do the same measures on these samples as described earlier. In place of trial therapy, the clinician should engage in relaxed, stress-free, noncompetitive play with the child, using proper fluency models. If the child's stuttering is reduced in this kind of interaction, that is a good sign. This child will do well in therapy. He might also be a candidate for spontaneous recovery, of course, but there are no guarantees that spontaneous recovery will occur. If we determine that the child is, in fact, a stutterer, we meet our professional responsibility best by recommending treatment, beginning as indirectly as possible. If we need to make therapy more direct, we make it only as direct as it needs to be.

If the stutterer is a child, the clinician should assess articulation/phonology and language. Fluency problems and problems in these areas often co-exist. If they do, the clinician is faced with decisions about how to address all the child's communication problems without exacerbating the stuttering. I personally believe that if language is involved, no matter the severity of the stuttering, language must be the priority. Even though stuttering is easier to treat in children than in adults, it can be effectively treated at any age. The window for language development does not remain open for a lifetime. In fact, it begins to close rapidly after the child's third birthday, so if the fluency client has a moderate or profound language delay, the treatment emphasis must be on language.

If the stutterer is a school-age child, the clinician will want to seek information from his teacher and from any other school specialist with whom he might be working. Stuttering, as I have pointed out many times, is not a disorder that exists in a vacuum. It is a communication problem that is inextricably connected to every dimension of the stutterer's life. The clinician needs to know as much as possible about the child's whole life, including his school life, in order to treat his stuttering effectively.

Acknowledgement: The author gratefully acknowledges Marisa Racette's contributions to this chapter. The material on assessment instruments was drawn from Ms. Racette's unpublished independent study, supervised by the author, and completed in partial fulfillment of the requirements for Ms. Racette's Master of Science degree at Illinois State University in Normal, Illinois (August, 2002).

REFERENCES

Andrews, G., & Cutler, J. (1974). S-24 Scale. In W. Manning (2000), *Clinical decision making in fluency disorders* (2nd ed.). San Diego, CA: Singular Publishing Group.

Bloodstein, O. (1995). *A handbook on stuttering* (5th ed.). San Diego, CA: Singular Publishing Group.

Bloodstein, O. (1993). *Stuttering, the search for a cause and cure.* Needham Heights, MA: Allyn & Bacon.

Brutten, G., & Dunham, S. (1989). The Communication Attitude Test: A normative study of grade school children. *Journal of Fluency Disorders, 14,* 371–377.

Erickson, R. (1969). The Scale of Communication Attitudes. In W. Manning (2000), *Clinical decision making in fluency disorders* (2nd ed.). San Diego, CA: Singular Publishing Group.

Griffin, J. (1960). *Black like me.* Boston: Houghton Mifflin.

Hulit, L. (1989). A stutterer like me. *Journal of Fluency Disorders, 14,* 209–214.

Hulit, L. (1985). *Stuttering therapy: A guide to the Charles Van Riper approach.* Springfield, IL: Charles C Thomas.

Hulit, L. (1985). *Stuttering: In perspective.* Springfield, IL: Charles C Thomas.

Johnson, W. (1961). *Stuttering and what you can do about it.* Minneapolis, MN: University of Minnesota Press.

Johnson, W., Darley, F., & Spriestersbach, D. (1963). *Diagnostic methods in speech pathology.* New York: Harper & Row.

Ornstein, A., & Manning, W. (1985). Self-efficacy scaling by adult stutterers. *Journal of Communication Disorders, 18,* 313–320.

Riley, G. (1994). *Stuttering severity instrument for children and adults* (3rd ed.). Austin, TX: Pro-Ed.

Sheehan, V. (1986). Approach-avoidance and anxiety reduction. In H. Shames & H. Rubin (Eds.), *Stuttering then and now.* Columbus, OH: Charles E. Merrill.

Starkweather, C. Talking with the parents of young stutterers. In *Counseling stutterers.* Memphis, TN: Speech Foundation of America, Publication No. 18.

Van Riper, C. (1992). *The nature of stuttering* (2nd ed.). Prospect Heights, IL: Waveland Press.

Van Riper, C. (1973). *The treatment of stuttering.* Englewood Cliffs, NJ: Prentice-Hall.

GLOSSARY

Abulia. A kind of *psychosomatic dyspraxia.* The stutterer feels as though he cannot move his articulators at will. There is sensory deprivation, especially auditory and visual. Abulia occurs very rarely and is usually associated with the most severe moments of stuttering, especially moments involving silent, prolonged postponements.

Adaptation. In this exercise, the stutterer is instructed to stutter constantly when he would normally avoid or postpone. Adaptation is often done on a quota basis. That is, the client is instructed to stutter a certain number of times or on every word for a specified period of time. The purpose is to desensitize. Also known as *flooding.*

Anticipatory Behavior. A behavior used when the stutterer perceives that stuttering is imminent. The purpose is to prevent overt stuttering. The categories of behavior considered *anticipatory* are avoidance and postponement.

Anticipatory Struggle Hypothesis. According to this view, the stutterer stutters when he *thinks* he will stutter. It is the anticipation of stuttering that prompts him to create the physiological conditions that make stuttering inevitable. The stutterer tries hard to not fail as he believes he will. The struggle to not stutter results in the very behaviors we recognize as *stuttering.*

Avoidance. A behavior used to prevent saying a certain word or entering a certain situation. The stutterer can avoid by simply *refusing* to say the word or enter the situation, by *substituting* a nonfeared word for a feared word or substituting a nonfeared situation for a feared situation (e.g., a letter or e-mail for a phone call), or by *circumlocuting.*

Block (Blockage). See *closure.*

Buffering. This exercise is used during stabilization. The clinician purposely exposes the client to specific communicative stresses that give the client difficulty. He is challenged to deal with the stresses by controlling his speech and his emotions.

Cancellation. The stutterer modifies a moment of stuttering *after* it has been produced. That is, he completes the stuttered word, pauses, and then repeats the word using the modification.

Circumlocution. Explaining a word rather than saying it. For example, the stutterer might say, "The elongated piece of upholstered furniture," instead of "couch."

319

Closure. A momentary closing or blockage somewhere in the speech mechanism. For example, the stutterer might forcefully close the vocal folds or lips so that air is interrupted. Usually occurs on plosives, but can occur on any phoneme.

Complemental Air. By the time the stutterer completes a series of repetitions or has struggled through a closure or postural fixation, he may have used all the air he would normally expire in a speech production and will actually begin his final speech attempt on complemental or residual air. More common on continuants than plosives and very common on /h/.

Core Behaviors. These are the most basic of stuttering behaviors. All other overt behaviors are directly or indirectly related to three core behaviors: *repetitions, closures,* and *postural fixations.* They are called *core* behaviors because they are the central behaviors around which are wrapped all the other behaviors.

Counterconditioning. Conditioning designed to replace a negative response to a stimulus with a positive response. *Deconditioning* is designed to replace a negative response with a neutral response. In some cases, the term *counterconditioning* is used when the term *deconditioning* would be more accurate.

Covert Features. The word *covert* means *hidden* or *unseen,* so the covert features of stuttering are the *hidden* or *unseen* aspects of the disorder. Covert features include the stutterer's feelings, attitudes, and perceptions.

Desensitization Therapy. This therapy is designed to reduce the anxiety component of stuttering. The goal is to disassociate stuttering responses from the stimuli that seem to evoke them.

Disguise Reaction. A behavior used to cover up a moment of stuttering. e.g., coughing, laughing, throat clearing, pretending to think.

Escape. See *interrupter.*

Etiological Factor. A cause that underlies a disorder, that explains its origin or genesis.

Fear (in stuttering). In relation to stuttering, fear is the expectation of fluency failure, ranging from doubt about the ability to produce speech without stuttering to absolute certainty that stuttering, and all the unpleasantness associated with stuttering, will occur.

Flooding. See *adaptation.*

Fluent Stuttering. A fluent stuttering, or *target behavior,* is a moment of stuttering characterized by minimal temporal alteration, easy unforced repetitions, or slight prolongations, with no struggle, avoidance, or postponement. During identification, we challenge the client to find *fluent stutterings* in order to impress upon him that he not only decides when he is going to stutter, he decides the degree to which we will stutter.

Incidence. In the context of stuttering, *incidence* is the number of people in a given population who were, are now, or will become stutterers.

Interrupter. Also called *escape.* A behavior used to end a moment of stuttering, an attempt to impose rhythm on arrhythmic speech, e.g., head jerk, foot stomp, finger snap.

Maintaining Factor. A maintaining factor causes a disorder to persist even when the etiological and precipitating factors are no longer operative.

Massed Practice. In *massed practice,* the client produces a given word about 100 times. The first few repetitions of the word are stuttered. The vast majority of the repetitions (80–90) are produced using modifications, and the last few are produced normally. This technique is used during stabilization to attack remaining linguistic fears.

Modification. A production of a stuttered word or a word on which the client believes he might stutter that has the following characteristics: (1) highly conscious motor act; (2) deliberate or preplanned articulation; (3) slower than normal production so that feeling is enhanced; (4) correct articulatory positions with gradual shifts to succeeding sounds and syllables; (5) easy, loose, unforced productions; and (6) calculated follow through.

Negative Practice. An unwanted behavior is produced on purpose so that a more appropriate behavior can be *discovered.* In stuttering therapy, negative practice is sometimes called *pseudostuttering.* The client stutters on purpose in order to reduce his anxiety about the behavior and in order to discover more appropriate production behaviors.

Negative Suggestion. The clinician offers predictions of failure, the kinds of predictions the stutterer himself makes, before he enters a threatening speaking situation. The client is challenged to resist being influenced by the suggestion.

Nonreinforcement. The client says a feared word over and over again until he can say it fluently. He is instructed to simply say the word, not to say it in any particular way. In the course of repeating the word, he will move from stuttering, to less severe stuttering, to normal production. He is encouraged to compare and contrast these productions.

Overt Features. The word *overt* means *observable,* so the overt features of stuttering are those behaviors that can be observed–seen and/or heard.

Pantomime. In *pantomime,* the movements of speech are made, but there is no sound production, not even a whisper. This technique is used to heighten the stutterer's tactile-proprioceptive awareness. It can be applied to stuttered productions, modified productions, and normal productions.

Postponement. A behavior used to delay an attempt on a feared word in the hope that the fear will subside enough to allow a fluent production.

Postural Fixation. A *postural fixation* is a core behavior of stuttering. When the stutterer produces a postural fixation, he severely constricts, but does not close, the flow of air through the speech mechanism. This behavior is most common on fricatives since constriction is a natural characteristic of fricatives.

Pragmatics. In linguistics, *pragmatics* is the study of how language is used to get things done.

Precipitating Cause. A precipitating factor does not account for the origin of a disorder, but it does *trigger* the disorder if the proper etiological factor is operative.

Preparatory Set. The client plans the modification when he *anticipates* a moment of stuttering. He produces the targeted word in a modified manner before he produces any overt behaviors.

Prevalence. In the context of stuttering, *prevalence* is the number of a people in a given population who are stutterers at the present time.

Propositionality. *Propositionality* is the technical term for *meaningfulness.* The term can be applied to words and to situations. That is, some words have greater propositionality than others, and some situations have greater propositionality than others. Content words (nouns, verbs, adjectives, adverbs) are more propositional than function words (articles, prepositions, conjunctions). Talking to a judge during a trial is more propositional than talking to a tree. Saying, "I love you," to a human being is more propositional than saying, "I love you," to a dog, cat, or goldfish.

Proprioception. Sensory feedback from the muscles and joints concerning position in space or the direction and extent of movement. Closely related to *tactile* feedback.

Prosody. Sometimes described as the *music of speech.* It includes the elements superimposed on the sequences of sounds that comprise speech—rhythm, stress, intonation, rate. Also called *suprasegmental phonology.*

Pseudostuttering. See *negative practice.*

Pull-out. The client makes the modification *during* the moment. In producing a word, as soon as he feels himself producing a moment, he stops, pauses, releases the excessive muscular tension, plans the modification, and completes the word using the modification.

Reciprocal Inhibition. A concept developed by Joseph Wolpe: "If a response incompatible with anxiety can be made to occur in the presence of anxiety-evoking stimuli, it will weaken the bond between these stimuli and the anxiety responses." *Reciprocals* of anxiety include eating, relaxing, being assertive, and sexual behavior.

Repetitions. The stutterer repeats sounds or syllables in order to find the appropriate degree of muscular tension and the correct articulatory position. Each repetition in a sequence reflects improvement in the position and/or degree of muscular tension.

Resistance Therapy. This exercise is used during the stabilization phase of therapy. The client speaks in unison with the clinician who stutters as severely as she can, or the client enters a speaking situation after the clinician has given him a powerful negative suggestion, or the client talks under DAF while the clinician fades the DAF in and out. The client is challenged to resist being manipulated into his old stuttering behaviors and to speak under control at all times, modifying as necessary in order to maintain fluency.

Restimulation. This technique is used with the *young beginning stutterer* to help prevent increased awareness. In *restimulation,* after the child produces a moment of stuttering to which he reacts, and after the child has completed the thought he was trying to express, the clinician or caregiver calmly reflects the child's message and expands upon it.

Scaling. Multiple productions of a given word, usually using a scale of 1–10, on which '1' is a production with *well below normal muscular tension* and '10' is a production characterized by *severe struggle.* The purpose of scaling is to challenge the client to become aware of the wide range of decisions that come into play when he produces a word, decisions that result in normal productions, mildly disrupted productions, and seriously disrupted productions.

Servosystem. A *servosystem* is an automatic, or semi-automatic, self-regulating system. Speech is a servosystem in that speech output is automatically regulated according to the feedback–auditory, tactile, and proprioceptive–the speaker receives as he talks. That is, by monitoring the feedback from his own speech, the speaker knows if he has made a mistake or is making a mistake. He corrects his output accordingly.

Spontaneous Recovery. In *spontaneous recovery,* a client gets better for reasons other than therapy. About half of all children who begin to stutter recover spontaneously–without treatment.

Starter. A behavior used to end postponement, or, in the absence of postponement, to make the speech attempt mandatory. It is often the same physical behavior as the interrupter and, like the interrupter, is used to impose rhythm on arrhythmic speech.

Superimposed Behaviors. A superimposed behavior is produced *on top of* a core behavior. This kind of behavior cannot exist on its own. For example, *vocal fry* is produced when the stutterer produces a laryngeal closure. In the process of fighting through the closure, he makes his vocal folds vibrate, but under enormous tension and strain. That effortful vocal fold vibration is *vocal fry,* a behavior that would not occur if there were no closure upon which it can be superimposed. There are four superimposed behaviors in stuttering: *vocal fry, complemental air, tremors,* and *interrupters.*

Tactile Feedback. The sense of touch. Closely related to *proprioception.*

Target Behavior. See *fluent stuttering.*

Timing Device. See *starter.*

Tremor. A rhythmic vibration of a muscle or group of muscles. Stuttering tremors develop in the speech mechanism–usually in the larynx, tongue, lips, or mandible when three physiological conditions are present: (1) localized hypertension of the muscles involved; (2) inappropriate positioning of the structure involved; and (3) a sudden movement, surge of muscular tension, or spurt of airflow to *trigger* the tremor.

Triad of Behaviors. A triad of behaviors consists of (1) a severely stuttered production of a word, (2) a *fluent stuttering* production of the word, and (3) a normal production of the word. Triads are used during the identification phase of therapy to help the stutterer recognize the physiological characteristics that differentiate stuttering from normal speech, and mild moments from severe moments.

Variation. Changing behaviors on purpose in order to break stereotypical patterns.

Vocal Fry. Also known as *glottal fry.* The vocal fry accompanying stuttering is a harsh, hypertense vibration produced when air is forced through tightly closed vocal folds. It is produced at the end of a laryngeal closure as the stutterer is fighting through the closure.